Neurogenetics
Principles and Practice

Neurogenetics

Principles and Practice

Roger N. Rosenberg, M.D.

Professor of Neurology and Physiology
Chairman, Department of Neurology
Southwestern Medical School
University of Texas Health Science Center at Dallas
Dallas, Texas

Raven Press ■ New York

To Adrienne, Jennifer, and Lara
with love and thanks
for your forbearance

Raven Press, 1140 Avenue of the Americas, New York, New York 10036

Library of Congress Cataloging-in-Publication Data

Rosenberg, Roger N.
  Neurogenetics.

  Includes bibliographies and index.
  1. Nervous system—Diseases—Genetic aspects.
2. Neurogenetics. I. Title. [DNLM: 1. Nervous
System Diseases—familial & genetic. WL 100 R813n]
RC346.R67 1985   616.8′0442   85-19280
ISBN 0-88167-151-7

The material contained in this volume was submitted as previously unpublished material, except in the instances in which credit has been given to the source from which some of the illustrative material was derived.

Great care has been taken to maintain the accuracy of the information contained in the volume. However, Raven Press cannot be held responsible for errors or for any consequences arising from the use of the information contained herein.

Materials appearing in this book prepared by individuals as part of their official duties as U.S. Government employees are not covered by the above-mentioned copyright.

Preface

The field of neurogenetics is developing rapidly both in the areas of enzyme defects associated with neurological disorders and with respect to the molecular genetics of brain development, neurooncology, the dementias, and inherited disorders. This book describes and summarizes this expanding literature and provides the clinician or basic neuroscientist with a comprehensive assessment of our current knowledge of neurogenetics.

Chapters are included that define the theory and principles of modern genetics, which are applied in later discussions of the clinical disorders. With the entry of recombinant DNA techniques in elucidating mechanisms of brain function and inherited disorders, every effort has been made to incorporate that new literature into the clinical discussions. The framework and foundation for the understanding of recombinant methods is presented in Chapter 4, providing insight into the various molecular defects involving clinical disorders described subsequently in Chapters 5 and 6. A look into the future with some speculation of the role of genetic engineering and neurological disorders is provided in Chapter 7.

It is hoped that the excitement evident in the disciplines of neurogenetics has been captured and conveyed in this volume. Biochemical and molecular differentiation of neurons and glia, the molecular basis of neuroneoplasia, and a molecular genomic understanding of inherited neurological disease represent a frontier of inquiry in biology and medicine that captures the imagination and stimulates the intellect. It is hoped that this undertaking presents both a factual statement and a sense of heightened inquiry about what is new and important in neurogenetics. This volume will be of interest, it is hoped, to neurologists, geneticists, pediatricians, internists, and neuroscientists who have an abiding interest in gene action and the nervous system.

Roger N. Rosenberg, M.D.

Acknowledgments

Genetics is one discipline that transcends every field of neurologic disease and research. A commitment to genetics has allowed me to pursue my interests in neuronal and glial differentiation and clinical syndromes. The possibility of developing this dual affinity was suggested to me as a resident by H. Houston Merritt, M.D., who was interested himself in the spinocerebellar degenerations and Huntington's disease and the altered cell lineages involved in their causation. I am most indebted to him for his guidance and support.

Marshall W. Nirenberg's influence was enormous in giving to a group of us in his laboratory in the late 1960s a quantitative system and an approach to molecular biological experiments with differentiating cell cultures of neuroblastoma, glioma, and their hybrids. He sensitized me and others to the need for and possibility of applying methods of molecular biology to genetic neurologic diseases. My hope is that this book reflects equally the clinical influence of Dr. Merritt and the scientific methods of Dr. Nirenberg.

I am particularly grateful to Fred Baskin, Marcelle Morrison, and Abraham Grossman, with whom I have collaborated scientifically in a series of papers during the past decade. We have thoroughly enjoyed one another's company and mutually benefited from our many scientific discussions and debates. Molecular differentiation was and is an enterprise that we thoroughly enjoy, and our camaraderie has made the special difference.

My clinical experience and travels with William L. Nyhan provided a unique opportunity to see patients and families in remote and difficult places with a master clinician, geneticist, and scientist. He showed me how to use patients in a small village on the Island of Flores in the Azores to solve a problem in variability of gene expression in a large family. His encouragement and interest in several genetic projects allowed our laboratory investigations to move forward. He truly is a remarkable physician-scientist, and my participation with him has been a privilege and honor.

I am truly indebted to Jay W. Pettegrew for his assistance in researching and writing with me a chapter on clinical genetics 7 years ago. An extensively expanded, revised, and updated version of our original effort is included in the book as Chapter 6. He is a fine child neurologist and neuroscientist with whom I thoroughly enjoyed interacting.

Lewis P. Rowland guided me through the writing of my first genetics paper as a resident and has been an inspiration and guiding light to me ever since. His clarity of expression and precision of thought have always served as a model, and I am forever in his debt for his literary guidance over the years and his sincere friendship.

Roscoe Brady urged me to compile a book such as this one covering both principles and clinical issues in neurogenetics. He is one of America's foremost molecular neurogeneticists, and it has been my pleasure to work with him on several clinical projects. His discussions on molecular approaches for therapy of those disorders are very much appreciated.

Amy and Lee Fikes have been good friends and supporters of my laboratory and research program for many years. They have made possible the initiation and development of several important research projects and their presence has made all the difference. They are a special couple, and I am indeed grateful.

I also thank Charles C. Sprague, M.D., President, Frederick Bonte, M.D., Dean-Emeritus, and Kern Wildenthal, M.D., Ph.D., Dean, University of Texas Health Science Center at Dallas, Southwestern Medical School, for their support in the development of the Department of Neurology and their friendship.

My students, residents, and patients have helped me immeasurably over the years to develop a keen awareness of the seriousness and complexity that these disorders represent. They have impressed me with a need to emphasize the importance of getting on with a molecular analysis of these disorders. An immediate goal is to obtain markers that are reliable and accurate to eliminate disease or to provide therapy with recombinant DNA techniques. It is hoped this book, which is a product of many influences already referred to, will provide a stimulus to future residents and graduate students to devote their academic careers to neurogenetics. It has been an exciting and rewarding endeavor for me, and I think the best is yet to come for our patients and the development of the field.

Roger N. Rosenberg, M.D.

Contents

Foreword

It is currently fashionable to employ the terms "explosion" or "revolution in neurogenetics" since answers to a myriad of baffling developmental and clinical neurological problems now may be approached in a systematic fashion. Chromosomal localization, gene cloning, and recombinant DNA technologies are expected to reveal mysteries heretofore completely unapproachable concerning many disorders.

These avenues are particularly appealing for understanding dominantly inherited neurological diseases, since, in most cases, the basis for these conditions is completely unknown. The techniques also will be used to determine the mutations that occur in recessively inherited disorders. For example, in Tay-Sachs disease, which is characterized by deficiency of hexosaminidase(s), various molecular alterations occur that can result in (a) impaired translation of enzyme subunits from messenger RNA, (b) abnormally large protein chains, (c) defective association of protein subunits, and (d) reduced protein synthesis. Related alterations have been reported concerning the abnormal biochemistry of metachromatic leukodystrophy where unstable enzyme (arylsulfatase A) is produced by some patients with the late-onset form of the disorder. These examples do not appear to be isolated events, and they indicate the complexity of molecular changes that can be presumed to occur in the majority of heritable neurologic disorders. Acquisition of such information is expected to lead to the development of useful strategies for the control and therapy of many of these conditions.

In order to provide clinicians and neuroscientists with a comprehensive source and awareness of the power of neurogenetics, Dr. Rosenberg has assembled a remarkable overview of the field in this volume. A text of this nature is not only timely, but essential for persons seeking a background in this area and for those who look to the applications that already have occurred and for an indication of others that are certain to follow from these investigations. Neurologists cannot escape the implications of being able to identify persons who carry mutations that cause recessive disorders and the serious consequence of harboring a dominant mutation whose expression is yet to appear. This is the coming state of the art and it behooves everyone involved with patients with neurogenetic diseases to be aware of these developments and their relevance. This book provides the essentials for present and future applications of these extraordinarily important breakthroughs.

Roscoe O. Brady, M.D.
Chief
Developmental and Metabolic Neurology Branch
National Institute of Neurological and Communicative Disorders and Stroke
National Institutes of Health
Bethesda, Maryland

Introduction

Gregor Mendel, the brilliant Augustinian monk of Brno, Czechoslovakia, published in 1865 (11) the first scientific quantitative basis for hereditary traits as expressed in his laws of uniformity, segregation, and free combination of genes. His work opened the first phase for a systematic investigation of human genetics. His contributions were forgotten for many decades but rediscovered in 1900 by Bateson (1) in the United Kingdom, Correns (4) in Germany, von Tschermak (18) in Austria, and de Vries (5) in the Netherlands. Equally brilliant were the observations in 1902 by Boveri (2) and Sutton (16) that chromosomes represented the physical basis of inheritance. Avery in 1944 is credited with demonstrating that DNA was the chemical basis of heredity. It is incredible to note that the first report in which the human chromosome number was established as 46 by Tjio and Levan (17) and Ford and Hamerton (6) did not appear until 1956. Lejeune et al. discovered trisomy 21 in Down's syndrome in 1959 (9), and Patau et al. identified trisomy 13 in 1960 (13). The first deletion syndrome, the cri du chat syndrome, was determined by Lejeune et al. in 1963 (10) to be caused by a partial deletion on the short arm of chromosome 5. In 1968 Casperson et al. (3) described chromosome banding techniques that permitted clear determination of all of the human chromosomes.

The one gene-one enzyme defect hypothesis for inherited disease was established by A. E. Garrod in 1902 (7) with the publication of his paper "The Incidence of Alcaptonuria: A Study in Chemical Individuality" in *Lancet*. He originated the term "inborn error of metabolism" and set the stage for the subsequent discovery of numerous recessively inherited diseases caused by enzyme defects, including the aminoacidopathies, leukodystrophies, gangliosidoses, and mucopolysaccharidoses.

Specific enzyme defects in several of these disorders made it possible to consider enzyme replacement therapy, even to the CNS by transient opening of the blood-brain barrier. Roscoe Brady was the unquestioned leader in the elegant elucidation of enzyme defects for the sphingolipidoses and was even able to show partial mobilization of stored substrate with enzyme replacement infusion as reviewed by Rosenberg (14,15). Elizabeth Neufeld and colleagues deciphered the enzyme defects in the mucopolysaccharidoses and demonstrated the presence of allelic genetic compounds (14).

1

Modern molecular genetics began with the discovery of the double helical model of DNA by Watson and Crick in 1953 (19), which readily provided an explanation for a replicating mechanism for DNA (20). The deciphering of the genetic code by Marshall W. Nirenberg and colleagues beginning in 1961 (12), which indicated 64 triplet codons for the 20 amino acids and initiation and termination signals, opened the door for the onrush of the subsequent molecular genetic revolution. By the early 1970s the stage was set for the discovery of elegant genomic mutations, deletions, inversions, and translocations to explain the basis of inherited disease at the molecular level.

Recombinant DNA techniques came next as a result of the innovative research of Paul Berg and colleagues (8), which made possible the establishment of genomic and complementary DNA (cDNA) libraries and gene cloning. On the horizon for genetic neurologic disease is the discovery of DNA polymorphism associations for prenatal or preclinical diagnosis of disease which will be discussed in detail. Somatic cell gene therapy and even germ cell gene therapy are contemplated in the not too distant future. The pace of genetic discovery is quickening and the future looks bright indeed (15).

REFERENCES

1. Bateson, W. (1902): *Mendel's Principles of Heredity*. Cambridge University Press, London.
2. Boveri, T. (1902): *Verh. Phys. Med. Gres. Wurzburg NF*, 35:67–90.
3. Casperson, T., de la Chapelle, S., Foley, G. E., Kudynowski, J., Modest, E. J., Simonsson, E., Wagh, V., and Zech, L. (1968): Chemical differentiation along metaphase chromosomes *Exp. Cell Res.*, 49:219.
4. Correns, C. (1900): *Ber. Dtsch. Botan. Res.*, 18:158–168.
5. de Vries, H. (1900): *Ber. Dtsch. Botan. Res.*, 18:83–90.
6. Ford, C. E., and Hamerton, J. L. (1956): The chromosomes of man. *Nature*, 178:1020–1023.
7. Garrod, A. E. (1902): The incidence of alcaptonuria: A study in chemical individuality. *Lancet*, 2:1616–1620.
8. Jackson, D., Symons, R., and Berg, P. (1972): Biochemical method for inserting new genetic information into DNA of simian virus 40; circular SV40 DNA molecules containing lambda phage genes and the galactose operon of *E. coli. Proc. Natl. Acad. Sci. USA*, 69:2904–2909.
9. Lejeune, J., Gautier, M., and Turpin, M. R. (1959): Etude des chromosomes somatiques de neuf enfants mongoliens. *CR Acad. Sci. Paris*, 248:1721–1722.
10. Lejeune, J., Lafourcade, J., Berger, R., Vialatte, J., Roeswillwald, M., Sering, P., and Turpin, R. (1963): Trois cas de deletion partielle du bras court d'un chromosome 5. *CR Acad. Sci. Paris*, 257:3098–3102.
11. Mendel, G. J. (1865): Versuche uber Pflanzen-hybriden. *Verhandl. Naturforsch. Vereins. (Brunn)*.
12. Nirenberg, M. W., and Matthaei, H. (1961): The dependence of cell-free protein synthesis in *E. coli* upon naturally occurring or synthetic polyribonucleotides. *Proc. Natl. Acad. Sci. USA*, 47:1588–1602.
13. Patau, K., Smith, D. W., Therman, E., Inhorn, S. L., and Wagner, H. P. (1960): Multiple congenital anomalies caused by an extra chromosome. *Lancet*, 1:790–793.
14. Rosenberg, R. N. (1981): Biochemical genetics of neurologic disease. *N. Engl. J. Med.*, 305:1181–1193.
15. Rosenberg, R. N. (1984): Molecular genetics, recombinant DNA techniques and genetic neurological disease. *Ann. Neurol.*, 15:511–520.

16. Sutton, W. S. (1902): *Biol. Bull.*, 4:231–248.
17. Tjio, H. J., and Levan, A. (1956): The chromosome numbers of man. *Hereditas*, 42:1–6.
18. von Tschermak, E. (1900): *Ber. Dtsch. Botan. Res.*, 18:232–239.
19. Watson, J. D., and Crick, F. H. C. (1953): Molecular structure of nucleic acids—A structure for deoxyribose nucleic acid. *Nature*, 171:737–738.
20. Watson, J. D. (1976): *Molecular Biology of the Gene; Third Edition*, Benjamin, New York.

1

Principles of Genetics

MENDELIAN GENETICS

A gene is defined as a specific linear segment of DNA that encodes for a single polypeptide. The phenotypic expression of that polypeptide may be transmitted in a dominant or recessive manner. In his 1865 paper Mendel expressed it this way: "The constant characters that appear in the group of plants may be obtained in all the associations that are possible according to the mathematical laws of combination. Those characters which are transmitted visibly, and therefore constitute the characters of the hybrid, are termed the dominant, and those that become latent in the process are termed recessive. The expression 'recessive' has been chosen because such characters withdraw or disappear entirely in the hybrids, but nevertheless reappear unchanged in their progeny in predictable proportions, without any essential alterations. Transitional forms were not observed in any experiment." Thus Mendel established the modern concept of genetics by stressing that there is a unit of heredity consisting of a factor that is transmitted from parent to child. His unit of heredity or "factor" is now termed the gene.

Mendel established three laws of heredity that remain the mainstay of modern clinical genetics.

The first law states that organisms that are homozygous for two different alleles (a gene existing in different forms at the same locus) at the same gene locus when crossed lead to genetically identical products that are heterozygous for this allele in the F_1 generation (Fig. 1).

The second law is an extension of the first and states that in a cross of the F_1 heterozygotes, there results a specific ratio of genotype products. One-quarter of the products are homozygous for each of the original parental types, and one-half remain heterozygous (Fig. 2).

The third law states that when organisms are crossed that differ in more than one gene pair, each individual gene pair segregates in an independent manner and follows the statistical law of independent segregation, also referred to as the law

Parts of this chapter were published previously by Rosenberg and Pettegrew in *Neurology*, Grune and Stratton, and in *The Clinical Neurosciences*, Churchill-Livingstone, Inc. and are reproduced with permission.

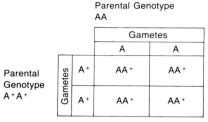

Parental Genotype
AA

FIG. 1.   Mendel's first law: law of uniformity and reciprocity.

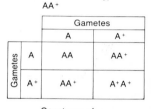

Parental Genotype
AA⁺

FIG. 2.   Mendel's second law: law of segregation and law of purity of gametes.

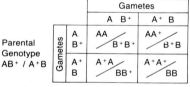

Parental Genotype:
AB⁺ / A⁺B

FIG. 3.   Mendel's third law: law of independent segregation or law of free combination of genes.

of free combination of genes. It is assumed that the third law applies in the case where no linkage is present (Fig. 3). The third law establishes the fact that a gene may exist in alternative forms and thus may express alternative phenotypes. Different forms of a gene existing at the same locus are referred to as alleles. Each parent, by contributing a single haploid ($1N$) gamete, provides one allele. The zygote, or product of both parental gametes that have fused to constitute a diploid ($2N$) organism, now has two alleles, one from each parent. The third law indicates that these alleles segregate independently and will not affect one another. Thus no transitional forms exist.

An individual or organism is said to be homozygous if the two alleles are identical and heterozygous if they are dissimilar. A dominant and a recessive allele present at the same gene locus in the same organism will express the appearance or phenotype only of the dominant allele.

It is now established that genes are sequenced in a linear manner like beads on a string on specific chromosomes. When homologous chromosomes independently separate and line up during the meiotic phase of gametogenesis, there is an exchange of chromosomal segments between the pairs. The reassortment of genes between homologous pairs of chromosomes is independent, and most rearrange without being influenced by adjacent genes. Some genes, however, always remain tightly associated during the interchromosomal exchanges and are said to be linked or show linkage. When there is macroscopic crossing-over of chromosomes, known as recombination, or the transfer of a piece of a chromosome from one chromosome to another, known as a translocation, the linked genes always move together. The closer the physical approximation of linked genes, the less the chance for their independent recombination. It was Sturtevant (29) who utilized the concept of a gene map distance based on the degree of recombination between genes to mark their relative positions on a linear scale.

The degree of map distance or separation between genes is measured as the percent recombination:

$$\text{Map distance} = \frac{\text{number of recombinants}}{\text{total number of progeny}} \times 100$$

In this case the degree of separation is expressed as map units in units of centimorgans (cM) and is equal to the percent of recombination.

ORIGINS OF BIOCHEMICAL GENETICS

It was Garrod (11) who proposed that hereditary factors were associated with enzymes and provided data in support of this idea. He specifically postulated that alcaptonuria was caused by an "inborn error of metabolism" resulting in the failure of an enzymatically determined reaction to occur. Beadle and Ephrussi (4) and Beadle and Tatum (5) made a compelling case for the association of gene action with enzymes by studying initially eye color development in *Drosophila* and subsequently radiation-induced mutants of *Neurospora* in which altered phenotypes could be related to specific mutations and lack of product synthesis. The mutations resulted in specific inactivities of enzyme protein. In 1945 Beadle (3) reviewed his concepts and proposed again the one gene-one enzyme hypothesis.

It was in 1957 that clear evidence was finally provided showing that a gene determined the structure of a protein. Vernon Ingram (14) in that year described the alteration in the β-globin gene product that resulted in sickle cell disease. A single amino acid change, valine for glutamate in position 6 of the β-globin peptide, was the necessary and sufficient molecular change to account for that genetic disease. This discovery made the one gene-one enzyme hypothesis even more specific, as it could now be expressed as one gene-one polypeptide. The field of biochemical genetics as traced from Mendel, Boveri and Sutton (chromosomal location of genes), Morgan and Sturtevant (measurement of gene loci), and Beadle and Ingram (one gene-one polypeptide) was established on the experimental foundation that the unit of heredity followed specific laws of inheritance, that this unit or gene was arranged linearly on chromosomes, and that gene action was expressed through enzyme or structural protein.

The molecular basis of gene action was established by three key discoveries: (a) Avery, MacLeod, and McCarty's (1) proof in 1944 that DNA and not nuclear protein was the chemical molecule responsible for bacterial transformation and infectivity; (b) Watson and Crick's (32,33) solving of the double helical structure of DNA in 1953, which offered a rational basis for cell replication by separation of the double strands; and (c) Nirenberg's (23) deciphering of the genetic code between 1961 and 1966 by showing that 64 triplet codons of nucleic acid bases encoded the 20 amino acids as well as providing start and stop signals for protein synthesis (Fig. 4). The stage was now set for molecular biological methods to be applied to genetic diseases.

The discovery of restriction endonucleases by H. Smith and D. Nathans of Johns Hopkins University provided a means of reducing DNA strands predictably to small restriction fragments. The unusual property of these enzymes of recognizing specific sequences of DNA and cutting DNA only at those points would have a major

	U		C		A		G	
	UUU	Phe	UCU	Ser	UAU	Try	UGU	Cys
	UUU	Phe	UCU	Ser	UAU	Try	UGU	Cys
U								
	UUA	Leu	UCA	Ser	UAA	Ochre	UGA	(Umber)
	UUG	Leu	UCG	Ser	UAG	Amber	UGG	Trp
	CUU	Leu	CCU	Pro	CAU	His	CGU	Arg
	CUG	Leu	CCC	Pro	CAC	His	CGC	Arg
C								
	CUA	Leu	CCA	Pro	CAA	Gln	CGA	Arg
	CUG	Leu	CCG	Pro	CAG	Gln	CGA	Arg
	AUU	Ile	ACU	Thr	AAU	Asn	AGU	Ser
	AUC	Ile	ACC	Thr	AAC	Asn	AGC	Ser
A								
	AUA	Ile	ACU	Thr	AAA	Lys	AGA	Arg
	AUG	Met	ACG	Thr	AAG	Lys	AGG	Arg
	GUU	Val	GCU	Ala	GAU	Asp	GGU	Gly
	GUC	Val	GCC	Ala	GAC	Asp	GGC	Gly
G								
	GUA	Val	GCA	Ala	GAA	Asp	GGC	Gly
	GUG	Val	GCG	Ala	GAG	Glu	GGG	Gly

FIG. 4. The genetic code after M. W. Nirenberg. These codons read in the 5′ to 3′ direction. Thus pUpUpU = phenylalanine. The termination codons (ochre, amber, and umber) are included.

impact on deciphering the molecular basis of many genetic diseases. Using these restriction enzymes, Paul Berg of Stanford University created a recombinant DNA molecule by splicing one segment of a viral genome into the genomic DNA of another virus. This work eventually led Stanley Cohen of Stanford and Herbert Boyer of the University of California San Francisco to utilize the bacterial plasmid, a circular DNA structure separate from the bacterial chromosome, as the vector for a segment of spliced DNA of human origin. Bacteria were transformed when they were transfected (transfer of exogenous DNA) with recombinant DNA plasmids containing both bacterial and human DNA. Their work made it possible to clone bacterial colonies containing a single human gene contained in a hybrid or recombinant bacterial plasmid. On December 2, 1980, Boyer and Cohen were awarded a patent (No. 4237224) entitled "Process for Producing Biologically Functional Molecular Chimeras," and the legal means were established to license corporations to clone and isolate genes and eventually gene products of human origin that would have tremendous commercial value. The techniques to clone potentially any human gene were also available for research into the molecular basis of any genetic disorder. It took a mere 40 years from Avery's discovery that DNA is the material of inheritance to the development of the techniques of Cohen and Boyer to clone any gene. The pace will quicken considerably as we approach the end of the twentieth century, and somatic cell gene therapy cannot be far behind (Table 1).

GENETIC PRINCIPLES OF DISEASE

Neurologic genetic diseases include (a) entities inherited in a mendelian dominant, recessive, or sex-linked manner, (b) polygenetic and multifactorial diseases, and (c) chromosomal defects. New clinical syndromes are being described yearly, and in McKusick's 1983 catalog *Mendelian Inheritance in Man* (22), for example, a total of 3,368 clearly defined and established diseases are listed, with a striking increase of 1,881 syndromes alone since 1966. The clinician must be knowledgable about the more common disorders, their mode of inheritance for genetic counseling and for their potential elimination. Further, the clinician-biologist must be familiar with genetic disease to appreciate and develop insight into the normal function of a gene. A genetic mutation is a unique, single lesion imposed on the nervous system and an opportunity to decipher normal gene action.

As emphasized by Harris (12), more than one-third of the proteins, and thus of the genes, in each person exist in a form that is different from that of the majority. These gene differences result in variations in the capacity of people to respond and deal successfully with environmental challenges. Diseases might be viewed as the interaction of a person's genetic constitution and the environment. When marked environmental factors are not necessarily responsible for evoking disease in an individual because of his or her unique genetic composition, such diseases are referred to as genetic diseases. Dietary levels of phenylalanine in persons deficient in phenylalanine hydroxylase (phenylketonuria or PKU), exposure to phenobarbital

TABLE 1. *Achievements in genetics and neurogenetics*

1865–Gregor Mendel establishes the laws of heredity.

1906–A. E. Garrod describes the first "inborn error of metabolism," alcaptonuria.

1934–A. Folling describes the metabolic derangement in phenylketonuria.

1944–O. T. Avery et al. discover that the structural basis of inheritance is DNA.

1952–G. T. Cori and C. F. Cori describe the first glycogen storage disorder as caused by an enzyme defect.

1953–James Watson and Francis Crick solve the molecular structure of DNA as a double helix of nucleotides with a backbone of ribose phosphates.

1957–Vernon Ingraham provides evidence for the one gene-one polypeptide model.

1961–M. W. Nirenberg deciphers the genetic code into triplet nucleotide codons.

1963–D. C. Gajdusek and C. Gibbs show that kuru, scrapie, and Creutzfeld-Jakob disease can be transmitted by brain inoculation into experimental animals and thus are caused by infectious pathogens producing slow viral-like diseases.

1965–R. O. Brady describes the major sphingolipidoses as being caused by catabolic enzyme defects and (1972) implements treatment with enzyme replacement therapy.

1967–J. E. Seegmiller describes the enzyme defect in Lesch-Nyhan syndrome.

1969–C. R. Scriver and Leon Rosenberg introduce the concept of treatment of inherited disease with megavitamin doses in specific disorders.

1970–E. F. Neufeld establishes the biochemical bases for the mucopolysaccharidoses as caused by discrete enzyme defects.

1970–David Nathans and Hamilton Smith develop the use of restriction endonucleases to cut DNA into specific restriction fragments.

1972–Paul Berg develops recombinant molecules of DNA by combining the DNA from two independent viruses to form a single hybrid one.

1973–Herbert Boyer and Stanley Cohen develop the means to insert a human gene into a bacterial plasmid, producing a unique bispecies recombinant molecule and ushering in the era of genetic engineering.

1974–M. S. Brown and J. L. Goldstein describe the molecular biological defect in hypercholesterolemia in heterozygotes; a deficiency in the low density lipoprotein receptor.

1977–Walter Gilbert and Frederick Sanger develop the techniques to determine the sequence of specific nucleotides in DNA.

1982–Richard Palmiter, using recombinant techniques, introduces the rat growth hormone gene into mouse zygotes and produces "gigantic mice" that are able to pass this characteristic on to the next generation.

1983–James Gusella describes a DNA polymorphism associated with Huntington's disease and maps the mutant gene to chromosome 4.

1984–S. Prusiner describes prions as infectious protein molecules responsible for kuru, scrapie, and Creutzfeld-Jakob disease. Prions may belong to a class of gene inducers that induce transcription of genes that carry the message to make more of the inducer. This raises the possibility of protoscrapie genes present normally in all cells.

1984–T. Friedman demonstrates possible somatic cell gene therapy for Lesch-Nyhan disease by showing expression of the human HGPRT enzyme in a mouse bone marrow cell with recombinant DNA techniques.

---

in persons deficient in uroporphyrinogen synthetase (porphyria), and possible viral agents with the presence of the DW-2 allele at the HLA-D locus on chromosome 6 (multiple sclerosis) are examples of environmental, multifactorial events that are concerned in the expression of genetic neurologic disease.

Dominantly inherited disorders are the most common form of genetic neurologic disease. A disease is *dominant* if the gene locus responsible for its production is expressed in a heterozygous individual. A *heterozygous individual* is one who has two different alleles or genes at the same locus on a homologous pair of chromosomes for a single trait or characteristic phenotype determined by that gene. An *allele* expressing a trait is dominant if it is evident in a heterozygous person. A *trait* or disorder is recessive if an allele is expressed only in the homozygous state, with both genes being identical at a given locus on a chromosomal pair. *Recessive disorders* rank second in incidence and sex-linked diseases third of the mendelian described neurologic diseases. *Sex-linked inheritance* refers to traits or disorders determined by genes on the X or Y sex chromosomes. For practical clinical purposes, sex-linked diseases refer to X-linked recessive genetic traits phenotypically expressed in hemizygous males; females, being XX, must be homozygous for a genetic trait for it to be completely expressed.

On the average, one-half of the children of an affected parent with an autosomal dominant disease will develop the disorder. Males and females are affected equally, with each sex transmitting the condition to male and female children, including male-to-male transmission. Clear vertical transmission of the dominant condition through successive generations is typical. New mutations in an individual rather than an inherited mutation are responsible for a certain percentage of dominant genetic disease. It has been estimated that there are 5×10^{-6} mutations per gene per generation, and thus one might expect 1 in 100,000 newborn persons to have a new mutation at a genetic locus. Neurofibromatosis and myotonic muscular dystrophy are examples in which new mutations make a considerable contribution to the total number of patients.

One-quarter of the children of two parents who are heterozygous for an autosomal recessive disorder will develop the disorder. Both parents will be "normal" carriers of the trait. Vertical transmission does not occur in recessive families, and males and females are affected equally. Although individuals who are heterozygous for a recessive gene appear "normal," biochemical abnormalities can be identified, with recorded levels of enzyme activity intermediate between the homozygote and noncarrier populations in examined cells *in vitro* such as leukocytes and cultured skin fibroblasts. Persons homozygous for a dominant gene are in general more affected than are heterozygous persons. Delay in age of onset and variability in clinical expression are typical of dominant disorders, and early age of onset and uniformity of phenotype are the case in the recessive disorders.

In an X-linked recessive disease, one-half of the daughters of a heterozygous mother will be asymptomatic, heterozygous carriers, one-half of her daughters will be genotypically normal, and one-half of her sons will be affected with the disease. Minor clinical features of the syndrome can be seen in the obligate female carrier of an X-linked recessive disorder. This phenomenon is caused by random inactivation of the X chromosome (Lyon hypothesis), rendering an excessive number of mutant X chromosomes active in a cross section of tissues in some females. Normal X chromosomes are rendered inactive in a high percentage of cells as a reciprocal event and are represented as Barr bodies. These clinically abnormal female carriers have been reported in such X-linked recessive disorders as Duchenne's muscular dystrophy, fragile X syndrome, adrenoleukodystrophy, and Fabry's disease. X-linked dominant diseases are inherited like the sex-linked recessive disorders, but the presence of a single mutant gene on one X chromosome is sufficient to express the trait in the heterozygous female. Distinction between an autosomal dominant and an X-linked dominant mode of inheritance can be difficult, as in both instances the disease is transmitted to one-half of the children of both sexes. Determination of the presence of disease in the children of an affected male is a good way to separate the autosomal dominant from the sex-linked dominant mode of inheritance. An X-linked dominant disease is being expressed if all of the daughters and none of the sons of an affected father develop the disorder. In an autosomal dominant condition, one-half of both the daughters and the sons of an affected father would develop the disease.

Polygenic and *multifactorial inheritance* also are involved in some genetic neurologic disease. A number of pairs of genes located in different loci that express a trait or single phenotypic characteristic of a disease represent polygenic inheritance. Multifactorial diseases result from the interaction of several genes and environmental factors. Some polygenic-multifactorial diseases include certain forms of epilepsy, cleft lip palate, spina bifida, anencephaly, and manic-depressive psychosis.

Penetrance refers to the degree of expression of a gene trait or characteristic of a disease. Penetrance is an important concept in dominant genetic neurologic disorders, such as Huntington's disease, acute intermittent hepatic porphyria, and neurofibromatosis. If a heterozygote demonstrates the complete form of a trait, the gene is said to be fully penetrant. Similarly, a homozygote for a recessive pair of genes is also penetrant when its encoded trait is clinically evident. Variations in penetrance within large families for several concordant traits may be marked and can present challenges in constructing pedigrees and determining the mode of inheritance. What appears to be generation skipping in an otherwise dominant pedigree may be in actuality minimal gene penetrance in minor family segments.

Variation in the type of clinical manifestations occurring rather than in their degree is referred to as *expressivity of gene function.* Some individuals in a large kindred with neurofibromatosis, minimal café au lait spots, and peripheral nerve tumors are said to exhibit minimal penetrance, and individuals manifesting only café au lait spots or only tumors are said to show variations in expressivity.

GENETIC HETEROGENEITY AND NEUROLOGIC DISEASE

Introduction to the Genetic Code

Modern biochemical genetics began in 1953 with the publication of the double-stranded helical model of DNA by Watson and Crick (33). The model provided an explanation for DNA replication, and therefore gene replication, and the potential for understanding gene specificity, and therefore gene mutation. In 1966 Marshall Nirenberg (23) provided the next cornerstone for the elucidation of the molecular basis of genetic disease by deciphering the genetic code. Nirenberg showed that the four nucleotide bases of DNA form the elements of a code in which 64 different triplet sequences each represent a protein amino acid, with some amino acids being represented by more than one triplet codon. A polypeptide molecule may be composed of 100 to 600 amino acids, and these are in turn encoded by 300 to 1,800 nucleotide molecules in a primary DNA and ultimately in a messenger RNA (mRNA) base sequence. Thus a single substitution of a base in the original DNA sequence, a point mutation, may lead to a substitution of an amino acid within the polypeptide chain.

It has been predicted theoretically before experimental data were available (6) that some amino acid substitutions will render a protein biologically less active or even inactive because of a change in the three-dimensional conformational state of the molecule or, in the case of enzyme protein, because of the inclusion of a defect in the substrate-binding or allosteric regulatory regions of the molecule. Other amino acid substitutions may have less severe consequences and, in fact, may not alter the biological efficiency of the molecule at all.

Point mutations that change the codon meaning are referred to as *missense* mutations. Other DNA mutations that control the regulation of protein synthesis (including the initiation or termination of protein synthesis) are called *nonsense* mutations. Note that premature induction or termination of protein synthesis can occur without changing the amino acid composition. More recently, intervening sequences of DNA *(introns)* situated between sequences of DNA that encode for the structure of a protein *(exons)* have been identified, and here mutations may produce more sophisticated effects on the processing of precursor mRNA species.

Mutations in intron DNA sequences responsible for regulation or coordination of protein synthesis or in exon DNA sequences needed for posttranslational mod-ification may result in reduced biological activity of a protein required for differ-entiated membrane transport, receptor affinity, or enzyme activity. Other mutations in DNA may provide a genetic diversity or heterogeneity that is part of the normal variation in the population and is not associated with disease. As Crick points out in a recent review, the molecular biology of processing of precursor mRNA by splicing out intron regions is an important regulatory step, but it is only the beginning. Regulation of initiation of transcription, intron splicing, capping, poly-adenylation, packaging of message, and the exit from the nucleus involves events that must be contributing to human genetic heterogeneity both in health and disease through point or frame shift mutations followed by their increase in frequency as a result of random genetic drift. (Random genetic drift refers to the entry and distribution of a new gene into a new population with a neutral effect on survival value.) These terms will be defined and discussed in detail in Chapter 4.

Normal Genetic Diversity in the Population

Careful estimates have indicated that the DNA in the nucleus of each human cell is able to encode for about 100,000 genes and thus for more than 100,000 poly-peptide chains. The DNA is arranged in a linear sequence and is associated with nucleosomes (a protein–nucleic acid regulatory complex) packaged into the chromosomes. Each human cell contains 23 chromosome pairs, separate sets being derived from each of the individual's parents. Thus a person has two copies of each chromosome and two copies of each gene. A gene locus refers to the precise location on the chromosome of each copy of a particular gene. An *allele* refers to a gene at a particular gene locus that exists in two or more different forms. A person is known as a *homozygote* for a particular gene when the two copies of the gene at a particular gene locus are identical. A person is a *heterozygote* when the two copies of the gene at a particular gene locus are different. *Genetic heterogeneity* occurs when there is a mutation at a specific gene locus, resulting in a mutant protein that may merely express a normal variation in the population but that may also result in genetic disease.

Genetic heterogeneity may be caused by the presence of a number of different mutations at a single genetic locus *(allelic mutations)* or at different genetic loci *(nonallelic mutations)*. As a general example, hemophilia is a clinical syndrome in which nonallelic mutations can produce a similar clinical picture. On the other hand, sickle cell anemia and certain hemoglobinopathies are examples of diseases arising from allelic mutations that involve various changes in the gene coding for the β chain of hemoglobin, but many of which result in a similar clinical picture. It is important to note that the mode of inheritance may also differ as a result of genetic heterogeneity caused by mutations at some genetic loci. For example, Charcot-Marie-Tooth disease and hereditary spastic paraplegia may be inherited as autosomal dominant traits in some families, as autosomal recessives in others, and occasionally as X-linked recessives. Thus a clear understanding of the molecular events involved in genetic polymorphism is important to appreciate the variations in clinical inheritance and clinical phenotype and to provide accurate genetic counselling (26).

NATURAL SELECTION AND GENETIC DISEASE

It is quite clear that if a mutation occurs that confers some advantage on individuals possessing that gene, then natural selection will cause the frequency of that gene to increase in the population. Indeed, if conditions remain stable, a situation will ultimately arise in which all members of the population carry the gene. In the case in which the mutation confers some disadvantage on the carrier, the outcome of natural selection is equally obvious.

However, in some cases the effect of the mutation on an individual's ability to survive and reproduce may depend on whether the person is *homozygous* (i.e., having identical genes derived from mother and father in the two corresponding loci of a pair of chromosomes) or *heterozygous* (i.e., inheriting different genes from the parents) for the mutant gene.

If we represent the mutant homozygote as *aa*, the heterozygote as *Aa*, and the normal genotype as *AA*, then if the heterozygote has an advantage over both homozygotes, a polymorphism will arise in which the mutant gene *a* remains at a stable frequency within the population, even though the homozygote *aa* may be lethal. In other words, genetic defects may not necessarily be sifted out from a population by the process of natural selection.

Effects such as this may become especially subtle when the defect does not express itself until late in life, i.e., when the reproductive life of the individual is over and natural selection can exert its least effect. Indeed, some theorists view aging itself as the final expression of defects that have been genetically suppressed during youth.

Under these circumstances natural selection may act on the gene frequencies only slowly, and other effects may predominate. One such effect is *genetic drift*. New populations are often started by small numbers of emigrants who carry only a small fraction of the genetic variability of the parental population and hence differ from it. If chance operates in the selection of founder individuals, new populations will tend to differ from the parent population and from each other. This *founder effect* is clearly of potential importance in establishing ethnic genetic differences.

Provided the population is small, then random fluctuations in gene frequencies will occur, which because of the size of the group in which these are occurring, may mean that particular genes are lost while others increase to fixation, i.e., all individuals in the population become homozygous for the gene.

Population Genetics in a Normal Population

Prior to 1966, the year of publication of *Enzyme Polymorphism in Man* by Harry Harris (12), the textbook presentation of population genetics dwelt extensively on problems concerning the spread of single-point mutations. Populations were divided into two groups: those individuals who possessed the mutant gene and those who did not. If the mutant gene resulted in an increase in darwinian fitness, as a measure of an individual's ability to survive and reproduce, then its frequency in the population would increase. If the mutation was disadvantageous, then the gene would be gradually eliminated from the population. This simplistic view of population genetics predicts that very little genetic heterogeneity should exist in populations that have been exposed to the same selective pressures for long periods of time. In other words, the degree of enzyme polymorphism should be very small.

However, in 1966 it became apparent that in real populations the situation was very much more complicated. This advance was made possible by the introduction of electrophoretic techniques that could distinguish between closely related protein molecules by measuring their migration through a gel under the influence of an electric field. Since a single amino acid mutation may alter the net charge on a protein molecule, the enzyme polymorphism within a population can be visualized, and, to some extent, quantified using this technique.

Harris first studied the red cell enzyme acid phosphatase to determine the presence of genetic polymorphism and found that several distinct enzyme phenotypes could be identified, which he referred to as A, BA, B, CA, and CB. They occurred in a British population with frequencies of 0.13, 0.43, 0.36, 0.03, and

0.05, respectively, and all involved very different levels of normal enzyme activity. Using electrophoresis, Harris identified the isoenzyme patterns of phosphoglucomutase, adenylate kinase, and placental alkaline phosphatase. The overall significance of this contribution was the description of an unexpectedly broad spectrum of enzyme variation in a normal human population.

Degree of Genetic Polymorphism

In 1972 Harris and Hopkinson (13) assayed for the occurrence of enzyme and protein polymorphism in 71 human enzymes. Their conclusions were dramatic. Of the 71 enzyme loci studied, 20 (28%) showed electrophoretic polymorphism. By summing the observed values for polymorphism at each locus and dividing by the total number of loci, they obtained an estimate of the average polymorphism per locus. The value obtained was 0.067 or 6.7% and implied that each individual in the population was heterozygous at least 6.7% of these 71 loci. However, their studies only took into consideration polymorphism measured as electrophoretic variance. Since only about one-third of all mutations are detectable by this technique, about two-thirds of mutations result in no change in the charge of the protein. This means that a more accurate estimate of the true degree of heterozygosity would approach 21%. This would therefore suggest that everyone in the population had a genetic variation or heterozygosity at more than 20% of his or her genetic loci, which in turn would mean that more than one-fifth of all enzymes in each normal person were present in a form different from that in the majority of the population. There is therefore only an extremely small chance that, with the exception of monozygotic twins, any two individuals will be genetically identical.

Both Harris and Kimura view mutations that result in genetic heterogeneity as playing a powerful role in molecular variation and evolution. Expressed slightly differently, there is growing evidence to suggest that very slightly deleterious mutations whose disadvantages, in the face of natural selection, are not excessively large may play a significant role in evolution. An important question that remains to be explained is the means by which this degree of polymorphism arises and is maintained within a population.

One view is that the polymorphism is caused by natural selection in the darwinian sense; another view suggests that multiple common alleles are caused by neutral or near-neutral mutations and random genetic drift. Many of the mutations alluded to are amino acid substitutions in the enzyme molecule that have little or no effect on its functional properties and thus are effectively neutral from the point of view of natural selection. This would bias the argument toward a random process and genetic drift. This concept is of great academic interest, as it predicts the evolution of new genetic neurologic disorders and possibly a changing isoenzyme pattern for the normal healthy brain.

Genetic Heterogeneity and Inborn Errors of Metabolism

Sanfilippo's syndrome, Gaucher's disease, generalized gangliosidosis, Tay-Sachs disease, Hurler-Scheie genetic compound syndrome, Hurler's and Hunter's diseases, and Lesch-Nyhan disease all represent clear examples of genetic heterogeneity in inherited neurologic disease.

Sanfilippo's syndrome has been described as being caused by several separate biochemical mutations. Sanfilippo-A is the result of a defect in heparan sulfate sulfatase and Sanfilippo-B is the result of a defect in N-acetyl-α-glucosaminidase. There are other genotypes as well. Both of these enzymes are primarily concerned with the degradation of the mucopolysaccharide heparan sulfate, but they act at different sites on the molecule. Here is an example, then, of a common clinical phenotype caused by two separate nonallelic mutations.

Gaucher's disease (7) occurs as three separate clinical syndromes, the adult, infantile, and juvenile (types 1, 2, and 3, respectively). The sphingolipid glucosyl-ceramide accumulates because of a defect in the enzyme glucosylceramidase. The enzyme deficiency in the infantile form has been reported to be more severe than in the adult form and correlates with a more rapid accumulation of the glycolipid in the infantile form of the disease. It is presumed that these two phenotypes are caused by an allelic state with different mutations occurring in the same enzyme molecule.

Infantile and juvenile forms of generalized gangliosidosis (8,24) have been described, and in both forms a defect in the enzyme β-galactosidase is present that leads to the storage of GM-1 ganglioside within the nervous system. The infantile form of the disease accumulates the glycolipid at a faster rate than the juvenile form, and this is correlated with differences in enzyme activity due to allelic mutations at different points within the same enzyme molecule.

A series of isoenzymes of N-acetylhexosaminidase-A (hex-A) have been described that correlate with the temporal course of classic Tay-Sachs disease, the occurrence of juvenile onset of Tay-Sachs disease, and the childhood or juvenile onset of cerebellar ataxia as a Tay-Sachs variant (15). The later occurrence of disease and its longer duration both correlate with an increasing level of enzyme activity. Presumably these forms represent allelic mutations at different points in the same molecule (hex-A). A variant of this syndrome known at GM-2 gangliosidosis, type II, or Sandhoff's disease results from a deficiency of both hexosaminidase-A and hexosaminidase-B and is clinically indistinguishable from classic infantile Tay-Sachs disease. These isoenzymes are multimeric in that hexosaminidase-A is composed of four polypeptides (alpha$_2$, beta$_1$, beta$_2$). Hexosaminidase-B consists only of the beta subunits. The genetic heterogeneity of this syndrome is complicated further by Sandhoff's and Jatzkewitz's discovery of another form of GM-2 gangliosidosis that is clinically indistinguishable from Tay-Sachs. The enzyme defect in the latter form involves both the A and B isoenzymes, but it cannot be detected with an artificial substrate. The enzyme defect is demonstrated utilizing the natural substrate GM-2 and is thus unique among forms of hex-A deficiency. This condition has been shown to be due to a missing activation required for the hydrolysis of GM-2.

Other interesting genetic compound diseases have been described that involve mucopolysaccharide metabolism. Hurler's syndrome and Scheie's syndrome result from different mutations in the same enzyme, α-iduronidase. These two syndromes are therefore the result of allelic mutations that result in very striking differences in the clinical syndrome. Classic Hurler's syndrome results in severe mental retardation with prominent skeletal deformities, hepatomegaly, and corneal clouding. Scheie's syndrome does not produce intellectual impairment and life-span is normal. We recently studied a patient with the Hurler-Scheie compound disease and were able to show that the patient's metabolism of ^{35}S-labeled mucopolysaccharide was not corrected with Hurler enzyme. The patient was also clinically intermediate between these two syndromes, as mental retardation and coarsening of facial features developed at 20 years of age. Examination of cerebral neurons at both the light and electron microscopic levels revealed the presence of pronounced mucopolysaccharide deposits. Thus this patient was a genetic mosaic for α-L-iduronidase, with each part of the enzyme being defective because of different mutations. The more common Hunter's syndrome, which is inherited as an X-linked recessive, bears a striking resemblance to Hurler's syndrome but is caused by an enzyme defect in sulfoiduronate sulfatase. Although heparan and dermatan sulfate are excreted in both Hurler's and Hunter's syndromes, the two diseases are caused by defects in two separate enzymes, and thus they represent examples of nonallelic mutations producing similar clinical phenotypes.

It is presumed that these allelic and nonallelic mutations have spread via the founder effect and genetic drift. That is, a mutation occurred in a member of a small ethnic population and during the course of subsequent generations spread through the group; the proportion of the population carrying the gene increased purely by mechanisms involving chance. Needless to say, genetic drift can occur only in very small populations and could equally well result in a decrease in frequency of a particular allele. The high incidence of Tay-Sachs disease among Ashkenazic Jews is a case in point. An alternative possibility is that the heterozygote confers some advantage on the carrier, as is the case for sickle cell anemia and resistance to malaria, for example. Under these circumstances a gene that is lethal as a homozygote can be maintained at appreciable levels within the population because of the advantage it confers on those heterozygous for it. In this particular case resistance against tuberculosis and the plague are postulated examples, but this thesis is as yet unproven.

Genetic heterogeneity has also been described in X-linked recessive neurologic diseases. Individual families have been described in which the Lesch-Nyhan syndrome (17) has been found to be caused by different defects in the enzyme hypoxanthine-guanine phosphoribosyltransferase. For example, Kelly in 1968 described the J family as having about 1% of normal enzyme activity when either hypoxanthine or guanine was used. Another family, family L, also showed much reduced enzyme activity, but this reduction was more marked with guanine as substrate than with hypoxanthine. Also the enzyme protein was more heat stable in the L family than the J family. Thus here is an additional example of allelic genetic heterogeneity on the X chromosome.

Pharmacodynamics of Drug Metabolism

It is well established and commonly appreciated that drugs are metabolized at different rates in individuals owing to genetic factors. When isoniazid was introduced, it was quickly appreciated that the rate at which it was metabolized by acetylation varied markedly between individuals but was fairly constant in any one person. It was demonstrated in 1959 that the rate of metabolism is the result of two alleles, with "slow inactivators" (acetyltransferase) being homozygous for one allele and "rapid inactivators" being either heterozygous or homozygous for the other.

Another example of the genetic basis of drug metabolism is the different rates of phenytoin metabolism. A family was carefully studied for the rate of phenytoin inactivation by *para*-hydroxylation. The mean half-life of urinary excretion of the principal metabolite, 5-*p*-hydroxyphenyl-5-phenylhydantoin, was 18 hr for the control population and 29, 31, and 43 hr for three family members, indicating a reduced rate of drug metabolism (26).

The induction of autosomal dominant, acute, intermittent, hepatic porphyria in some patients by specific drugs is well known. For example, barbiturates, phenytoin, sulfur drugs, and estrogens, among others, can precipitate an acute porphyric attack in some individuals. It is presumed that in these genetically susceptible individuals there is induction of the enzyme δ-aminolevulinic acid synthetase. The primary enzyme defect in this disorder is porphobilinogen deaminase (uroporphyrinogen synthetase), resulting in a reduction in the cellular level of porphyrins. It is suggested that a mutation in the enzyme δ-aminolevulinic acid synthetase separate from the primary defect may be responsible for the drug-induced induction in susceptible patients.

Treatment of Genetic Disease

Enzyme replacement therapy for autosomal recessive neurologic disease resulting from an enzyme defect is clearly in an experimental phase and its future is uncertain. Barranger et al. (2) have been able experimentally to "open" the blood-brain barrier for short periods of time to maximize enzyme transport into the nervous system. It is speculated that in the distant future genes encoded for the defective enzyme might be incorporated into a virus phage with a tropism for neurons and glia, thus correcting the biochemical defect at the cellular level.

Selected genetic disorders, however, have been treated on the basis of current knowledge of genetic heterogeneity, by coenzyme infusions. Leon Rosenberg et al. have demonstrated two allelic forms of methylmalonicaciduria involving the enzyme methylmalonyl-CoA carbonylmutatse (25). Some patients respond to high doses of the coenzyme vitamin B_{12}. Responsive patients apparently have a defect in the biosynthetic pathway for the generation of vitamin B_{12}, whereas the nonresponders have a defect in the apoenzyme itself. Thus, although clinically indistinguishable in these two groups of patients, the disease is the result of mutations at different loci. In a similar fashion, patients having a defect in the enzyme cystathionine synthetase express the clinical syndrome homocystinuria. Patients have been described who are responsive to large infusions of vitamin B_6 with an increase in enzyme activity, whereas other patients do not respond. This result may be an example of allelic mutations for different points in the same enzyme. There are many other examples of treatment of disease by cofactor vitamin enzyme induction, and it is the principle of a possible form of treatment which is emphasized here. Somatic cell and germ line gene therapy are discussed in Chapter 7.

Environmental Factors and Genetic Disease

It is clear that environmental factors may constantly modulate the clinical expression of genetic defects. Three genetic diseases illustrate this point. Phenylketonuria (PKU), an autosomal recessive disorder caused by a deficiency in the enzyme phenylalanine hydroxylase, is associated with mental retardation resulting from the presence of high levels in serum and brain of phenylalanine. In a strict sense this disease occurs because our Western diet contains a high amount of protein which is rich in phenylalanine. If for cultural or economic reasons the diet were very low in phenylalanine, as is the case for the diet used to treat these patients, then the disease would not manifest itself in society. The absence of mental retardation in some patients with PKU further suggests the presence of genetic heterogeneity as a crucial factor in modifying the etiological expression of genetic disorders.

Galactosemia is another autosomal recessive disorder in which the enzyme galactose 1-phosphate uridyltransferase is deficient, and if the infant is fed a diet high in galactose, cataracts will form. A diet free of galactose results in reversal of this syndrome, and, indeed, if galactose-containing foods were eliminated, this genetic disease would no longer exist.

Finally, a late mutation in evolution producing a deficiency of the enzyme L-gulonolactone oxidase resulted in the inability of our species to synthesize L-ascorbic acid (vitamin C). Scurvy is thus an environmental disease caused by the absence of dietary vitamin C, an essential metabolite.

A more controversial example is schizophrenia, in which a hypothesized defect results in an increased density of dopamine receptors in the frontal lobe of the brain that may predispose a person to develop this mental illness under excessive stress by the environment.

Autosomal Dominant Neurologic Disease

Great progress has been made in understanding genetic polymorphism in autosomal recessive and X-linked recessive neurologic disease. However, the molecular mechanisms underlying autosomal dominant, inherited, neural disease are not nearly so well understood, as has been shown recently in a review by Brady and Rosenberg (9). In most crosses between individuals showing contrasting characters controlled at a single locus, the heterozygote is indistinguishable from one of the homozygotic forms. In other words, one of the allelomorphs exercises its full effect regardless of whether or not it is partnered by an identical gene. This effect is termed "dominance" (Fig. 5). A nonallelic mutation involving a regulator gene could produce an abnormal repressor substance that binds irreversibly to two distant alleles and inhibits their transcription. This is one theoretical model whereby a single mutation could result in the inhibition of two separate alleles. More simply, a mutation concerned with the regulation of a metabolic pathway could raise enzyme activities to a critical level that might significantly disturb the metabolic pathway and result in a disease process in the heterozygote, as in porphyria.

It is even conceivable theoretically that the patient might be homozygous and mutant at both alleles of a gene locus and express a clinical pattern of disease that is autosomal dominant (Fig. 5). This model for clinically apparent autosomal dominant genetic disease of the nervous system caused by a homozygous genotype has been elegantly worked out for dominantly inherited retinoblastoma, in which chromosome 13 shows a deletion mutation at both esterase D loci (Fig. 5). The pedigree indicates a dominantly inherited disorder, and yet genotypically the patient is homozygously affected. One mutation is inherited from the patient's parent as a germ line mutation and the second mutation is an acquired secondary one. A modifier gene could alter penetrance and expressivity of the clinical disorder by interacting with either the germ-line-derived or the secondary mutation. Ultimately, it is the production of disease in the heterozygote that distinguishes dominantly inherited disease from recessively inherited disease where only the homozygote is clinically affected (Fig. 5).

Autosomal recessive disease is typified by the regularity of the clinical syndrome for a given level of enzyme deficiency. The disease is quite stereotyped, with little variation in severity or in the various forms or features the disease may have within a kindred. In contrast, dominantly inherited neural disease is associated with wide variations in severity and in the types of clinical involvement, even within a single

(a) Heterozygous Patient: One Allele Mutant

Mutant gene 1
————✕————   ---▶   Autosomal dominant
clinical disease

(b) Effect of Modifier:

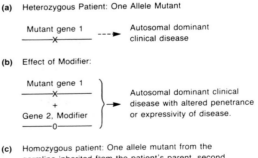

FIG. 5. Mechanisms of clinically autosomal dominant disease. Dominantly inherited disease **(a)** is expressed in the heterozygous patient and can be altered by a modifier gene **(b)**. It is possible that pedigrees showing dominant disease could actually be genotypically homozygous as in dominantly inherited retinoblastoma.

Mutant gene 1
————✕————
+   ⎫
Gene 2, Modifier   ⎬ ▶   Autosomal dominant clinical
————0————   ⎭   disease with altered penetrance
                           or expressivity of disease.

(c) Homozygous patient: One allele mutant from the germline inherited from the patient's parent, second allele mutant as an acquired somatic cell mutation.

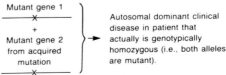

Mutant gene 1
————✕————
+   ⎫   Autosomal dominant clinical
Mutant gene 2   ⎬ ▶   disease in patient that
from acquired   ⎭   actually is genotypically
mutation   homozygous (i.e., both alleles
————✕————   are mutant).

family. A case in point concerns our recent studies with Joseph disease (27). Type I Joseph disease has its onset in the first to third decades of life with progressive spasticity and rigidity with subsequent dystonia and ophthalmoparesis. Type II disease begins in the second to fifth decades of life and is associated with both cerebellar deficits and pyramidal and extrapyramidal findings. Type III disease begins in the fifth to seventh decades with slowly progressive cerebellar deficits and atrophy. It is important to note the occurrence of type I disease in our propositus, Antone Joseph, and type III disease in his grandson. Similar variations in gene expression and penetrance are found in neurofibromatosis, myotonic muscular dystrophy, and Hungtington's disease. Variation may be best explained as being due to modifier genes (reviewed in the next section). Neurofibromatosis may be related to allelic mutations involving nerve growth factor, as described by Fabricant et al. in 1979 (10). Huntington's disease and myotonic muscular dystrophy may relate to receptor-membrane defects involving the subunit of a specific receptor. It may be that dominant neurologic disease relates to nonenzymatic structural or membrane proteins involving tissues and organs. Genetic heterogeneity involving a particular protein subunit in a receptor or membrane protein may express the various differences characteristic of dominantly inherited disease.

Dominantly inherited disease probably in the majority of instances will turn out to be caused by structural protein gene defects. Genes that encode for a protein subunit for a membrane, receptor, or organelle structure will be responsible for dominant diseases as distinct from the recessive disorders, which are caused by enzyme protein defects. Osteogenesis imperfecta is a case in point, as it is autosomal dominant, and in type 2 disease there is a deletion of about 500 base pairs in the DNA for the gene that encodes a procollagen peptide. It results in a shortened peptide, which, when it combines with peptides of normal size to form an oligomer, still results in a biologically functionless molecule. A heterozygous mutation here produces inactivity of 75% of the trimer polypeptides and clinical disease in the heterozygote.

A clearer emerging understanding of genetic heterogeneity involving neurologic genetic disease, it is hoped, will lead to more effective forms of treatment. In addition, through amniocentesis and determination of the presence of abnormal gene products in high-risk pregnancies, it is now possible to restrict significantly the clinical incidence of about 70 genetic diseases, and, theoretically, in the near future eliminate several of them.

Modifying Genes

Genetic diseases, whether recessive, dominant, or X-linked, refer to a single gene defect. When another gene has the ability to modify the penetrance or expressivity of the primary gene responsible for the clinical entity, then the second gene is referred to as a modifier gene (Fig. 5). The best-described types of modifying genes in man are in the ABO blood groups. ABH antigens in secretions depend on the *Se/se* secretor gene. Nonsecretors are homozygous *se/se* and secretors are either heterozygous *Se/se* or homozygous *Se/Se*. Thus *Se* is a recessive suppressor gene (31).

We have found evidence for a modifier gene in autosomal dominant spinocerebellar degeneration of the Joseph disease type. This discovery may have far-reaching consequences that can explain the variation encountered in penetrance and expressivity typical of many common dominantly inherited neurologic disorders. The occurrence of skipped generations in large pedigrees may also be caused by the presence of this type of modifier (Fig. 6) (A. Grossman and R. N. Rosenberg, *unpublished data*). The presence of the BA isoenzyme type of erythrocyte acid phosphatase was associated with the absence of clinical disease in one of our California families (Fig. 7) (A. Grossman and R. N. Rosenberg, *unpublished data*). The gene map location for this enzyme is chromosome 2,p23, (p refers to the chromosomal short arm and 23 refers to a specific locus on the p arm defined by banding patterns) which is presumably linked to the locus for the proposed modifier gene. In an analysis of almost 200 families with the Joseph disease type of spinocerebellar generation, 10% of the families were found to have a significantly reduced number of affected persons, i.e., less than the 50% of affected children that are expected when a parent is affected. Several families show classic skipped generations of this dominantly inherited disease (Fig. 6), presumably because of the full expression of the modifier gene on the primary mutant gene. The possibility that

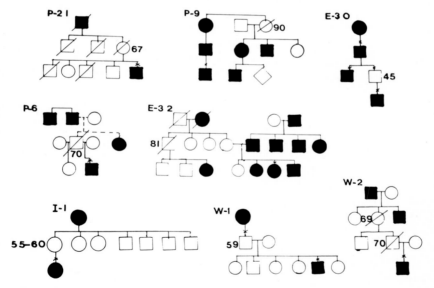

FIG. 6. Autosomal dominant Joseph disease type of spinocerebellar degeneration can result in a variation in clinical expressivity and penetrance of the mutant gene. Early onset aggressive disease or late onset mild development can occur. In fact, several families show a skipped generation, as shown here. This phenomenon is postulated to be caused by a modifier gene that is interacting with the primary mutant gene or its product to reduce the degree of gene penetrance (A. Grossman, G. Sequeiros, and R. N. Rosenberg, *unpublished data*).

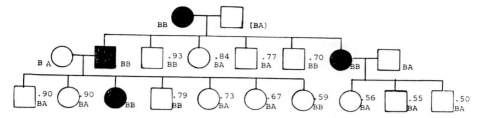

FIG. 7. The C family of California with Joseph disease type of spinocerebellar degeneration is illustrated. The distribution of BB and BA genotypes of erythrocyte acid phosphatase-1 among the members of the family is illustrated. The numbers represent the calculated probabilities of never expressing disease as a function of each member's current age. There is a strong correlation between the BA haplotype of the enzyme and absence of disease, indicating linkage between the chromosome 2p23 locus for acid phosphatase-1 and the postulated suppressor gene locus (A. Grossman, G. Sequeiros, and R. N. Rosenberg, *unpublished data*).

modifier genes in dominantly inherited neurologic diseases may explain variation in penetrance and expressivity of disease has not been fully explored. This postulate is more precise and directly assayable than the explanation of clinical variation as due to normal background genetic heterogeneity involving many genes.

Linkage

Thomas Hunt Morgan established that genes were linked to each other on chromosomes and formulated gene maps in the fruit fly *Drosophila melanogaster*. Genes that are on the same chromosome and are closely physically associated will move together when exchanges of chromosomal segments occur during the meiotic stages of gametogenesis. The units of measurement, as worked out by Sturtevant in 1925 (29), are referred to as centimorgans (cM) in honor of Morgan; 1 cM refers to one map unit, about 10^6 base pairs of nucleotides and 1% recombination frequency. Recombination is defined as the independent segregation of genes that occurs when chromosomal segments exchange. In a sense, linkage between two adjacent genes is measured by the percent recombination between loci.

For practical clinical purposes, two genes are linked if they are less than 5 cM and preferably 2 cM apart. Thus a percent recombination frequency of between 2 and 5% is acceptable for clinical linkage studies. It is the goal of several research teams to locate marker genes either by classic erythrocyte enzyme methods, isoenzyme antigen studies, or complementary DNA (cDNA) probes linked to the mutant gene for a neurologic disorder. In this manner a marker gene is useful to predict clinical disease in the at risk person and also to isolate the mutant gene and determine the altered primary gene product. Linkage is also measured statistically by the use of lod scores (log value of the odds); a lod score greater than 3, i.e., 10^3, for two genes is significant for linkage with a probability of 1,000:1.

The gene map is growing rapidly due mainly to the techniques of somatic cell genetics and *in situ* hybridization. Using a radiolabeled DNA copy of a gene, direct hybridization of the probe to chromosomal DNA will indicate the precise gene location, as hybridization will occur only between DNA sequences. This point is illustrated in Figs. 8 and 9, which show the precise assignment of the human ornithine transcarbamylase locus on the X chromosome using the *in situ* hybridization technique with a cDNA probe for the gene (18).

It is believed that the gene map will be completely deciphered by the year 2000. The rate of progress in assigning gene loci is great, and a doubling of assignments is occurring about every 5 years. As more assignments are made, new linkages and new potential marker genes for mutant genes responsible for genetic disease will

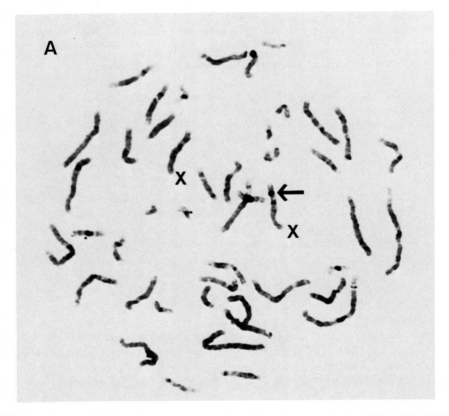

FIG. 8. Wright-stained chromosomes after *in situ* hybridization with plasmid pHO-731. The 1.5-kb Pst I fragment of OTC DNA cloned into pBR332 was labeled with the tritiated triphosphates of deoxyadenosine, deoxycytosine, and thymidine, by nick translation to a specific activity 1.6×10^7 cpm/μg. The probe was hybridized to chromosome spreads overnight at a concentration of 25 ng/ml at 37°C. Photographic emulsion was applied to the slides, which were then exposed for 9 to 13 days. Chromosomes were stained with quinacrine mustard dihydrochloride and photographed with a fluorescence microscope. The slides were then treated with Wright stain and, under bright light, a second photograph was taken of the cells previously chosen for analysis. **A:** Representative normal human metaphase spread (46,XX) with a silver grain over the short arm of an X chromosome in the region of band p21 (*arrow*). (From ref. 18, with permission.) (*Continued.*)

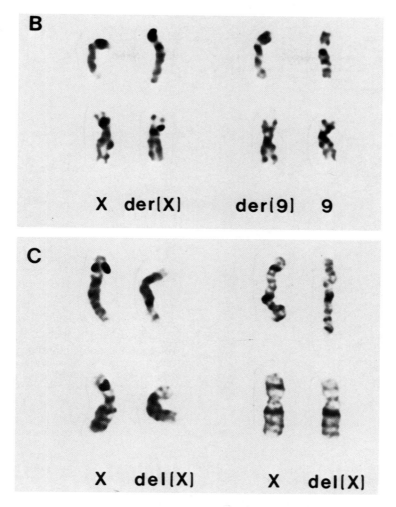

FIG. 8. (*Continued.*)   **B:** Partial karyotypes of two cells from lymphoblastoid cell line GM 6007 [46,*X*,t(X:9) (p21) (p22)], illustrating typical labeling of the der(X) and the X chromosomes in the region of band Xp21.   **C:** On the **left**, X chromosomes from two GM 7773 [46,X,del(X) (p21.1p21.3)] cells, showing labeling of the normal X short arm but not of the deleted X short arm. On the **right**, for comparison, are the X chromosomes from two GTG-banded cells that were not hybridized with the probe. (From ref. 18, with permission.)

be found. One cannot overemphasize the importance of linked marker genes in localizing the gene responsible for a genetic disease of the nervous system in which the mutant gene and its product are not known. By making a linkage association, it is possible to assign the approximate chromosomal location for the mutant gene and with cDNA probes develop a DNA linkage association between the marker and mutant loci. This approach will yield impressive results in the next several

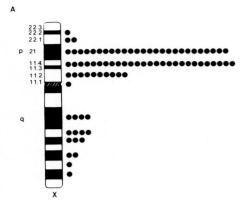

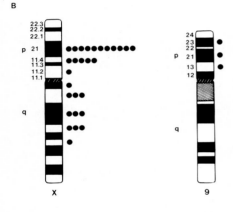

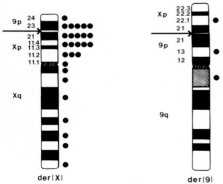

FIG. 9. Ideogrammatic representation of the distribution of silver grains after *in situ* hybridization with the OTC probe. Chromosomes were unambiguously identified on photographs of quinacrine-stained preparations, and then grains were scored at the microscope with the aid of bright-field photographs of the same cells. Although chromosome length varied between the 400- (metaphase) and the 850- (prophase) band stages, grains over chromosomes were conservatively scored on these 400-band-stage ideograms. **A:** Distribution of grains over structurally normal X chromosomes from 46,XX cells and 48,XXXX cells (54 of each). Twenty-two of 214 grains (10.3%) in the 46,XX cells were over bands Xp11.2 to p21, and 41 of 199 grains (20.6%) in the 48,XXXX cells were over the same region. **B:** Ideograms showing the grain distribution over the normal X and the normal 9 chromosomes, as well as over the reciprocal products of a translocation between chromosomes 9 and X from GM 6007 [46,Xt(X:9) (p21) (p22)]. *Arrows* designate the breakpoints on the rearranged chromosomes. Seventeen (7.3%) of the total 234 grains scored in 66 cells were over bands Xp11.2 to Xp21; 18(7.7%) were over the region Xp11.2 to 9p23 of the der(X). In contrast, only two grains (0.9%) were over the der(9) short arm, and three (1.3%) were over the short arm of the normal 9. (From ref. 18, with permission.) (*Continued.*)

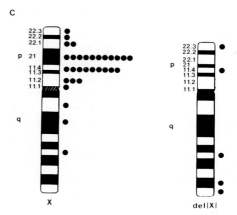

C

FIG. 9. *(Continued.)* **C:** Grain distribution over the normal and deleted X chromosomes of GM 7773 (46,Xdel (X) (p21.1p21.3)). In 41 cells analyzed for grains over all chromosomes, 13 of 129 grains (10.1%) fell in the region Xp11.2 to p21 of the normal X, but only 1(0.8%) fell in this (partially deleted) region of the abnormal X. The grains over the X chromosomes of 23 additional cells, scored only for X and deleted X, are included in this diagram. (From ref. 18, with permission.)

decades in attempts to clone mutant genes, as Gusella et al. are now attempting for Huntington's disease. The approach depends on establishing gene linkages.

NEUROETHOLOGY

The chicken is only an egg's way of making another egg.

Samuel Butler

The organism is only DNA's way of making more DNA. More to the point, the hypothalamus and limbic system are engineered to perpetuate DNA.

Edward O. Wilson

A discussion of neurogenetics could not be complete without reference to neuroethology, which is the study of the genetic basis of behavior. Edward O. Wilson (34) has advanced the body of knowledge in the field under the term sociobiology. Surely our attention as students of the nervous system has been fixed on learned or acquired knowledge. Information storage and retrieval mechanisms are the *sine qua non* of brain function, and the implication that the brain has stored information innately and genetically and that we act on it in an almost preconscious manner has not been widely acclaimed. Wilson cites the view that altruism is a central driving force behind ethological behavior. Parents risk their lives to save their children ostensibly out of love or altruism, but also perhaps because of a genetically determined compulsion to save the pool of DNA inherent in the children, which is next closest to that of the parents. It is a behavioral gene or genes that compel the organism to perpetuate the gene pool or the family line.

Analyses of animal behavior have dissected out the cellular basis and even genetic basis of nonlearned, genetically fixed, ethological behavior. In fact a Nobel Prize has already been awarded to Konrad Lorenz, Karl von Frisch, and Niko Tinbergen for their pioneering work to establish this field (19–21,30). Seymour Benzer's studies with mutagenized gynandromorph fruit flies have been especially compelling. X-Linked mutations in the fruit fly have produced flies that are photophobic, phototropic, sluggish fliers, and even epileptic. Complex social behaviors in ant or bee colonies are excellent examples of genetically determined complex behaviors. The distinctive songs of birds are unique to a species, and only birds of the opposite sex of that species will respond to that characteristic song.

Boys with Lesch-Nyhan syndrome represent an excellent example of a genetic defect involving purine metabolism in the brain that can explain a profound defect in behavior. Inactivity of the X-linked enzyme hypoxanthine guanine phosphoribosyl transferase (HGPRT) results in an abnormally high level of oxypurines in brain. The oxypurine guanosine probably acts as a primary neurotransmitter and also alters receptor functions by modulating adenyl cyclase in neurons and glia. Thus the severe self-mutilation and retardation that these boys experience if not restrained is an example of genetically determined altered behavior.

However, more common behaviors, such as pair bonding (marriage), group bonding (villages), incest taboos, cleanliness, religious feelings, and funeral rites, among many other common daily behaviors, are found in highly primitive tribes throughout the world and were practiced as such long before contact with modern civilization. It is conjectured that such common behaviors were not actually learned by aborigines in Australia or natives in the highlands of New Guinea or in the depths of the Congo or Amazon rain forests. Rather, these basic behaviors are the result of behavioral genes that compel us to act, just as analogous genes cause ants and bees to carry out their complex tasks.

Seymour Kety (16) has shown with his twin studies in Denmark that there is a primary important genetic factor that influences the occurrence of schizophrenia. Monozygotic twins raised in different foster homes by nonbiological parents had a 70% degree of concordance for schizophrenia. These studies minimized the importance of common environmental influences on the disease and convincingly demonstrated powerful genetic influences as causes of this complex behavioral syndrome.

Chromosomal Defects

Neurologic disorders caused by chromosomal abnormalities are few in number and are a result of (a) deletion defects owing to loss of a piece of a chromosome, (b) translocation defects owing to transfer of a piece of one chromosome to another, and (c) nondisjunction defects in which an additional chromosome during early meiosis is acquired, resulting in an autosomal trisomy. Trisomies 22, 21, 18, and 13 all result in mental retardation in varying degree, with trisomies 13 and 18 producing other skeletal malformations and failure to thrive; death often occurs before 1 year of age. The overall frequency of chromosomal defects as determined in karyotypes of unselected newborn infants is 1 in 200, and it is 50% in spontaneous abortions occurring during the first trimester. Most chromosomal defects are therefore not compatible with life.

Trisomy 21 (Down's syndrome) is the most common autosomal trisomy, with a population frequency of 1 in 600; trisomy 18 has a population frequency of 1 in 5,000; and trisomy 13, 1 in 15,000. Trisomy 21 may be a result of nondisjunction occurring in early meiosis in either spermatogenesis or oogenesis or in the first mitotic cleavage of the zygote, and it can also result because of a 14/21 (D/G) or 21/22 (G/G) translocation event (the D and G refer to specific groups of chromosomes). Either a translocation event or nondisjunction results in excess material of chromosome 21 and can produce Down's syndrome with motor and mental retardation and characteristic facial and dermal changes; there is also increased risk of leukemia. It is important to note that karyology must be carried out in parents having one child with Down's syndrome, because if one parent is a carrier of a chromosomal rearrangement as a translocation defect, the recurrence risk in future children may be as high as 20%. It must also be reemphasized that the incidence of trisomy 21 increases drastically in mothers over the age of 35 years. Mental retardation syndromes are also described in rare deletion syndromes 5q (cri du chat), 18q (de Grouchy's syndrome), and 22q (the G deletion syndrome) (q refers to the long arm of the chromosome).

Genetic Counseling

Genetic counseling is an extremely effective means of allaying anxiety and guilt and of containing disease. Counseling is sought by members of large families having dominantly inherited disease and by couples who have had one child with a presumed genetic disorder. The patients want to know the risks for future children, the availability of prenatal diagnosis, or the possibility of heterozygote detection for a known familial genetic disorder by amniocentesis and measurement of a marker for the disease.

The first and most important step in providing counseling is to determine exactly the proper diagnosis, the degree of its penetrance and expressivity, the mean age of onset, the natural history of the disease, and finally the mode of inheritance. Once these data have been compiled, it is then possible to determine risk factors for individuals and subsequent progeny. In a positive manner, counseling can determine who is not at risk so that anxiety is allayed and family planning can be undertaken. It is clear that counseling can avoid sociologic chaos, convert ignorance of a genetic disease process in a family into insight and understanding, and provide a rational constructive approach to family planning.

The combined approach of counseling and determining risk factors by utilizing metabolic or biochemical markers is a powerful tool in eliminating genetic disease. Prenatal detection of fatal genetic disease is one means of containing these disorders and ensuring the birth of normal children. Indications for prenatal diagnosis include the following: (a) couples who have previously had a child with anencephaly or spina bifida (5% recurrence risk); (b) couples who have previously had a child with a chromosomal aberration, such as the trisomy 21 form of Down's syndrome (2% recurrence risk); (c) couples in which either husband or wife carries a balanced translocation chromosome for Down's syndrome (up to 20% recurrence risk); (d) couples at risk for having a child with a detectable metabolic defect (25% risk for an autosomal recessive disorder and 50% risk for a dominantly inherited disorder);

(e) pregnant women 38 years of age or older, who have a 2% chance of having a child with Down's syndrome; and (f) women whose male fetuses could have a 50% risk of being affected with a serious X-linked disease, such as Duchenne's type muscular dystrophy or Lesch-Nyhan syndrome.

REFERENCES

1. Avery, O. T., MacLeod, C. M., and McCarty, M. (1944): Studies on the chemical nature of the substance inducing transformation of pneumococcal types. *J. Exp. Med.*, 79:137–158.
2. Barranger, J., Rapoport, S., Frederick, W., et al. (1979): Modification of the blood-brain barrier: Increased concentration and fate of enzymes entering the brain. *Proc. Natl. Acad. Sci. USA*, 76:481–485.
3. Beadle, G. W. (1945): Biochemical genetics. *Chem. Rev.*, 37:15–96.
4. Beadle, G. W. and Ephrussi, B. (1936): The differentiation of eye pigments in *Drosophila* as studied by transplantations. *Genetics*, 21:225–247.
5. Beadle, G. W., and Tatum, E. L. (1941): Genetic control of biochemical reactions in *Neurospora*. *Proc. Natl. Acad. Sci. USA*, 27:499–506.
6. Brady, R. O. (1966): Sphingolipidoses. *N. Engl. J. Med.*, 275:312–318.
7. Brady, R. O. (1983): Genetic errors and enzyme replacement strategies. In: *Genetics of Neurological and Psychiatric Disorders*, edited by S. Kety, L. P. Rowland, R. L. Sidman, and S. W. Matthysse. Raven Press, New York.
8. Brady, R., O'Brien, J., Bradley, R., and Gal, A. E. (1970): Sphingolipid hydrolases in brain tissue of patients with generalized gangliosidosis. *Biochem. Biophys. Acta.* 210:193–195.
9. Brady, R., and Rosenberg, R. N. (1978): Autosomal dominant neurological disorders. *Ann. Neurol.* 4:548–553.
10. Fabricant, R., Todaro, G., and Eldridge, R. (1979): Increased levels of a nerve-growth factor cross-reacting protein in "central" neurofibromatosis. *Lancet*, 1:4–6.
11. Garrod, A. E. (1923): *Inborn Errors of Metabolism*. London; reprinted by Oxford University Press, 1963.
12. Harris, H. (1966): Enzyme polymorphisms in man. *Proc. R. Soc. Biol.*, 164:298.
13. Harris, H., and Hopkinson, D. A. (1972): Average heterozygosity per locus in man: An estimate based on the incidence of enzyme polymorphisms. *Ann. Hum. Genet.*, 36:9–20.
14. Ingram, V. M. (1957): Gene mutations in human haemoglobin: The chemical difference between normal and sickle cell hemoglobin. *Nature*, 180:325–328.
15. Johnson, W. G. (1981): The clinical spectrum of hexosaminidase deficiency disorders. *Neurology*, 31:1453–1456.
16. Kety, S. S. (1976): Genetic aspects of schizophrenia. *Psychiatr. Ann.*, 6:14–32.
17. Lesch, M., and Nyhan, W. L. (1964): A familial disorder of uric acid metabolism and central nervous system function. *Am. J. Med.*, 36:561–570.
18. Lindgren, V., et al. (1984): Human ornithine transcarbamylase locus mapped to band Xp21.1 near the Duchenne muscular dystrophy locus. *Science*, 226:698–700.
19. Lorenz, K. (1958): Evolution of behavior. *Sci. Am.*, 199(6):67–78.
20. Lorenz, K. (1965): *Evolution and Modification of Behavior*. University of Chicago Press, Chicago.
21. Lorenz, K. (1970): *Studies in Animal and Human Behavior*. Harvard University Press, Cambridge.
22. McKusick, V. A. (1983): *Mendelian Inheritance in Man*, 6th ed. Mosby, St. Louis.
23. Nirenberg, M., Caskey, T., Marshall, R., Brimacombe, R., Kellog, D., Doctor, B., Hatfield, D., Levin, J., Rottman, F., Pestka, S., Wilcox, M., and Anderson, F. (1966): The RNA code and protein synthesis. *Cold Spring Harbor Symp. Quant. Biol.*, 31:11–24.
24. O'Brien, J. (1983): The gangliosidoses. In: *The Metabolic Basis of Inherited Disease; Fifth Edition*, edited by J. Stanbury, pp. 945–969. McGraw-Hill, New York.
25. Rosenberg, L. E. (1972): Disorders of propionate, methylmalonate and vitamin B12 metabolism. In: *The Metabolic Basis of Inherited Disease*, 3rd ed., edited by J. B. Stanbury, J. B. Wyngaarden, and D. S. Fredrickson, pp. 440–458. McGraw-Hill, New York.
26. Rosenberg, R. N. (1984): Genetic variation and neurological disease. *Trends Neurosci.*, 3:144–148.
27. Rosenberg, R. N. (1984): Molecular genetics, recombinant DNA techniques and genetic neurologic disease. *Ann. Neurol.*, 15:511–520.

28. Sloan, H., and Fredrickson, D. (1972): Rare familial diseases with neutral lipid storage. In: *The Metabolic Basis of Inherited Disease*, 3rd ed., edited by J. B. Stanbury, J. B., Wyngaarden, and D. S. Fredrickson, pp. 808–832. McGraw-Hill, New York.
29. Sturtevant, A. H. (1925): The effects of unequal crossing over at the bar locus in *Drosophila*. *Genetics*, 10:117.
30. Tinbergen, N. (1965): Behavior and natural selection. In: *Ideas in Modern Biology*, edited by J. A. Moore. *Proc. 16th Int. Zool. Congr., Washington, 1963*, 6:529–542.
31. Vogel, F., and Motulsky, A. G. (1982): *Human Genetics.* Springer-Verlag, Berlin.
32. Watson, J. D. (1976): *Molecular Biology of the Gene*, 3rd ed. Benjamin, New York.
33. Watson, J. D., and Crick, F. H. C. (1953): Molecular structure of nucleic acids—A structure for deoxyribose nucleic acid. *Nature*, 171:737–738.
34. Wilson, E. O. (1975): *Sociobiology, The New Synthesis*. Belknap Press of Harvard University Press, Cambridge.

2

Genetic Program of Neuronal and Glial Differentiation

In 1907 Ross G. Harrison published "Observations on the Living Developing Nerve Fiber," the first published account of the maintenance and growth of neural tissue *in vitro*. He explanted a small portion of neural tube from a frog embryo and demonstrated the development of an axis cylinder from perikaryon over clotted lymph. The great importance of this experiment was that (a) it indicated that neuronal morphologic differentiation could be continued and studied for prolonged periods *in vitro*, and (b) it provided unambiguous data to support the Cajal neuron doctrine, as the evolving naked fibers in his cultures were processes of neuronal units and not syncytial in origin. Since Harrison's paper, a voluminous body of literature has accumulated documenting the development of explants *in vitro* from central and peripheral nervous systems. This has been comprehensively reviewed by Murray (29) and includes the following topics: cellular morphology and movements, neurite outgrowth, neurophysiologic properties, neurosecretion, effect of drugs and nerve growth factor, the electron microscopic appearance of long-term cultured neurons, maintenance and formation of new synapses *in vitro*, myelination *in vitro*, axoplasmic flow, and experimental allergic encephalomyelitis and neuritis *in vitro*. The quantitative biochemical characterization of neuronal differentiation *in vitro* has been developed more recently.

The development of highly sensitive radioisotopic microassays for enzymes involved in neurotransmitter biosynthesis has allowed characterization of enzyme activities in small amounts of neural tissue during stages of differentiation in cell culture. It has become possible with these new techniques to move beyond morphologic and histochemical descriptive characterizations of *in vitro* neuronal differentiation. The enzymology of neurotransmitter synthesis and degradation in cell culture has opened an exciting new chapter in the quantitative understanding of developmental processes in the nervous system. The cell culture system provides a highly dynamic approach to the study of neuronal differentiation, as rates of cell

---

This chapter is modified from material published previously in *Tissue Culture of the Nervous System*, edited by G. Sato, Plenum Press, New York, 1973, with permission of the publisher.

growth, cell density, and growth environment can be varied at will to study their effects on specific enzymatic events.

Dissociated newborn Balb/C mouse brain and the cloned C1300 Ajax mouse neuroblastoma are two distinctly different cell culture systems that have provided interesting quantitative enzymatic information about the differentiation of nervous system tissue. The Balb/C mouse brain approach allows dissociated neurons, glia, fibroblasts, histiocytes, and blood vessel endothelial cells to interact as single cells and re-form into a monolayer on a Petri dish or into an aggregate of mixed cells in a suspension-rotation culture. The cell culture of mouse neuroblastoma utilizes a pure population of cloned, transformed neuroblasts and allows the study of enzymatic and morphologic development of neurons devoid of the effect of any other cell type. This chapter describes experiments in which I participated as a Research Associate for Marshall Nirenberg of the National Institutes of Health and then subsequently in my own laboratory.

DISSOCIATED PRIMARY MOUSE BRAIN CULTURES

Monolayer Cultures

Newborn Balb/C mouse brain was cultured as single cells after serial trypsin dissociations (38,52). Ten million viable brain cells as determined by exclusion of nigrosin stain were placed in 150-mm Petri dishes and incubated in 10% CO_2, 90% air, 100% humidity, 37°C in Dulbecco's modified Eagle's medium with 10% fetal calf serum, 50 U/ml penicillin, and 10 μg/ml streptomycin. The ontogeny of the cultures was followed by assays of cell number, DNA and protein content, and activities of three enzymes considered to be markers of neuronal differentiation.

Choline-*O*-acetyltransferase (CAT) (E.C. 2.3.1.6) and acetylcholinesterase (AChE) (E.C. 3.1.1.7), two important enzymes in acetylcholine metabolism, and glutamic acid decarboxylase (GAD) (E.C. 4.1.1.15), responsible for the synthesis of the inhibitory neurotransmitter γ-aminobutyric acid (GABA), were chosen for characterization. CAT, AChE, and GAD activities were assayed according to the methods of Wilson et al. and Schrier et al. Enzyme activities per milligram of protein were measured for three enzymes approximately every 3 days in culture for a 2-week period (38,54).

Single-cell populations were obtained from intact newborn Balb/C mouse brains by serial exposure to 0.25% trypsin in Puck's Ca^{2+}, Mg^{2+}-free D_1 salt solution at 37°C for three 15-min intervals. This yielded about 100×16^6 viable brain cells/g wet weight of brain, or 7.4×10^6 cells from the dissociation of a single mouse brain. The dissociation yielded 21% of the DNA present in an intact brain, as measured quantitatively by fluorometric measurement, and if this represented about 21% of the total number of cells, then the Balb/C newborn mouse brain contains about 35×10^6 cells.

As shown in Fig. 1, about 10% of the initially plated cells remained viable by day 3 in culture, and it was the rapid division of these surviving cells that produced

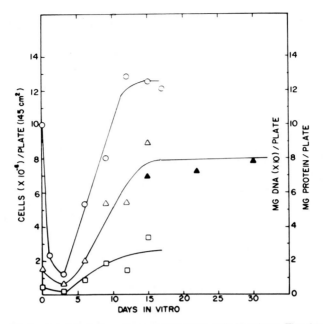

FIG. 1. Growth characteristics of newborn mouse brain cells in culture. The day 0 values represent the DNA and protein content of the initially plated cells. On day 0, 10^7 viable cells were placed in each dish. ○, Cell count; △,▲, protein content; □, DNA content per plate. ▲, Protein content for an extended time period. (From refs. 38 and 52 with permission.)

a monolayer of about 12×10^6 cells after 2 weeks in culture. There was a parallel rise in total plate protein and DNA content during the growth period.

Aliquots of the freshly dissociated newborn mouse brain cells were assayed for CAT, AChE, and GAD activities and compared with newborn mouse brain homogenate, cultured nonneuronal brain cells, and cultured nonbrain cells (Table 1). The remainder of the freshly dissociated cells were placed in culture, and enzyme assays were performed every 3 days. Assay conditions are described in Tables 2 and 3.

A summary of the changes in enzyme activities as the cultures grew and differentiated is given in Fig. 2. It is of great interest that each of the marker enzymes selected followed a different pattern of induction of activity. The "signal" for induction of CAT was present as the cells were rapidly dividing and persisted into the postconfluent phase. Although there were increasing amounts of acetylcholine being synthesized as the cultures approached and became confluent, there remained persistent low levels of AChE activity. Apparently, the "signal" for its induction was independent of the concentrations of acetylcholine present under these culture conditions or the AChE activity expressed was adequate to hydrolyze available acetylcholine. GAD activity, i.e., synthesis of GABA, remained low during the period of rapid cell division, and only with confluency and restricted cell division

TABLE 1. *Enzyme specific activities in newborn mouse brain and cultured cells*

Determination	Newborn mouse brain homogenate	Cultured cells							Newborn mouse brain cells
		Brain, nonneuronal				Nonbrain			
		C6	C12	CHB	RC179	L929	Hcla	3T3-S	
GAD									
By CO$_2$ production	487	79	71	84	43	55	13	8	93
By GABA production	496	8	5	1	3	0.2		6	86
CAT	75	9			2	10	3	5	16
AChE	25,900	732	701		280	625	299	102	1120

Specific activities of GAD, CAT, and AChE were determined on extracts of cultured cells. An uncentrifuged homogenate of newborn Balb/C mouse brain was used for comparison. The maximum content of homogenate protein in the assays was 237 μg for mouse brain homogenates, 110 μg for C6, 906 μg for C2$_1$, 852 μg for CHB, 258 μg for RG179, 1,306 μg for L929 (B82 clone), 939 μg for HeLa, 533 μg for 3T3-S (Swiss mouse 3T3), and 580 μg for mouse brain cells cultured 30 days. Formation of GABA was determined in assays with 1-[u-^{14}C]glutamate as substrate, followed by electrophoresis and chromatography. All determinations on cultured cells were 7 to 20 days after confluency. GAD activity shows for C6 represents the highest activity (at 31.5 mg of cell protein per 150-mm dish) found among four separate points on a growth curve.

From ref. 38, with permission.

TABLE 2. *Range and sensitivity of assays*

Assay	Source of homogenate	Incubation time (min)	Radioactive product	Usual range and sensitivity, amount of ^{14}C or ^{3}H product/ reaction (pmol)	Average amount of ^{14}C or ^{3}H product/ min/mg protein (pmol)
AChE	Neuroblastoma clone	10	[^{2}H]Acetate	1,000 14,000	75,000
			[^{14}C]Acetate	75 14,000	75,000
CAT	Mouse brain (age 35 days)	10	[^{14}C]Acetylcholine	5 700	1,500
GAD	Mouse brain (newborn)	10	[^{14}C]CO$_2$	20 3,000	150
Catechol-*O*-methyltransferase	Neuroblastoma clone N18	20	3-[^{14}C]Methoxy-4-hydroxyben-zoic acid	10 1,200	75

From ref. 52, with permission.

was there induction of GABA formation. GAD activity in brain cultures was at least 10-fold higher than in nonneuronal cell cultures.

The morphologic appearance of the cultures changed dramatically during this 2-week culture period. At first cells were rounded-up and appeared as nonspecific undifferentiated cells. During the first week in culture, cells developed processes

TABLE 3. *Enzyme stability and product recovery*

Modification	CAT (%)	AChE (%)	GAD (%)	Cathechol-*O*-methyltransferase (%)
Enzyme stability				
Complete reaction	100	100	100	100
Minus enzyme	2	9	8	9
Enzyme frozen and thawed three times	98	99	109	108
Enzyme held at 1°C for 2–3 hr	100	100	116	104
Enzyme held at 100°C for 10 min	2	9	8	8
Reaction incubated at 1°C				
Product recovery	9	31	10	7
Radioactive product added instead of substrate	95	110	94	83

The amounts of radioactive product formed (pmol) per complete reaction corresponding to 100% were 610, 300, 630, and 114 for CAT, AChE, GAD, and catechol-*O*-methyltransferase reactions, respectively. Product recovery was tested by adding the following compounds to reactions in place of radioactive substrate: CAT assay, 28 nmol X-[^{14}C]acetylcholine iodide (1.53 × 10 dpm); AChE, 205 nmol [^{14}C]sodium acetate (8.05 × 10^5 dpm); GAD, 35 nmol [^{14}C]NaHCO$_3$ (3.97 × 10^5 dpm) and 0.015 nmol 4-[^{14}C]methoxy-3-hydroxybenzoic acid (350 dpm).
From ref. 52, with permission.

and several cell types were recognized only as being polygonal or spindle shaped, but no characteristic cell resembling a neuron could be identified. By day 9 in culture, phase-dark large multipolar cells could be seen (Fig. 3), and during the next 2 weeks many more phase-dark cells became evident, with the elaboration of many long, complex-appearing neurites (Fig. 4), suggesting circuit formation. A culture maintained for 42 days and then stained with a Bodian protargol silver stain, which has high affinity for neuronal processes, contained many cells that stained positively and looked like characteristic neurons (Fig. 5).

Thus the monolayer culturing of mixed, dissociated newborn Balb/C mouse brain cells resulted in the organization of a new network of cells. Most important is that this approach provided simultaneous direct morphologic and enzymatic data of neuronal redifferentiation *in vitro* and that changes in activities of enzymes concerned with acetylcholine and GABA metabolism were selective.

Suspension-Rotation Cultures

Recently a suspension-rotation brain cell culture system derived from embryonic dissociated mouse brain was developed by Seeds (42) and Seeds and Gilman (43). Dissociated cells from embryonic mouse brain reaggregated in suspension-rotation cultures, and between days 4 and 14 in culture there were significant increases in specific activities of CAT, AChE, and GAD. Also within hours of rotation culturing, an aggregate of cells was produced that was capable of producing a four- to sixfold increase in the intracellular level of cyclic AMP (adenosine-3′,5′-mono-

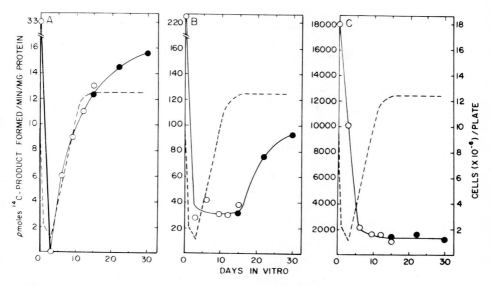

FIG. 2. The specific activities of **(A)** CAT, **(B)** GAD, and **(C)** AChE plotted against the time that cells were in culture. Initially, 10^7 viable newborn Balb/C mouse brain cells were placed in each 150-mm Petri dish. The day 0 points represent the specific activity of the enzyme in the initially plated cells. ---, Cell count; ○, activity of the culture/mg protein/min; ●, the same activity for an extended time period. (From refs 38 and 52, with permission.)

phosphate) due to a brief incubation with 10^{-4} M norepinephrine or isoproterenol (43). The cyclic AMP response to these sympathomimetic agents did not occur with freshly dissociated brain or in cultures 15 hr old, but was present in 9-day cultures. This response could be considered a developmental event, as a similar nonresponsiveness was observed in brains of newborn rats and appeared only after 4 days of age.

Synaptogenesis has been observed to occur in dissociated embryonic brain cells that reassociate in rotation culture to form aggregates (45). Synapse formation was not evenly distributed with the aggregate but rather was found in groups, making it difficult to compare directly the number of synapses made in 12- and 33-day-old rotation aggregates. However, between days 12 and 33 *in vitro*, it was estimated that there were a fivefold increase in the number of synapses, increased numbers of vesicles per synapse, and increased electron density adjacent to the postsynaptic membrane. These observations by Seeds and Vatter are indeed important, as they provide a model *in vitro* system for approaching directly for the first time the molecular events involved in synapse formation, and for approaching the question of whether cell-cell interaction is highly specific and under genetic control or more flexible and random.

In summary, the sequence of events occurring during neural differentiation of primary dissociated brain cells in rotation-suspension or monolayer culture includes

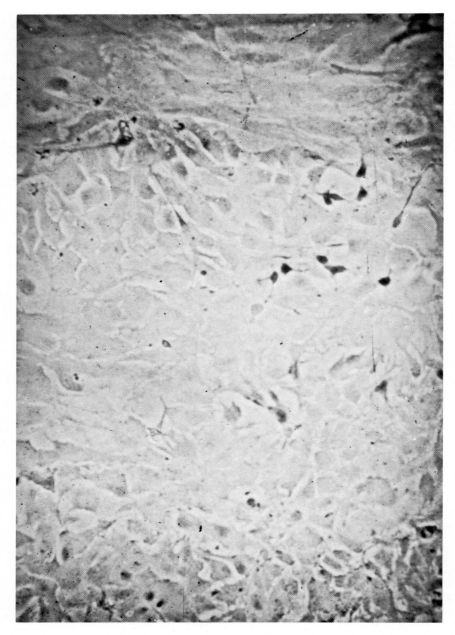

FIG. 3. Photomicrograph of a culture 9 days *in vitro*. There is a layer of flat, polygonal-shaped cells, and there are occasional phase-dark pyramidal-shaped cells with multipolar processes which morphologically resemble neurons. × 50. (From refs. 38 and 52, with permission.)

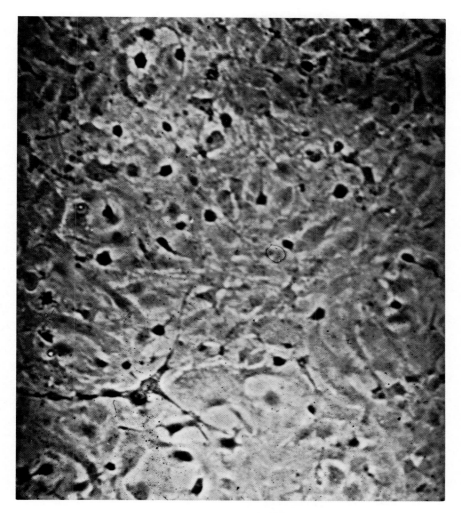

FIG. 4. Photomicrograph of a 25-day-old culture. The increased number of phase-dark pyramidal-shaped neuron-like appearing cells is evident compared with that in Fig. 3. Note one large multipolar-appearing phase-dark cell with long discrete neurites. ×35. (From refs. 38 and 48, with permission.)

(a) morphologic dedifferentiation with loss of cell processes and formation of nonspecific-appearing cells; (b) cellular attachment to a flat surface or cell-cell aggregation in rotation culture; (c) establishment of a confluent monolayer of cells or an enlarging clump of aggregated cells in rotation; (d) emergence after a variable latent period of morphologically recognizable neurons; (e) expression of biochemically differentiated neuronal functions, i.e., increased specific activities of CAT, AChE, and GAD for the synthesis of acetylcholine, hydrolysis of acetylcholine,

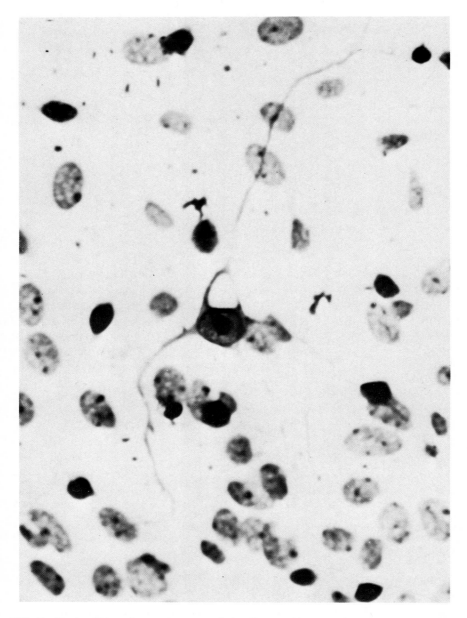

FIG. 5.   By day 43 in culture, many phase-dark cells are evident containing long processes, as seen in the cell illustrated in Fig. 4. A neuron-like appearing cell is shown here after staining of the culture with a modified Bodian protargol silver stain, which has affinity for neurites of neurons. The cell demonstrates long neurites by this technique, which suggests that it is a neuron, and its uniqueness is readily appreciated by comparing it with surrounding cells. Note the pyramidal-shaped soma and a large central nucleus, which also suggests that it is a neuron. × 420. (From refs. 38 and 48, with permission.)

and formation of GABA from glutamate, respectively; (f) neurotransmitter induction of $3',5'$-cyclic AMP; and (g) *de novo* formation of synapses in culture.

NEUROBLASTOMA C1300 AJAX MOUSE CELLS IN CULTURE

The distinct advantage of culturing cloned neuroblastoma rather than dissociated whole brain in suspension-rotation or monolayer cultures is that neuroblastoma is a cell line of pure neuroblasts devoid of nonneural cells. Although neuroblastoma C1300 cells are tumor cells and have been in culture for 5,000 to 8,000 cell generations, they have retained many properties of differentiated *in vivo* mammalian neurons. These properties include the presence of (a) CAT (4), AChE (5), tyrosine hydroxylase (4), and catechol-O-methyltransferase (5); (b) neurites containing microtubules, neurofilaments, and dense-core vesicles (40); (c) catechol formation (40); and (d) membranes capable of generating action potentials in response to electrical stimulation or acetylcholine (30).

The C1300 neuroblastoma cell line derived from the Ajax mouse was originally adapted to cell culture by Augusti-Tocco and Sato (4). They demonstrated that the monolayer cell cultures of neuroblastoma were capable of metabolizing acetylcholine and also possessed tyrosine hydroxylase. Human neuroblastoma also has been cultured *in vitro* and has been shown to contain enzymes concerned with norepinephrine synthesis and degradation. Here then is a powerful system for studying neuronal differentiation of enzymes needed for neurotransmitter metabolism.

Blume et al. (5) demonstrated that AChE activity in neuroblastoma cells could be regulated and that enzyme activity was inversely related to rate of cell division. The specific activity of mouse neuroblastoma AChE increased 25-fold when the rate of cell division was restricted, whereas catechol-O-methyltransferase (E.C. 2.1.1.6) did not change significantly (Fig. 6).Thus when cultures were confluent, when cell division was restricted, and when neurite formation was evident, the highest levels of AChE activity per milligram of protein were present. The rate of cell division could be regulated by adjusting the serum concentration. When fetal calf serum was removed during the growth period, cell division ceased and AChE activity was significantly and rapidly induced. Readdition of serum to the culture medium resulted in a brisk reestablishment of cell division and a reduction in AChE activity (Fig. 7).

Clones of neuroblastoma have been recently described (2) that had high levels of either CAT or tyrosine hydroxylase or that had neither enzyme. Thus three types of clones of neuroblastoma cells were found to exist with respect to neurotransmitter synthesis: cholinergic, adrenergic, and clones that did not synthesize acetylcholine or catechols. All the clones contained AChE and apparently cannot be used as a specific marker of cholinergic neurons. Thus this elegant contribution by Amano et al. points out that at the single-neuron level, despite thousands of generations in culture, distinct classes of neuroblastoma cells exist that have retained the genetic expression for a single neurotransmitter. Further, it was suggested that the expression of a gene required fór the synthesis of one transmitter may restrict the

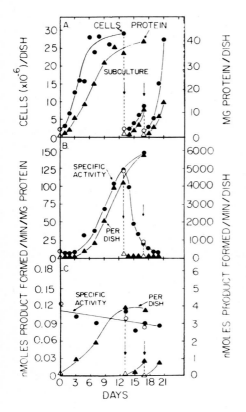

FIG. 6. Neuroblastoma cells in logarithmic growth were subcultured without trypsin. On days 13 and 17 of incubation, some of the cells were dissociated with trypsin (indicated by the vertical dashed lines). Filled and open symbols represent the values obtained before and after subculture, respectively. **A:** ●, Cells/dish; ▲, mg protein/dish. More than 85% of the cells were viable throughout the experiment. **B:** ●, AChE specific activity; by the filled circles; ▲, AChE activity/dish. **C:** ●, Catechol-*O*-methyltransferase specific activity; ▲, activity/dish. (From ref. 5, with permission.)

expression of genes for alternate neurotransmitters. Thus a gene product of CAT might inhibit gene expression for tyrosine hydroxylase, and the simultaneous expression of both these genes might in turn inactivate them, with the formation of a cell with both low cholinergic and low adrenergic activities. These indeed are provocative concepts and important problems for future investigation.

Neurite formation can also be regulated, as shown by Seeds et al. (44), with length and rapidity of their development being inversely proportional to serum concentration in the growth medium. Seventy percent of cultured neuroblasts developed neurites in a few hours in the absence of serum, compared with less than 10% of cells cultured for 70 hr in the presence of 10% fetal calf serum. Cycloheximide experiments using up to 1.8×10^{-4} M, a concentration that inhibits proline incorporation into protein by more than 97%, had little effect on neurite outgrowth. The antimitotic drugs vinblastine and colchicine inhibited neurite outgrowth completely at 10^{-7} and 10^{-6} M, respectively. Seeds et al. (44) suggested that neurite formation depended on the assembly of microtubules from preformed protein subunits and did not require protein synthesis as long as the subunit pool was maintained.

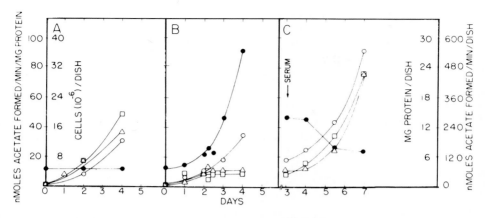

FIG. 7. The rate of cell division was regulated by adjusting the serum concentration. Neuroblastoma cells were incubated for 24 hr prior to 0 time in 150-mm dishes containing the medium described in the text (Dulbecco's modified Eagle's medium plus 10% fetal calf serum). At 0 time, the medium was removed and cells were washed once with growth medium; then fresh medium with **(A)** or without **(B)** 110% fetal calf serum was added. Some cells were incubated for 3 days without serum, as shown in B; nondividing cells were then shifted up to the rapidly dividing state by addition of 10% fetal calf serum **(C)**. The medium was changed and fresh medium containing 10% fetal calf serum was added at 4 and 5.5 days. ●, AChE specific activity; ○, AChE activity/dish; △, cells (10^6/dish); □, mg protein/dish. (From ref. 5, with permission.)

NEUROBLAST-GLIOBLAST BIOCHEMICAL RELATIONSHIPS

Neurobiologists have fixed their interests mainly on the neuron and less on the other major cell type in brain, the glial cell. Processes of astroglial cells *in vivo* are found extensively along the soma and axons of neurons and the endothelial cells of capillaries and thus are strategically positioned to provide transport of anabolites and catabolites between plasma and neuron and between neurons. The other important glial cell type, the oligodendroglia, synthesizes the axonal myelin sheath.

Cyclic AMP

Tumor glioblastoma cells have been grown in monolayer culture as a means of investigating various biochemical parameters that may be affected by neuroblasts or neurotransmitters to provide a better understanding of these events in the intact brain. Gilman and Nirenberg (18) demonstrated a 200-fold induction in cyclic AMP in a clonal line of rat glial tumor cells (C6 cells) by norepinephrine. Clark and Perkins (12) also showed a rapid increase in the concentrations of cyclic AMP induced by norepinephrine, epinephrine, and histamine in a tumor astrocyte cell line derived from a primary culture of a human glioblastoma multiforme. A similar 50- to 100-fold inductive effect by catecholamines on cyclic AMP formation occurred in primary monolayer cultures from embryonic rat brain, and there was a four- to sixfold increase in cyclic AMP in rotation-reaggregated brain cultures induced by norepinephrine, suggesting that in these mixed cultures the induced cyclic AMP might be of glial origin (43).

Prashad et al. (34) showed that cyclic AMP-binding proteins from mouse neuroblastoma cells were purified by cyclic AMP-affinity sepharose resin and were analyzed by two-dimensional polyacrylamide gel electrophoresis. The two cyclic AMP-binding proteins R1 and R2 were identified on the second-dimensional slab gels. The isoelectric points of these proteins are 5.4 (R1) and 5.2 (R2), and both proteins have a molecular weight of 48,000 to 50,000. These two cyclic AMP-binding proteins, identified in the cellular fractions by photoaffinity labeling techniques, are located above actin (pI = 5.4, MW = 43,000) on the second-dimensional slab gels. Analysis of cellular fractions of cytoplasmic, particulate, and nuclear nonhistone proteins from [^{35}S]methionine-labeled cells on two-dimensional gels shows the presence of proteins R1 and R2. $N^6,O^{2'}$-Dibutyryladenosine 3′,5′-monophosphate (Bt$_2$ cyclic AMP) induced only one cyclic AMP-binding protein, R1, from three- to eightfold in these fractions. Bt$_2$ cyclic AMP stimulated the synthesis of cyclic AMP-binding protein R1 without affecting R2. Cyclic AMP-binding protein R1 is 0.06 and 0.2% of the total cytoplasmic proteins in the control and Bt$_2$ cyclic AMP-treated cells, respectively, and R2 is 0.06% in both cells. Chromatin isolated from Bt$_2$ cyclic AMP-treated cells also showed an increase in [^{3}H] cyclic AMP binding. Bt$_2$ cyclic AMP also affected the levels of 42 nuclear nonhistone proteins: 23 proteins increased and 19 proteins decreased. The increase in the nuclear cyclic AMP-binding protein and the changes in other nonhistone proteins may affect the transcriptional activity of some specific genes, thus causing biochemical changes in neuroblastoma cells.

Morrison et al. (28) demonstrated the relative rates of synthesis and turnover of poly(A)-containing messenger RNAs (mRNAs) in the S-20 (cholinergic) and NIE-115 (adrenergic) neuroblastoma clones after 3 days of treatment with dibutyryl cyclic AMP or the phosphodiesterase inhibitor N-4-(3-butoxy-4-methoxybenzyl)-2-imidazolidinone (Ro20-1724) in an attempt to correlate transcriptional and posttranscriptional changes with observed cyclic AMP-induced changes in the differentiated state. Treatment of S-20 cells with dibutyryl cyclic AMP for 3 days caused a fourfold increase in intracellular cyclic AMP and a 30% decrease in growth rate compared with the levels in control cells. However, there was no difference in the synthesis of the poly(A)-containing RNAs, relative to the ribosomal RNAs, after either 2 or 18 hr of labeling with [^{3}H] adenosine. There was also no increase in the steady-state mRNA levels. Treatment with Ro20-1724 caused only a transient twofold increase in intracellular cyclic AMP level when S-20 cells were plated at a low density and no increase at higher densities, although growth was inhibited by 60%. There was, again, no increase in the relative synthesis of poly(A) mRNAs with 2 hr of labeling in cells treated with Ro20-1724, but there was a twofold increase after labeling for 18 hr. Optical density measurements, however, showed that this increased incorporation of [^{3}H]adenosine did not result in an increase in the absolute amount of unlabeled poly(A)-containing mRNAs. NIE-115 cells showed an eightfold increase in intracellular cyclic AMP after 3 days of treatment with Ro20-1724 and an 80% inhibition of growth rate. However, the relative rates of synthesis of the poly(A)-containing mRNAs were identical to those obtained using

S-20 cells. These results show that neither increased intracellular cyclic AMP levels nor growth inhibition necessarily results in a relative increase in the synthesis of the poly(A)-containing mRNAs in these neuroblastoma clones. These was no change in the synthesis or processing of the poly(A) regions of the mRNAs in the S-20 control and treated cells. In contrast to results with other cells, the poly(A) profiles were heterogeneous, even after 1 h of labeling. The average size of the poly(A) region decreased similarly in control and drug-treated cells after 1, 2, and 18 hr of labeling.

Neurotransmitter Inactivation

Henn and Hamberger (22) obtained enriched fractions of neurons and glia from rabbit brain and investigated accumulation of norepinephrine, serotonin, dopamine, and GABA. Both neurons and glia were able to concentrate monoamine transmitters about fourfold from an incubating medium containing 0.1 to 1 μM concentrations. Glial cell fractions were able to concentrate GABA over a hundredfold from the medium as compared to only fourfold for the neuronal fraction. This suggests that glial cells in the intact brain might serve as an important buffer reservoir for inactivation of neurotransmitters that might otherwise increase in concentration in the synaptic cleft, and that glia might be essential for maintenance of rapid, prolonged chemical neurotransmission.

Glucose Transport

Galambos postulated in 1961 (17) that neuron-glia synapses occurred in addition to neuron-neuron synapses (Fig. 8). A metabolic interrelationship between these two cell types was suggested by the finding by Gilman and Nirenberg (18) that the neurotransmitter norepinephrine caused an increase in cyclic AMP in rat glioblastoma cells in culture. Further, it was known that glycogenolysis was increased by cyclic AMP due to an activation of a protein kinase that converts phosphorylase *b* to phosphorylase *a*, the active form of the enzyme. On the basis of these results, Newburgh and Rosenberg (31) examined the effect of norepinephrine on the transport of glucose in cloned glioblastoma cells (clone C6) isolated from a rat astro-

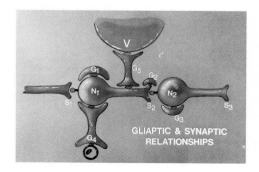

FIG. 8. Neuronal glial anatomic relationships are illustrated showing potential sites of interaction. Direct neuronal-neuronal interactions occur at synapses S_1–S_3. Neuronal-glial interactions can potentially occur at gliapses G_1–G_3. Specialized glia allow capillary-neuronal interaction (G_4) and ventricular (v) CSF neuronal interaction (G_5).

cytoma and in mouse neuroblastoma cells (clone C46) in cell culture. These cell lines were the gift of Dr. Gordon Sato.

Petri dishes (60 mm) were incubated with 3×10^6 cells for 2 days in Dulbecco's modified Eagle's medium (DMEM) with 10% fetal calf serum at 37°C in an atmosphere of 10% CO_2 and 90% air at 100% humidity. The medium was then changed to 2 ml of fresh DMEM or Earle's balanced salt solution containing the radioactive glucose desired and incubated for 30 min. For the studies with theophylline, the cells were incubated for 1 hr in the culture medium plus 1×10^{-3} M theophylline prior to adding the radioactive medium. Norepinephrine (0.017 mg/ml) was added where indicated. In the experiments in which cells were prelabeled with radioactive glucose, the cells were incubated for 2 hr in a radioactive medium, washed twice with a nonradioactive medium, and then incubated for 30 min in a nonradioactive medium. After the incubation the cells were scraped from the Petri dish, filtered through a millipore filter (HaWP 0.025, HA 0.45 μ, 25 mm), and washed twice with 0.32 M sucrose, and the filter was counted in a Beckman scintillation counter.

For the studies of the effects of norepinephrine on the uptake of D-[^{14}C] glucose, glioblastoma cells were grown for 2 days in DMEM plus 10% fetal calf serum. The growth medium was removed and replaced with the same medium plus 1×10^{-3} M theophylline. After 1 hr the medium was replaced with Earle's balanced salt solution containing various radiolabeled compounds, incubated for 20 min, and filtered. When the cells were not preincubated in theophylline, there was an inhibition by norepinephrine of from 20 to 50% of the incorporation of glucose. Less inhibition (10–30%) was found when the cells were preincubated in theophylline. If the cells were incubated as previously described, except that Earle's balanced salt solution was replaced with DMEM plus 10% fetal calf serum plus the radioactive substrate, similar results were obtained.

In another series of experiments, the cells were incubated for 2 hr in the presence of radioactive glucose and then washed, and the medium was changed to Earle's balanced salt solution. The cells were then incubated for 30 min in the presence of 1×10^{-3} M theophylline and norepinephrine. Norepinephrine caused an increase in the release of isotope from the cells as evidenced by the presence of less radioactivity in these cells. The evolution of [^{14}C]CO_2 from specifically labeled [^{14}C]glucose was determined. The addition of norepinephrine caused an increase in [^{14}C]CO_2 evolution from 1-[^{14}C]glucose, 2-[^{14}C]glucose, and 6-[^{14}C]glucose.

The effect of norepinephrine on glucose metabolism in neuroblastoma cells was also studied. The cells were grown for 2 days in DMEM plus 10% fetal calf serum. The growth medium was removed and replaced by Earle's balanced salt solution containing various radiolabeled compounds, incubated for 30 min, and filtered. Norepinephrine had no effect on the incorporation of label from radioactive glucose in these cells.

The question examined in these experiments was whether norepinephrine affects the uptake of radioactive glucose, the release of radioactive compounds derived from radiolabeled glucose, or the metabolism of radioactive glucose in glioblastoma and neuroblastoma cells in culture. From the results presented, it appears that the addition of norepinephrine does not have an effect on these processes in glioblastoma cells and not in neuroblastoma cells in cell culture.

It is of interest to speculate that what is occurring in glioblastoma cells can be explained as shown in Fig. 9. The breakdown of glycogen is activated by norepinephrine as a result of an increase in cyclic AMP, which activates the protein kinase for conversion of phosphorylase *b* to phosphorylase *a*. This then results in an increase of glucose within the cell. If radioactive glucose is added to the medium, less will be taken into the cell because of an increase in an intracellular pool of glucose or compounds derived from glucose. This is the result that was obtained. If the cells are prelabeled with glucose and the radioactive medium is removed, then it might be expected that radioactivity would be lost from the cell in the presence of norepinephrine. This was found to occur. In addition, it might be expected that if norepinephrine causes an increased conversion of glycogen to glucose, increased oxidation of the glucose might also occur. The results are consistent with this postulate.

Although it is interesting to speculate that the effect of norepinephrine is on the breakdown of glycogen, the nature of the experiments does not permit an unequivocal conclusion in this regard. This would require determination of the products derived from the radioactive glucose and the nature of the compounds lost from the cell in the presence of norepinephrine.

Nevertheless, it is of interest to propose that *in vitro* these products from glial cells are made available to neurons and used for metabolic processes in the latter cells, assuming the present experiments might have relevance to the intact brain. Thus one can envision the relation of neurons and glial cells to be one whereby a neurotransmitter from neurons triggers a reaction in glial cells that results in the latter providing metabolites to the neurons for various synthetic reactions or for the generation of energy for cellular processes.

Somatic Cell Hybrids and Possible Genetic Complementation

Somatic cell hybrids of neuroblastoma and glioblastoma cells have been used to investigate the genetic regulation that may exist between their genomes. Thus hybrid

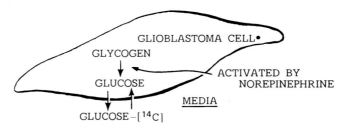

FIG. 9. Diagram of a glioblastoma cell, showing that norepinephrine affects glucose metabolism by activating glycogenolysis and subsequently inducing CO_2 production by glycolysis. (From ref. 31, with permission.)

cells serve as a model system for exploring neuronal-glial genetic regulation, which, analogously, may be in effect in the intact brain. These hybrids resemble parent neuroblastoma cells in many of their properties, including acetylcholinesterase activity (2), dopamine-b-hydroxylase activity (20), clear and dense-core vesicle formation (19), the ability to extend long neurites (13,41,44), and possession of electrically excitable membranes (19). It is noteworthy that some hybrid clones possess activity of CAT that is 500 times greater than that of the parent neuroblastoma or glioblastoma in individual cultures (2). This argues that genetic complementation between the genomes of the neuroblastoma and glioblastoma cells may induce high steady-state levels of choline acetyltransferase in the hybrid cell, and that this may be the mechanism for enzymic induction in the intact mammalian brain. Klee and Nirenberg (23) have found a high density of opiate receptors on hybrid cells, which again argues for genetic complementation. Christian et al. (11) found a soluble factor produced by neuroblastoma-glioblastoma hybrid cells that results in the aggregation of acetylcholine receptor molecules to form mature aggregates capable of generating miniature endplate potentials *in vitro*. This finding suggests that genetic complementation between neuroblasts and glioblasts may be required for the production of a soluble factor, which may in part be responsible for the aggregation of specific proteins to form an active acetylcholine receptor and thus maintenance of neuromuscular transmission. The glial genome may also be important in forming acetylcholine receptor aggregates, thus providing a better target for synapse formation during embryogenesis and after denervation. Similar genetic cooperativity exists between peripheral nerve Schwann cells and motor axons, as described by Aguayo et al. (1), who showed that Schwann cells of the superior cervical ganglion do not receive the appropriate signal from associated axons to induce myelination. However, these Schwann cells, when transplanted into a nerve where axons are normally myelinated, result in myelination of regrowing axons by grafted superior cervical ganglion Schwann cells. Thus the Schwann cells of this sympathetic ganglion have the potential to cause myelination of motor axons but depend on an appropriate neural signal for this to occur.

Rosenberg et al. (36) examined the species of proteins synthesized by parent individual cultures of neuroblastoma and glioblastoma cells. The patterns for proteins synthesized by neuroblastoma or glioblastoma cells, as identified on two-dimensional polyacrylamide gels, were very different. Proteins were identified that were dominant for one cell type and not expressed in the other. A hybrid cell line,

---

FIG. 10. Protein species from differentiating neuroblastoma (N18TG2; **middle**), glioblastoma (C6-BU-1; **bottom**), and hybrid (NG105-15; **top**), cell lines in culture were separated and identified initially in the first dimension by the use of isoelectric focusing gels and were further separated in the second dimension by sodium dodecyl sulfate (SDS)-acrylamide gels. A specific protein species (Z) was identified in hybrid cells that was not present in either parental neuroblastoma or glioblastoma cultures. Protein Z was expressed, however, by the co-culturing of neuroblastoma and glioblastoma cells, suggesting its induction is dependent on a soluble factor. It is suggested that similar neuronal-glial interaction may be functional in the intact brain, and that similar reciprocal modulation between neurons and glia may be a central mechanism of differentiation in the nervous system. The *arrow* refers to where albumin migrates on these gels as an internal control. (From ref. 36, with permission.)

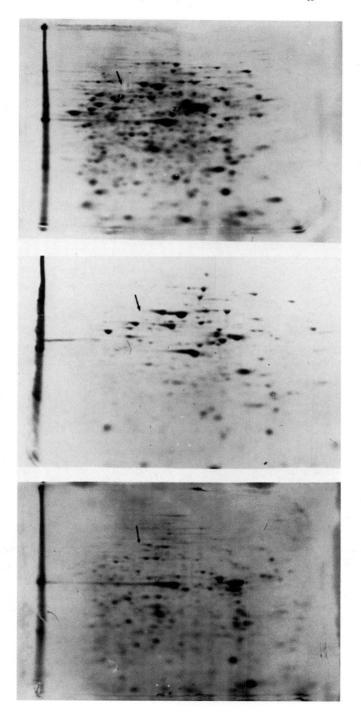

NG 108-15, composed of parent mouse neuroblastoma and rat glioblastoma genomes, expressed many of the neuroblastoma type of proteins and relatively fewer of the glioma type of proteins. A specific protein species, referred to as Z protein, was identified in hybrid cells but was not present in either parental neuroblastoma or glioblast cultures (Fig. 10). The Z protein (MW-53,000) was expressed, however, by the coculturing of neuroblastoma and glioblastoma cells, suggesting that its induction is dependent on a possible soluble factor.

The Z protein in hybrid cells was demonstrated both on stained gels and by autoradiography. Chromosome analysis of hybrid cells confirmed the presence of both rat and mouse chromosomes.

The expression of the Z protein induced in hybrid cells or by coculture of parents, but not by the individual culture of either parent alone, is good evidence in favor of the concept of reciprocal genetic regulation between neuroblastoma and glioblastoma genomes. The reexpression of the Z protein in hybrid cells is presumably a glioblastoma-induced function of a repressed neuroblastoma character, as Z protein is present in the original parent N18 clone, which in turn is the parent of the cell line N18TG2, one of the parents of the hybrid cell line (Fig. 11). Z protein was also found in homogenates of intact Ajax mouse brain, the strain of mouse from which the parent neuroblastomas were obtained. Thus it is possible that the Z protein synthesized by Ajax mouse brain may be due to genetic complementation between glia and neurons (36).

In view of these data, the occurrence of trophic interaction between neurons and glia in the intact brain must also be considered as a possible mechanism for differentiation. The dominance of neuroblast genetic expression in the hybrid cell suggests the possibility of similar regulation and inhibition of glial function by neurons *in vivo*. Neuronal-glial interaction may be necessary for the genetic expression of differentiated functions that are absent from, or weakly expressed by, either cell type alone, as, for example, the presence of opiate receptors (23), increased choline acetyltransferase activity in hybrid cells (2), and the showing of a unique protein species, the Z protein, in hybrid cells (36). Could a trophic interaction also

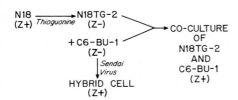

FIG. 11. The presence or absence of protein Z is shown in relation to the clonal cell line assayed or coculture conditions. It is expressed in hybrid cells and cocultures but not parental cultures of neuroblastoma or glioblastoma. It is of interest that it was expressed in line N18, from which N18TG-2 was derived. Thus this protein's expression is dependent on neuroblastoma-glioblastoma interaction, suggesting similar functions may be in effect for protein expression in the intact brain. It is indicated from these studies that it is an N18 gene repressed in N18TG-2 that is activated by a C6-BU-1 gene product either in the hybrid or in cocultures, which finally expressed protein Z. (From ref. 36, with permission.)

The description of the molecular biology of certain aspects of neuronal differentiation in cell culture was acquired in a very short period of time and allows speculation that this *in vitro* approach may have brought us closer to appreciating the brain code than we currently realize.

NEURAL ADHESION RECOGNITION MOLECULES

The precise architectonic, histologic formation of the nervous system requires the presence of orienting recognition molecules under genetic control. They function to sort out neurons into unique classes, regulate neuronal and glial migrations, and control precise synapse formation. The order of magnitude of these events is considerable, as there are perhaps 10^{12} neurons in the human brain and several thousand times that number of glia and synapses. Marshall Nirenberg's and Gerald Edelman's laboratories have been approaching these issues and have identified several classes of neuronal recognition molecules.

Under precise genetic control, there is early in embryogenesis an overproduction of neurons followed by a programmed cell death. This is followed by neuronal migrations to form specific nuclear groups and then by synapse formation. The growth of axons to their targets is accomplished by pathfinding mechanisms that probably include several types, including mechanical guidance by pioneer axons or by glial fibers, and chemical guidance, by diffusible substances or by nondiffusible molecular cues on cell surfaces. These molecular cues on the surface of unique classes of neurons provide for specific adhesions, for migration caused by gradients of these molecules, and for "area code-type molecular address systems" (50).

Cajal and Sperry suggested that a chemotropism or chemoaffinity system, respectively, existed for specific neuronal migrations. Sperry indicated initially that each retinal ganglion cell had a specific cell surface molecule that recognized its tectal complementary marker. He broadened the concept later by proposing that the retinal map was based on two molecules in orthogonal gradients in the retina and they were complementary to separate molecular gradients in the tectum. This theme has been taken up anew by Nirenberg and Edelman.

Trisler et al. (51), using monoclonal antibodies that bound preferentially to small regions of the chick retinal ganglion cells, identified a topographic gradient of cell surface molecules. A 35-fold gradient of one antigen extended from dorsoposterior to ventroanterior margins of the retina. The gradient is based on the number of antigen molecules per cell rather than the proportion of cells bearing the antigen. The purified cell surface antigen is a protein with a molecular weight of 46 to 49 kD and an isoelectric point of pI 4.0 to 4.1. On the basis of these data they conclude that the gradient of topographic molecules is involved in the coding of positional information for the eventual establishment and maintenance of synaptic formation (50,51).

Edelman refers to cell adhesion molecules (CAMs) as cell surface determinants that result in specific cellular interactions. A specific neural cell adhesion molecule (N-CAM) was identified by generating fluorescent-tagged antibodies to a unique neural cell surface antigen. N-CAM molecules differ in embryonic and adult brain in their sialic acid composition; thus there is some developmental processing, which becomes important in discussing the staggerer mutant (see Chapter 3). A neural-glial adhesion molecule (Ng-CAM) has also been identified that mediates the binding of neurons selectively to glia and not neurons. The Ng-CAM binds to an adhesion molecule on glia that is yet not isolated and identified. An adhesion molecule found on embryonic liver cells (L-CAM) has also been identified. The formation of the embryonic nervous system is dependent on the functional expression of these molecules. The central N-CAM regions that develop into the neural plate, notochord, somites, and lateral plate mesoderm are surrounded by a ring of regions that express L-CAM-positive cells. Further, there is a head-to-tail gradient of N-CAM staining, with fluorescent antibody-mediated staining being most intense in the neural plate. Thus N-CAM and L-CAM have clear anatomic boundaries that must be functionally critical to normal embryonic development.

The conversion of embryonic N-CAM (E form: 200 kD) to the adult forms (A forms: 180, 140, and 120 kD) proceeds so that there is little of the E form at 21 days and virtually none at 180 days in most regions of the mouse brain. In the autosomal recessive mouse mutant staggerer, this conversion is greatly delayed in the cerebellum. At 21 days there is still abundant E form of N-CAM and less than normal amounts of the A form. Thus a major architectonic, histologic defect in the cerebellum of these mutant mice is associated with a functional defect in this class of adhesion molecules (14–16).

These neuronal, glial, and nonnervous system cell surface adhesion recognition molecules are involved in the molecular bases for neuronal and glial migration and subsequent histologic formation of the brain. Their recent elucidation represents a major new set of findings in understanding genetic mechanisms of brain development. It is clear that many more such recognition molecules will be discovered and their role defined in this process. The molecules that then become functional, which have been alluded to above, are responsible for information storage and retrieval. These molecules represent the next level of molecular complexity, which remains totally unexplored.

NEURONAL AND GLIAL MITOGENS

Neuronal and glial interactions can result in the proliferation of glia. In cocultures of Schwann cells with sensory or autonomic neurons, or with neuronal processes, Schwann cells are stimulated to divide (37,49). It is important to note that only those Schwann cells close to neuronal processes are stimulated to proliferate, and the effect is prevented by interposing a thin collagen membrane between neuron and Schwann cell. Thus it is presumed the neuronal Schwann cell mitogen is a plasma-membrane-bound factor and must be allowed to interact directly in contact with the Schwann cell (49). These experiments on the regulatory effect of neurons on glial proliferation and differentiation can be added to the previous observations that neurons initiate myelin synthesis by Schwann cells (1,10) and by oligondendroglia (46,53), induction of type IV collagen synthesis and basal lamina deposition by Schwann cells (8,9), and glucocorticoid induction of glutamine synthetase in retinal Müller cells (25,26).

Sobue and Pleasure (48) also demonstrated the specificity of the target cell response to the coculturing of neuronal processes. Although neuronal axonal fragments stimulated mitotic activity in cultured Schwann cells, these fragments markedly inhibited rat astroglial mitosis in culture as estimated by tritiated thymidine uptake. Neuronal fragments also produced a phenotypic alteration of cultured astroglia, producing cells that were star-shaped with thick cable-like glial fibrils.

Brockes and coworkers (6,7,24) have described a protein growth factor purified from bovine pituitaries (glial growth factor) that induces proliferation in glia. The laboratories of Pleasure and Brockes are in the process of more fully characterizing this factor and determining its primary biochemical effect.

The genetic control of glial proliferation and differentiation during brain development relates directly to these brilliant studies of Pleasure, Bunge, Brockes, and their colleagues. It is a vital area of neurobiological research that needs intensive further scrutiny and support. These observations also have direct clinical relevance, as Pleasure's laboratory recently reported that both human and rat axolemma is capable of stimulating human Schwann cell replication *in vitro* (47). In my view, genetic diseases analogous to the trembler mouse model, involving neuronal-glial interactions that result in hypomyelination, will be found in humans. These studies will elucidate the molecular events potentially involved in demyelination and identify the primary altered gene product. Mitotic factors for astroglia and Schwann cells may become clinically useful as well to treat demyelinating disorders of the central and peripheral nervous systems in the future.

CONCLUSION

The program of neuronal differentiation in the intact brain includes an early phase of proliferation of those cells that migrated from the paraventricular subependymal germinal region to form cortex or basal ganglia. Mitotic neuroblasts can also be produced in culture by retaining high levels of fetal calf serum in the culture medium. Mitotic cultures can be converted to postmitotic cultures by simply lowering the protein content of the culture medium. This simple signal of protein reduction, which induces a postmitotic population of neuroblasts with neurite formation, might also be part of the program of *in vivo* differentiation as a result of the maturation of the blood-brain barrier and the exclusion of serum proteins from brain extracellular space.

A later phase in neuronal differentiation *in vivo* after axonal and dendritic proliferation and synapse formation is the induction of neurotransmitter biosynthesis and metabolism. Neuroblastoma and glioblastoma cells in culture can be induced to differentiate by the addition of a variety of agents, including 5-bromodeoxyuridine, dibutyryl cyclic adenosine 3'-5' monophosphate (db-cyclic AMP), and prostaglandins (PGE_1 and PGE_2), with the simultaneous induction of choline acetyltransferase or tyrosine hydroxylase. These events involve the activation of protein kinases with subsequent phosphorylation of nuclear histone protein. Further, there are changes in the concentration of the four species of nuclear histone proteins during development in culture. These changes occur before increases in specific activity of the neurotransmitter synthetic enzymes in the cytoplasm and thus may be important regulatory phenomena. Both neuroblastoma and glioblastoma cell lines possess high-affinity uptake permeases for the ultimate inactivation of norepinephrine, dopamine, serotonin, taurine, glutamate, glycine, and GABA. *De novo* synapse formation between neuroblastoma and muscle cells has been demonstrated and has proved a valuable model system to investigate neurotransmitter biochemistry.

Recently the regulation of glycogen metabolism in astrocytoma and neuroblastoma cell cultures has been elegantly investigated. The regulation of the concentrations of intracellular glycogen and of the predominant forms of glycogen phosphorylase and glycogen synthase varies with (a) the available energy supply and (b) altered intracellular concentration of cyclic AMP. When glucose levels are high intracellularly, glycogen is synthesized, glycogen phosphorylase *a* decreases, and glycogen synthase *a* increases. When glucose in the medium decreases to a critical level, phosphorylase *a* increases and glycogen concentration in the cells decreases in parallel with the medium glucose. These events are of great value, as they show that the neuroblast itself, devoid of glia, is capable of synthesizing appreciable amounts of glycogen and that defects in this pathway impairing glycogen synthesis and metabolism might result in neurologic disease of primary neuronal origin. In this regard it is of note that insulin promotes the conversion of phosphorylase to the *b* form and synthase to the *a* form in both cell lines. Modulation of glucose metabolism by trophic interaction has also been shown when neuroblastoma and glioblastoma cells are cocultivated, as compared with higher rates of glycolysis by either cell line separately.

The ultimate differentiated function of nervous system tissue is to encode, store, and retrieve information. The neurophysiologic and biochemical principles and mechanisms that have evolved from simple metazoans to the mammalian brain are enormously complex and incompletely understood. The systems for handling vast amounts of motor, sensory, language, perceptual, and cognitive functions inherently present in the human brain are indeed detailed but perhaps decipherable if reduced to elementary units. The code or codes by which the brain fixes experience and recalls it might be approachable through study of simple systems potentially capable of learning, such as the cell culture of neurons and glia under controlled conditions. A cell culture containing both neurons and glia and capable of learning would be an ideal one for studying the code, for it would utilize small numbers of the two important brain cell types, allow study of the biochemical interrelationships between glia and neurons, and permit a direct correlation between physiologic events and the synthesis and turnover of specific macromolecules.

The important role of neuronal and glial adhesion and recognition molecules in normal brain architectonics is just beginning to be appreciated. Cell surface molecular gradients mediate neural migraton, as shown by Marshall Nirenberg and colleagues. Cell adhesion molecules for neuron-neuron and neuron-glia groupings are now known from the work of Gerald Edelman's group, and a defect in an N-CAM maturation step is associated with a mouse cerebellar mutant. Pleasure, Bunge, and Brockes and their co-workers have opened an exciting and important new molecular approach to characterizing mitogenic factors in the nervous system. Neurally mediated glial mitogens have been identified and characterized by them, and their work will provide the means to explore the molecular mechanisms of defective neuronal-glial interaction that underlie genetic disorders.

REFERENCES

1. Aguayo, A., Charron, L., and Bray, G. (1976): Potential of Schwann cells from unmyelinated nerves to produce myelin: A quantitative ultrastructural and radiographic study. *J. Neurocytol.* 5:565–573.
2. Amano, T., Hamprecht, B., and Kemper, W. (1974): High activity of choline acetyltransferase induced in neuroblastoma × glia hybrid cells. *Exp. Cell Res.*, 85:399–408.
3. Amano, T., Richelson, E., and Nirenberg, M. (1972): Neurotransmitter synthesis by neuroblastoma clones. *Proc. Natl. Acad. Sci. USA*, 69:258–263.
4. Augusti-Tocco, G., and Sato, G. (1969): Establishment of functional clonal lines of neurons from mouse neuroblastoma. *Proc. Natl. Acad. Sci. USA*, 64:311–315.
5. Blume, A., Gilbert, F., Wilson, S., Farber, J., Rosenberg, R., and Nirenberg, M. (1970): Regulation of acetylcholinesterase in neuroblastoma cells. *Proc. Natl. Acad. Sci. USA*, 67:786–792.
6. Brockes, J., Fryxell, K., and Lemke, G. (1981): Studies on cultured Schwann cells: The induction of myelin synthesis and the control of their proliferation by a new growth factor. *J. Exp. Biol.*, 95:215–230.
7. Brockes, J., Lemke, G., and Balzer, D. (1980): Purification and preliminary characterization of a glial growth factor from the bovine pituitary. *J. Biol. Chem.*, 255:8374–8377.
8. Bunge, M., Williams, A., and Wood, P. (1982): Neuron-Schwann cell interaction in basal lamina formation. *Dev. Biol.*, 92:449–460.
9. Bunge, M., Williams, A., Wood, P., Vitto, J., and Jeffrey, J. (1980): Comparison of nerve cell and nerve cell plus Schwann cell cultures, with particular emphasis on basal lamina and collagen formation. *J. Cell Biol.*, 84:184–202.
10. Bunge, R. P., and Bunge, M. B. (1978): Evidence that contact with connective tissue matrix is required for normal interaction between Schwann cells and nerve fibers. *J. Cell Biol.*, 78:943–950.
11. Christian, C., Daniels, M., Sugiyama, H., Vogel, A., Jacques, L., and Nelson, P. (1978): A factor from neurons increases the number of acetylcholine receptor aggregates on cultured muscle cells. *Proc. Natl. Acad. Sci. USA*, 75:4011–4015.
12. Clark, R., and Perkins, J. (1971): Regulation of adenosine 3':5'-cyclic monophosphate concentration in cultured human astrocytoma cells by catecholamines and histamine. *Proc. Natl. Acad. Sci. USA*, 68:2757–2760.
13. Daniels, M. P., and Hamprecht, B. (1974): The ultrastructure of neuroblastoma glioma somatic cell hybrids. *J. Cell Biol.*, 63:691–699.
14. Edelman, G. M. (1983): Cell adhesion molecules. *Science*, 219:450–457.
15. Edelman, G. M. (1984): Cell-adhesion molecules: A molecular basis for animal form. *Sci. Am.*, 250(4):118–129.
16. Edelman, G. M., and Chuong, C.-M. (1982): Embryonic to adult conversion of neural cell adhesion molecules in normal and staggerer mice. *Proc. Natl. Acad. Sci. USA*, 79:7036–7040.
17. Galambos, R. (1961): A glia-neural theory of brain function. *Proc. Natl. Acad. Sci. USA*, 47:129–136.
18. Gilman, A., and Nirenberg, M. (1971): Effect of catecholamines on the adenosine 3':5'-cyclic monophosphate concentrations of clonal satellite cells of neurons. *Proc. Natl. Acad. Sci. USA*, 68:2165–2168.

19. Hamprecht, B. (1974): Cell cultures as model systems for studying the biochemistry of differentiated functions of nerve cells. *Hoppe Seylers Z. Physiol. Chem.*, 355:109–110.

20. Hamprecht, B., Traber, J., and Lamprecht, F. (1974): Dopamine-beta-hydroxylase activity in cholinergic neuroblastoma × glioma hybrid cells; increase of activity by N^6, O^2-di-butyryl adenosine e′:5′-cyclic monophosphate. *FEBS Lett.*, 42:221–226.

21. Harrison, R. G. (1907): Observations on the living developing nerve fiber. *Anat. Rec.*, 1:116–124.

22. Henn, F., and Hamberger, A. (1971): Glial cell function: Uptake of transmitter substances. *Proc. Natl. Acad. Sci. USA*, 68:2686–2690.

23. Klee, W. A., and Nirenberg, M. (1974): A neuroblastoma × glioma hybrid cell line with morphine receptors. *Proc. Natl. Acad. Sci. USA*, 71:3474–3477.

24. Lemke, G., and Brockes, J. (1983): Glial growth factor: A mitogenic polypeptide of the brain and pituitary. In: *Fed. Proc.*, 42:2627–2629.

25. Linser, P., and Moscona, A. (1979): Induction of glutamine synthetase in embryonic neural retina: Localization in Muller fibers and dependence on cell interactions. *Proc. Natl. Acad. Sci. USA*, 76:6476–6480.

26. Linser, P., and Moscona, A. (1983): Hormonal induction of glutamine synthetase in cultures of embryonic retina cells: Requirement for neuron-glia contact interactions. *Dev. Biol.*, 96:529–534.

27. Lowry, O. H., Rosebrough, N., Farr, A., and Randall, R. (1951): Protein measurement with the Folin phenol reagent. *J. Biol. Chem.*, 193:265–275.

28. Morrison, R., Hall, C. L., Pardue, S., Brodeur, R., Baskin, F., and Rosenberg, R. N. (1980): The synthesis and degradation of poly(A)-containing mRNAs in mouse neuroblastoma cells treated with dibutyryl cAMP or with Ro20-1724. *J. Neurochem.*, 34:50–58.

29. Murray, M. R. (1965): Nervous tissues *in vitro*. In: *The Biology of Cells and Tissues in Culture, Vol. II.*, edited by E. N. Willmer, pp. 373–455. Academic Press, New York.

30. Nelson, P., Ruffner, W., and Nirenberg, M. (1969): Neuronal tumor cells with excitable membranes grown *in vitro*. *Proc. Natl. Acad. Sci. USA*, 64:1004–1010.

31. Newburgh, R. W., and Rosenberg, R. N. (1972): Effect of norepinephrine on glucose metabolism in glioblastoma and neuroblastoma cells in cell culture. *Proc. Natl. Acad. Sci. USA*, 69:1677–1680.

32. Nirenberg, M., Caskey, T., Marshall, R., Brimacombe, R., Kellogg, D., Doctor, B., Hatfield, D., Levin, J., Rottman, F., Pestaka, S., Wilkox, M., and Anderson, F. (1966): The RNA code and protein synthesis. *Cold Spring Harbor Symp. Quant. Biol.*, 31:11–24.

33. Nirenberg, M., Jones, O. W., Leder, P., Clark, B. F. C., Sly, W. S., and Pestaka, S. (1963): On the coding of genetic information. *Cold Spring Harbor Symp. Quant. Biol.*, 28:549–557.

34. Prashad, N., Rosenberg, R., Wischmeyer, B., Ulrich, C., and Sparkman, D. (1979): Induction of adenosine 3′,5′-monophosphate binding proteins by N^6, $O^{2'}$-dibutyryladenosine 3′,5′-monophosphate in mouse neuroblastoma cells. Analysis of two-dimensional gel electrophoresis. *Biochemistry*, 13:2717–2725.

35. Rakic, P., and Sidman, R. (1968): Supravital DNA synthesis in the developing human and mouse brain. *J. Neuropathol. Exp. Neurol.*, 27:246–276.

36. Rosenberg, R. N., Vance, C. K., Morrison, M., Prashad, N., Meyne, J., and Baskin, F. (1978): Differentiation of neuroblastoma, glioma, and hybrid cells in culture as measured by specific protein species synthesized; evidence for neuroblast-glioblast reciprocal genetic regulation. *J. Neurochem.*, 30:1343–1355.

37. Salzer, J. L., and Bunge, R. P. (1980): Studies of Schwann cell proliferation. I. An analysis in tissue culture of proliferation during development, wallerian degeneration, and direct injury. *J. Cell. Biol.*, 84:739–752.

38. Schrier, B. K., Rosenberg, R. N., Thompson, E., and Farber, J. (1970): Enzyme markers in mouse brain cell culture. *Fed. Proc.*, 29:480.

39. Schrier, B. K., Wilson, S. H., and Nirenberg, M. (1974): Assay of enzymes of transmitter metabolism of neuroblastoma and other cultured cells from the nervous system. *Meth. Enzymol.*, 32:765–788.

40. Schubert, D., Humphreys, S., Baroni, C., and Cohn, M. (1969): *In vitro* differentiation of a mouse neuroblastoma. *Proc. Natl. Acad. Sci. USA*, 64:316–323.

41. Schubert, D., Humphreys, S., Debitry, F., and Jacob, I. (1971): Induced differentiation of a neuroblastoma. *Dev. Biol.*, 25:514–546.

42. Seeds, N. W. (1971): Biochemical differentiation in reaggregating brain cell culture. *Proc. Natl. Acad. Sci. USA*, 68:1858–1861.
43. Seeds, N. W, and Gilman, A. (1971): Norepinephrine stimulated increase of cyclic-AMP levels in developing mouse brain cell cultures. *Science*, 174:292.
44. Seeds, N. W., Gilman, A., Amano, T., and Nirenberg, M. (1970): Regulation of axon formation by clonal lines of a neural tumor. *Proc. Natl. Acad. Sci. USA*, 66:160–167.
45. Seeds, N. W., and Vatter, A. E. (1971): Synaptogenesis in reaggregating brain cell culture. *Proc. Natl. Acad. Sci. USA*, 68:3219–3222.
46. Seil, F., and Blank, W. (1981): Myelination of central nervous system axons in tissue culture by transplanted oligodendrocytes. *Science*, 212:1407–1408.
47. Sobue, G., Brown, M. J., Kim, S., and Pleasure, D. (1984): Axolemma is a mitogen for human Schwann cells. *Ann. Neurol.*, 15:449–452.
48. Sobue, G., and Pleasure, D. (1984): Astroglial proliferation and phenotype are modulated by neuronal plasma membrane. *Brain Res.*, 324:175–179.
49. Sobue, G., and Pleasure, D. (1985): Adhesion of axolemmal fragments to Schwann cells: A signal- and target-specific process closely linked to axolemmal induction of Schwann cell mitosis. *J. Neurosci.*, 5:379–387.
50. Trisler, D. (1982): Are molecular markers of cell position involved in the formation of neural circuits? *Trends Neurosci.*, 5:306–310.
51. Trisler, D., Schneider, M. D., and Nirenberg, M. (1981): A topographic gradient of molecules in retina can be used to identify neuron position. *Proc. Natl. Acad. Sci. USA*, 78:2145–2149.
52. Wilson, S. H., Schrier, B. K., Farber, J. L., Thompson, E. J., Rosenberg, R. N., Blume, A. J., and Nirenberg, M. W. (1972): Markers for gene expression in cultured cells from the nervous system. *J. Biol. Chem.*, 247:3159–3169.
53. Wood, P., Okada, E., and Bunge, R. (1980): The use of networks of dissociated rat dorsal root ganglion neurons to induce myelination of oligodendrocytes in culture. *Brain Res.*, 196:247–252.

3

Mouse Neurogenetics

One has only to spend some time at the extraordinary Jackson Laboratory in Bar Harbor, Maine, and witness the enormous diversity in their inbred mouse colonies to realize what an important role mouse genetics has played in understanding the biology of neurogenetic disease. Preeminent in this field has been Richard Sidman, Bullard Professor of Neuropathology at Harvard Medical School. His 1965 monograph with M. C. Green and S. H. Appel *Catalog of the Neurological Mutants of the Mouse* (10) was a landmark contribution listing the repertoire of mouse neurogenetic syndromes, which provided an organized means to develop experimental animal models of human genetic disease. As Dr. Sidman pointed out in 1983, however, his main interest in mouse mutations is not in how closely they simulate the exact features of human neurologic and genetic disease, but rather in the "correspondence on the deeper, and fundamentally more interesting levels of formal genetics (chromosomal map position, neighboring genetic loci, and intragenic structure), homologous gene products and target cells, and equivalence of the developmental or physiologic event that is perturbed" (9).

Sidman has recently reviewed his extensive experience in this field (9) and has described mutations that affect (a) behavior and (b) cerebellar structure, including homologous cerebellar mutations in mouse and man; the latter mutations affect mainly Purkinje neurons, granule cell neurons, cerebellar cortex, and deep cerebellar nuclei.

Tottering (gene symbol *tg*) is a behavioral mutant inherited as an autosomal recessive and mapped to chromosome 8. These mice at about 2 to 3 weeks of age develop absence and focal motor seizures. Their electroencephalographic recordings show bursts of bilaterally synchronous and symmetrical spike-and-wave discharges. These epileptiform discharges are associated with a cessation of movement and a fixed posturing. According to Sidman (9) these murine seizures bear a striking resemblance to the common absence seizures of children and, importantly, represent a single gene mutation that results in a complex and stereotyped form of behavior that is due to a molecular alteration that may underlie a form of human epilepsy.

The mutant diabetes *(db)* is an autosomal recessive in which homozygous mice become obese, have poor temperature regulation, and are sterile. Johnson and Sidman (3) found that *db/db* ovaries grafted to histocompatible wild-type females became fertile, indicating that their sterility is caused by functional abnormality of the hypothalamus. The *db/db* mice responded normally to exogenous gonadotropin-releasing hormone, but gonadotropin release from the pituitary was lower than normal (3,9). Further, endogenous hypothalamic gonadotropin-releasing hormone was significantly higher in castrated affected females than controls. Sidman concludes that infertility of *db/db* females is caused by inadequate gonadotropic stimulation because of inadequate hormone release from the hypothalamus.

The mouse mutation mocha *(mh)*, an autosomal recessive disorder named for the coat color, is a behavioral mutant associated with a mild axonal degenerative disorder involving the peripheral and central nervous system. Affected females at parturition become unduly aggressive and attack and kill their own young as well as attacking and injuring adult mice in their midst.

Mutations affecting cerebellar structure have been of primary interest to Sidman and his colleagues, and they have described about 18 independent genetic loci in the past twenty years.

Three diseases that probably affect the same genetic locus in both human and mouse have been described. Mottled *(Mo)* is known to be expressed as several different alleles at this locus on the X chromosome. The brindled phenotype, Mo^{br}, is similar to the human Menkes's kinky hair syndrome. $Mo^{br/y}$ mice have growth arrest by day 12, become poorly coordinated, and usually do not survive after day 20. It is thought the phenotypic abnormalities are due to defective intracellular copper transport and thus to a secondary reduction in activity of copper-dependent enzymes. Other mottled loci described by Sidman and associates include the original mottled, *Mo*, which is an embryonic lethal; Mo^{blo}, blotchy, in which males may survive weaning; and pewter, Mo^{pew}, in which males do reach adulthood and can reproduce (3).

Both mouse and Menkes's kinky hair patients show variable granule cell neuronal loss in the cerebellar cortex and abnormalities in Purkinje cell morphology. Mo^{br} male mice can be saved and the neuropathologic consequences minimized by therapeutic injections of cupric chloride (3,6).

The mouse beige *(bg)* mutation is homologous with Chediak-Higashi disease associated with ballooned lysosomes in Purkinje cells and Schwann cells. Patients develop infections, lymphomas, a peripheral neuropathy, and sometimes variable mental retardation and cerebellar ataxia. Affected mice demonstrate a significant reduction in Purkinje cells (9).

The autosomal recessive disorder wasted, *wst*, produces in the homozygous animal tremor, hypotonia, and early death. It bears a resemblance to human ataxia telangectasia. Both *wst/wst* mice and humans show a loss of Purkinje cells (9).

There are five major autosomal recessive or semidominant inherited mutations in the mouse that predominantly affect the Purkinje cell: reeler, staggerer, lurcher, Purkinje cell degeneration, and nervous.

In the reeler mutation *(rl)* the primary defect appears not to be an abnormality in Purkinje cell morphology but rather in its position in the cerebellar cortex. The cerebellar cortical histologic pattern and regularity of form are grossly disturbed, with the Purkinje cell location being markedly disturbed.

The staggerer mutation *(sg)* results in a hypoplastic cerebellum with a striking reduction in granule cell neurons, as originally described in 1962 by Sidman et al. (11). More recently it has been determined that the number of Purkinje cells is reduced to 25% of normal (1,2), and from study of chimeras it is believed that the Purkinje cell is the primary direct target of the staggerer *(sg)* gene, with granule cell loss perhaps, but not definitely, a result of Purkinje cell loss (1,2,9) or of inability to form stable synapses with the defective Purkinje cells (4).

Lurcher *(lc)* is an autosomal semidominant mutation that results in total loss of all Purkinje cells followed by about a 90% loss of granule cells and 80% loss of inferior olivary neurons. Studies with chimeras indicate that the lurcher gene locus acts directly and intrinsically on Purkinje cells and that the granule and olivary cell loss is extrinsic owing to a loss in their postsynaptic target, the Purkinje cell (9,13).

Purkinje cell degeneration *(pcd)* is an autosomal recessive mutation that acts intrinsically in the Purkinje cell (5) and results in their degeneration and loss. In addition retinal photoreceptor cells also degenerate. Mitral neurons of the olfactory bulb and thalamic neurons also undergo a pathologic loss, but the relationships of these other cellular degenerations to the Purkinje cell loss is not clear.

Nervous *(Nr)* is an autosomal recessive disease, and chimeric studies have not clearly shown whether the nervous locus acts intrinsically or extrinsically (secondarily) on Purkinje cells (9). There is a severe loss of Purkinje cells and also a loss of retinal photoreceptor cells.

Autosomal recessive mutations that primarily affect the granule cell neuron include weaver *(wv)* and tortured *(tor)*. Weaver animals become ataxic because of a failure in neurons in the external granular layer of the cerebellum to migrate inward to form the internal granular layer. Rakic and Sidman (8) described this degeneration as being caused by a failure of the Bergmann glial fibers to provide a radially arranged guide for granule cell migration; thus it is a defect extrinsic to the granule cell (9). Tortured is also an autosomal recessively inherited mutation in which homozygous animals develop abnormal postures and involuntary movements associated with a severe loss of granule cells (9).

Other mutations have been described in recent years that have not been characterized as well as the ones already referred to. They include leaner, meander tail, swaying, kreisler, stumbler, hyperspiny Purkinje cell, vibrator, and cerebellar outflow degeneration (9). Perhaps the most interesting of these is vibrator, which is an autosomal recessive on chromosome 11 and which produces a picture similar to spinocerebellar degeneration, with degeneration of dorsal root sensory ganglion cells, spinal cord neuronal loss, brainstem reticular neuronal loss, and degeneration of neurons in the lateral vestibular nucleus, the red nucleus, the deep cerebellar nuclei, and, in older animals, the cerebellar cortex and posterior vermis. These animals develop a fine rapid tremor of the head, trunk, limbs, and tail that causes them to "vibrate," hence its name. Eventually they become unstable because of muscle weakness and ataxia (9,12).

These observations of genetic neurologic disease involving both behavior and cerebellar development will provide the framework for subsequent work to decipher the molecular alteration in each of them. Each disorder is the result of a single gene mutation and a single altered gene product that specifically has altered neural function.

These accidents of nature will yield the necessary information to understand the brain codes for the normal architectonics of brain development necessary for a normal phenotype. Each mutation described will yield one new insight into a molecular step required for normal histogenesis. These inbred lines described by Dr. Sidman, his students, and others are of vital importance for molecular neuroscience to make progress in understanding the mechanisms for brain development and certain human genetic disorders, especially of the spinocerebellar type. Dr. Sidman has given us a very rich legacy to build on.

REFERENCES

1. Herrup, K., and Mullen, R. J. (1979): Regional variation and absence of large neurons in the cerebellum of the staggerer mouse. *Brain Res.*, 172:1–12.
2. Herrup, K., and Mullen, R. J. (1979): Staggerer chimeras: Intrinsic nature of Purkinje cell defects and implications for normal cerebellar development. *Brain Res.*, 178:443–457.
3. Johnson, L. M., and Sidman, R. L. (1979): A reproductive endocrine profile in the diabetes (db) mutant mouse. *Biol. Reprod.*, 20:552–559.
4. Landis, D. M. D., and Sidman, R. L. (1978): Electron microscopic analysis of postnatal histogenesis in the cerebellar cortex of staggerer mutant mice. *J. Comp. Neurol.*, 179:831–863.
5. Mullen, R. J. (1977): Genetic dissection of the CNS with mutant-normal mouse and rat chimeras. *Soc. Neurosci. Symp.*, 11:47–65.
6. Nagara, H., Yajima, K., and Suzuki, K. (1981): The effect of copper supplementation on brindled mouse. A clinico-pathological study. *J. Neuropathol. Exp. Neurol.*, 40:428–446.
7. Noebels, J. L., and Sidman, R. L. (1979): Inherited epilepsy: Spike wave and focal motor seizures in the mutant mouse tottering. *Science*, 204:1334–1336.
8. Rakic, P., and Sidman, R. L. (1973): Sequence of developmental abnormalities leading to granule cell deficit in cerebellar cortex of weaver mutant mice. *J. Comp. Neurol.*, 152:103–132.
9. Sidman, R. L., (1983): Experimental neurogenetics. In: *Genetics of Neurological and Psychiatric Disorders*, edited by S. Kety, L. P. Rowland, R. L. Sidman, and S. W. Matthysse, pp. Raven Press, New York.
10. Sidman, R. L., Green, M. C., and Appel, S. H. (1965): *Catalog of the Neurological Mutants of the Mouse.* Harvard University Press, Cambridge.
11. Sidman, R. L., Lane, P. W., and Dickie, M. (1962): Staggerer, a new mutation in the mouse affecting the cerebellum. *Science*, 137:610–612.
12. Weimar, W. R., and Sidman, R. L. (1978): Neuropathology of "vibrator"—a neurological mutation of the mouse. *Soc. Neurosci. Abstr.*, 4:401.
13. Wetts, R., and Herrup, K. (1980): Lurcher-wild type chimeric mice: Cerebellar Purkinje cells are primary site of gene action. *Soc. Neurosci. Abstr.*, 6:142.

4

Molecular Genetics and Neurologic Disease

Rapid advances have occurred in the past decade in our understanding of the biochemical basis of inherited neurologic disease, primarily resulting from detection of enzyme defects (39,40). In the rest of the twentieth century the pulse of development in this area will quicken considerably because of the recent introduction of molecular biological and, more particularly, recombinant DNA techniques for joining together or recombining DNA from two separate sources to attack problems in neurobiology and clinical neurology. These approaches will provide powerful and precise definitions for all inherited neurologic disorders and define genetic regulatory events that underlie cellular differentiation and tissue development in brain embryogenesis (41,42,46). This chapter discusses the issues and explains how and why recombinant DNA techniques will have a profound impact on neurobiology and clinical neurology. The coming significant revolution in the understanding of gene action in the nervous system using these techniques is inevitable and very welcome.

There have been major increases in the number of diseases recognized as inherited in a mendelian form in the past several years, as documented with each of the catalogs published by McKusick (25). Between 1978 and 1982 almost 200 dominantly inherited, 60 autosomal recessive, and eight X-linked recessive disorders were identified. There has been a proportional increase in identified inherited neurologic diseases. Further, of the total 1,637 documented genetic disorders, over half are inherited in an autosomal dominant manner. In genetic disorders of the nervous system, dominant diseases are also in the majority. Paradoxically, however, the greatest degree of molecular understanding of genetic diseases involving the nervous system comes from those that are recessively, not dominantly, inherited. The reason is that the recessive disorders, including the mucopolysaccharidoses, leukodystrophies, aminoacidopathies, and gangliosidoses, are all associated with the accumulation of a metabolite that can be related to a well-established biochem-

This chapter has been modified from a paper published previously in the *Annals of Neurology* (15:511-520, 1984,) and is reproduced with the permission of the publisher.

ical pathway (40). Recently the abnormal accumulation of the metabolites in serum or urine or of the storage products in neurons has been identified, quantitated, and then related to specific potential enzyme defects for these disorders. This scheme was the approach, for example, that Roscoe Brady and his colleagues brilliantly pursued in deciphering the inherited sphingolisidoses, in each of which a catabolic enzyme defect was found that was associated with the increase in the metabolic product (40).

The problem that one faces in dominantly inherited diseases such as neurofibromatosis, myotonic dystrophy, Huntington's disease, the spinocerebellar degenerations, and tuberous sclerosis is that there presently exists no metabolic clue, no storage product to indicate a potential biochemical basis of disease. In these disorders, in general, there is neuronal degeneration with a compensatory increase in glial cells. Even the finding of specific protein abnormalities on two-dimensional gels or of specific changes in mRNA in brain samples from a dominantly inherited neurologic disorder such as Joseph disease is not precise enough evidence to warrant the conclusion that these changes are primary gene product mutations rather than the result of disease (30,43). Therefore, new research strategies must be developed to answer the two questions, What is the molecular basis of the autosomal dominant disorders (those present on chromosomes 1 to 22, not on the X or Y chromosome), and What is the molecular basis for the clinical variation in gene expressivity and penetrance seen in dominantly inherited neurologic disease? A dominantly inherited disorder is one inherited from an affected parent. Sons and daughters are at risk at a 50% rate, and the pedigree indicates at least some male-to-male transmission of disease. Such questions are of great importance to the neurologists, perhaps more particularly to the child neurologist, because such diseases will affect an average of 50% of the children of an affected parent. Early diagnosis is important for genetic counseling, so that individuals can be identified as being affected and this information can be used in family planning. Further, the incidence of disease in a family will decrease significantly with good genetic counseling, as has been documented clearly in several large families that we have investigated. Future molecular research depends on identifying the children in large families who are affected with the disease. The clinician is important in these events, because he or she must provide the kind of clinical pedigree information that is indispensable to developing a molecular marker for these diseases (41).

MOLECULAR BASIS FOR CLINICAL VARIATION IN DOMINANTLY INHERITED NEUROLOGIC DISEASE

The second question, which concerns the molecular basis for clinical variation in dominantly inherited disease, should be addressed first, because it provides a natural introduction to the genetic code. The genetic code, as originally described and defined by Nirenberg and colleagues between 1961 and 1966, comprises 64 nucleic acid triplet codons for the 20 individual amino acids. A codon represents three nucleotides in DNA or mRNA that encode for a single amino acid and determine its precise location during protein synthesis. There is degeneracy, or multiplicity, in the code, as evidenced by the existence of multiple codons for a single amino acid (39,41). For example, UUU, three nucleotides of uridylate, represents one codon, and it signals for phenylalanine to be incorporated during protein synthesis. However, UUC (uridylate-uridylate-cytidylate) may also signal phenylalanine incorporation, and this duplication of coding is what is referred to as codon degeneracy. Further, if one nucleotide in the third position is changed by mutation, changing the codon from UUA (uridylate-uridylate-adenylate) to UUG (uridylate-uridylate-guanylate), leucine becomes incorporated into the newly synthesized polypeptide rather than phenylalanine; other examples abound. Another mutation may result in a so-called termination codon UGA (uridylate-guanylate-adenylate) rather than the tryptophan codon UGG (uridylate-guanylate-guanylate), which terminates the protein synthetic process. Such background mutations that change codon signals occur frequently and potentially can affect the primary amino acid sequence of many brain proteins (54). It has been estimated that between 70,000 and 100,000 proteins are expressed in a brain cell from about 3×10^6 genes (41). This variation in the primary amino acid sequence of brain proteins resulting from these codon point mutations provides genetic diversity, or heterogeneity, in the normal population and may affect the one mutation that causes dominant disease. Enzyme activity, receptor binding affinity, or structural protein functions may be slightly altered, albeit still within a normal range, and modify the gene expression of the one abnormal gene responsible for dominant disease.

In 1966 Harris (16) demonstrated gene variation (polymorphism) in humans, altering the concept of a normal genotype. He showed that humans have marked variation in enzyme activity—i.e., enzyme polymorphism—with about one-third of the enzymes he assayed from normal individuals showing a broad range of specific activity. These findings can now be extrapolated to the nervous system by looking at two important brain enzymes, dopamine β-hydroxylase (DBH) and catechol-*O*-methyltransferase (COMT) (56). Each enzyme expresses its activity through two separate alleles; one allele is obtained from each parent. DBH^L-DBH^L or COMT^L-COMT^L results in a low level of enzyme activity. DBH^H-DBH^H or COMT^H-COMT^H results in high activity. Allelic heterozygosity, which is seen in 50% of the population, results in intermediate levels of activity (56).

If one extrapolates from this kind of variation in biological activity that results from background codon mutations involving up to 10^5 different enzymes, receptors, and structural proteins in a brain cell, one can envision the enormous number of combinations of biological pressures that can affect the one mutation responsible for the dominant disease. Gene penetrance (the clinical variation in severity of any given characteristic) and gene expressivity (the different kinds of clinical features seen among affected individuals within a large pedigree or between large families with presumably the same genetic disease) must be in part explained by this type of normal genetic diversity (16,39,41,56).

MOLECULAR BASES FOR DOMINANTLY INHERITED
NEUROLOGIC DISEASE

The research needed to explain the molecular bases of dominantly inherited neurologic diseases will require the use of recently developed recombinant DNA techniques. The molecular structure of the gene and gene processing must first be defined. Genes are complex structures that are split between structural coding regions called exons (which code for the structure of protein) and nonstructural coding regions called introns (which code for regulatory events and not the structure of the protein) (10). The primary transcript (the initial RNA complementary copy) from DNA is referred to as hnRNA and includes both the exon and the intron regions. The hnRNA is then processed by adding a tail of up to 200 adenylic acids at the 3' end (the part of the molecule synthesized last), a process known as polyadenylation, and is capped with guanylic acid at the 5' end (the part of the molecule synthesized first). The final processing is accomplished by the splicing out of the introns to produce the mature mRNA, which is then translocated into the cytoplasm and assembled onto the polysome for protein translation (41).

Introns may exert a major influence on the overall size of the hnRNA. For example, the ovalbumin gene, representing some 7,000 bases, has only 1,859 bases that encode for the exons and thus for actual structural protein. Introns represent the majority of bases in this gene, with approximately 5,000 bases present in seven introns (1,22). The function of an intron is not fully understood, but it is thought that it may regulate mRNA stability and thus increase the efficiency of message production and length of message half-life, thereby increasing the level of the translated gene product. For example, one intron mutation that produces an in-phase termination codon sequence (terminates protein synthesis prematurely) causes an unstable mRNA for the β-globin gene product and results in severe clinical thalassemia (13). Intron mutations identified only in hnRNA and not in mRNA may yield a class of dominantly inherited diseases of the nervous system analogous to thalassemia. Similarly, frame shift mutations resulting from nucleotide deletions or insertions may occur in exon or intron coding areas and result in a major misreading of the code downstream from that site, because DNA is not being read in its correct sequence. Frame shift mutations also may become an important class of mutations for genetic neurologic disease.

Not only are genes split into exons (structural coding regions) and introns (nonstructural regulatory regions), but genes also occur in multiple copies (3). Genes coding for one function may occur as compact families of multiple copies on the same chromosome, such as the prolactin gene on chromosome 6 in a discrete area. Genes may also occur as dispersed families representing multiple copies on several different chromosomes, as has been described for argininosuccinic acid synthetase and the β-tubulin genes. It should be stressed that not all of these gene copies will be transcribable; many may be defective, nontranscribed copies, the so-called pseudogenes. Also, isogenic (different genes coding for the same function) copies may have tissue specificity, and perhaps only two such gene copies of many copies in a dispersed family may be expressed in brain. Multiple gene copies may also be expressed on double minute chromosomes, multiple copies of miniature chromosomes found in cells amplifying gene action that we have described in our laboratory (2). Defects in interchromosomal regulation of multiple isogenic copy expression may occur and result in dominantly inherited neurologic disease. Thus, genes are split and may occur in multiple copies dispersed on several chromosomes for the same gene product.

Chaudhari and Hahn (8) recently reported using scDNA as a probe or signal for hybridization or bonding against total hnRNA and polyadenylated [poly(A)] hnRNA in newborn and adult mice, opening a new area for neurogenetic investigation. When they hybridized scDNA against poly(A) hnRNA and total hnRNA in newborn mice, they obtained about the same degree of hybridization for both kinds of hnRNA. When the same experiment was done with adult mice, the degree of hybridization for total hnRNA was about one-third greater than for poly(A) hnRNA. When the comparison was made between adult and newborn mice, it was found that the degree of hybridization for total hnRNA was about one-third greater in adults than in newborns, and the degree of hybridization for poly(A) hnRNA was the same for adults and newborns. It was therefore concluded that a complex class of non-poly(A) hnRNA (hnRNA that does not have a tail of adenylic acids) appeared postnatally. This unique non-poly(A) hnRNA class appeared at a time when the brain is virtually fully formed and when learning, memory, and cognitive events are beginning. The findings raise the intriguing possibility that a class of nonadenylated hnRNA or mRNA species will be found in which an impairment in synthesis, half-life, transport, or assembly to the ribosome could be responsible for a class of dominantly inherited mental retardation syndromes in which the structure of the nervous system is entirely normal.

Thus, not only are genes split, not only are genes dispersed, not only is there a special class for nonadenylated mRNA in brain, but genes may also move as transposons (genes that can transpose, or move) or as mobile insertable segments of DNA. The 1983 Nobel Prize in Medicine was given to Barbara McClintock, who described such transposons in the 1940s in maize; they have now been identified in yeast and in invertebrate and mammalian cells (50). Transposons when incorporated into the genome (linear sequence of DNA in the chromosome) are actively transcribed, but when they are deleted and appear in the nuceloplasm they are not transcribed. Transposon activation-deactivation, gene shuffling, and rearrangements are emerging as important events in cell differentiation. Defects in these mechanisms may produce a class of dominantly inherited neurologic diseases. Thus, dominantly inherited forms of brain tumors may be related to abnormal gene transpositions (32,47,55).

RECOMBINANT DNA TECHNIQUES

The approaches to understanding dominantly inherited neurologic disease (summarized in Table 1) will be productive only through the use of the recombinant

TABLE 1. *Research strategies in dominantly inherited neurologic disease*

Possible molecular bases of dominantly inherited disease (see text for details)
  Mutation in gene for structural protein: cell membrane, receptor, not enzyme
  Mutation in gene for primary transcript (hnRNA) processing events: intron splicing;
    capping of 5′ end, polyadenylation of 3′ end, mRNA transport into cytoplasm and
    binding to ribosome
  Mutation in regulatory gene(s) for compact and dispersed gene family interactions for
    gene amplification
  Mutation in gene for complex class of nonpolyadenylated RNA
  Mutation in gene(s) for activation or deactivation and movement of transposons
    (insertable DNA segments)
Possible molecular basis for clinical variation in gene expressivity and penetrance in
  dominantly inherited disease: normal background genetic heterogeneity resulting from
  degeneracy in genetic code

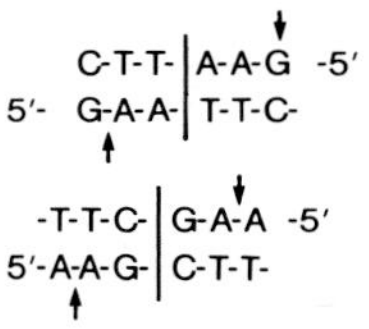

FIG. 1. Restriction endonucleases named Eco RI and Hind III are enzymes that identify a unique sequence of nucleotide bases in DNA and cut DNA within that sequence into restriction fragments. Recognition sites of Eco RI *(top)* and Hind III *(bottom)*.

DNA techniques that have been so powerfully applied to other, nonneurologic genetic disorders. The development of this technology began with the identification of restriction endonucleases, which are enzymes that recognize specific sites on DNA and cut or restrict DNA at these points into restriction fragments (Fig. 1) (20,51). The joined-together fragments of DNA from different sources are referred to as recombinant DNA. A segment of DNA containing a gene from a human inserted into a virus λ phage, and this unit, having DNA from two sources, is referred to as a segment of recombinant DNA. The λ phage containing a segment of human DNA serves as a vector or shuttle, carrying the recombinant DNA into a bacterial host. This approach produces a genomic library with unlimited numbers of the inserted genes in a bacterial host (Fig. 2). The entire human genome, split into individual fragments, incorporated into phage, and then into bacterial hosts, results in what is called a human genomic library. Selecting the one bacterial colony containing the single human gene of interest is known as gene cloning (21).

Restriction endonucleases usually recognize four to six base pair sequences and yield fragments of DNA about 4,000 bases long. Human genomic DNA, the total DNA from the chromosome of any cell, produces about 7×10^5 separate fragments. A probe or complementary copy of radioactive DNA can be copied for isolated mRNA by the enzyme reverse transcriptase. The resulting DNA is called cDNA because the constituent bases are complementary to the template mRNA. Adenine and uridine, as well as guanine and cytosine, are complementary to each other. This cDNA can be used to construct a library, matching the total number of mRNAs transcribed in that tissue (Fig. 2). The bacterial colony of interest can be identified and cloned by hybridization with a radiolabeled probe complementary to the human gene that has been inserted into the vector (26,29,41) (Fig. 3).

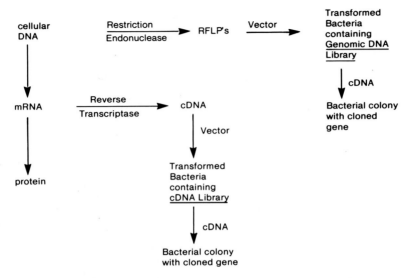

FIG. 2. Genomic DNA and cDNA libraries are produced from genomic DNA (DNA at the chromosomal level) and mRNA, respectively, using recombinant DNA techniques. RFLPs are fragments of DNA that are produced by cutting or restricting DNA with enzymes known as restriction endonucleases.

Using these techniques the following genes of neurologic interest have been cloned: among proteins, actin, tubulin, and the acetylcholine receptor protein; among neurotransmitter-dependent enzymes, phenylalanine hydroxylase, tyrosine hydroxylase, and dopamine-β-hydroxylase; among neuropeptides, calcitonin, dynorphin, enkephalin, gastrin, growth hormone, prolactin, proopiomelanocortin, somatostatin, vasopressin, and others (27,28,36,38). The revolution in molecular biology started by Watson and Crick in defining the structure of DNA and by Nirenberg and colleagues in deciphering the genetic code has clearly entered the arenas of neurobiology and clinical neurology. The genetic language of the brain is becoming as easy to read and understand as that of *Escherichia coli*, and the details of its genetic story are as compelling as any good novel (41).

Fragments of DNA produced by cutting the DNA with enzymes are called restriction fragment length polymorphisms (RFLPs) or length variations. These fragments of DNA of varying length are separated by molecular weight on agarose gels. The sized DNA fragments are identified by blotting them onto nitrocellulose filters (52). Using specific radiolabeled cDNA probes, a specific fragment on the blot can be identified by the specific cDNA complementary to it (Fig. 4). A band of density on the autoradiogram shows the location of the desired fragment of DNA. These RFLPs vary from individual to individual because of the normal variation in the primary DNA sequence, as discussed previously. Single base changes may introduce or delete restriction sites, i.e., sites of DNA sensitive to the restriction endonuclease cleaving enzyme. Sequence deletions, additions, or

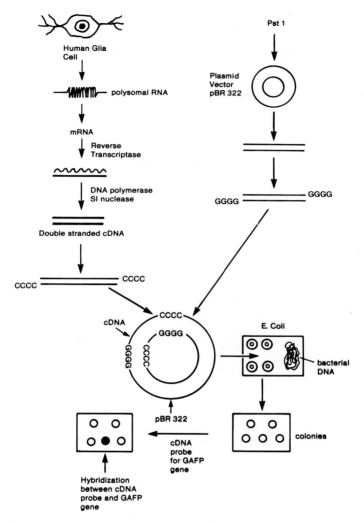

FIG. 3. The theoretical cloning of the glial gene, glial acidic filamentous protein (GAFP) subunit. mRNA for this protein subunit is isolated; a double-stranded cDNA copy is made against this mRNA population, placed into a plasmid vector, and incorporated into a bacterium. The bacterial colony containing this gene is selected by using a radiolabeled cDNA probe complementary to the gene of interest. SI nuclease, a single-stranded specific nuclease used to clip the hairpin formed during the synthesis of double-stranded cDNA.

translocations of several segments of nucleotides may affect the length of DNA between restriction sites. The number of polymorphic sites in a human cell has been estimated as about 20,000, and about 120 to 150 sites, or about 0.6% of potential polymorphic genetic loci, have been identified using current endonucleases and probes (5,17). These restriction loci do not occur at random but, rather,

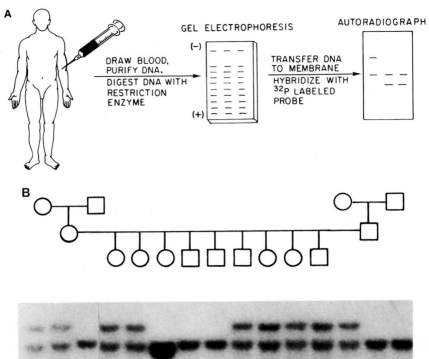

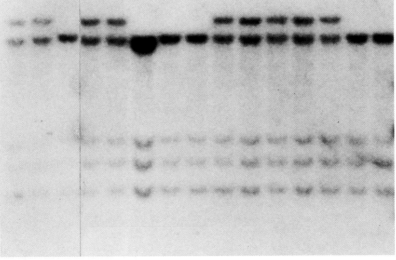

FIG. 4. Inheritance of restriction fragments within a family. **A:** From a small amount of peripheral blood, DNA representing all of an individual's DNA sequences can be purified biochemically and digested with site-specific nucleases. Different size fragments produced by the enzymatic digest can then be arrayed according to size by agarose gel electrophoresis. Differences in DNA sequences are revealed as differences in fragment size when hybridized to a specific cloned segment of human DNA. The hybridization is easily followed on X-ray film when the cloned segment is made radioactive. **B:** Autoradiograph of fragment sizes revealed by hybridization of a cloned human gene sequence, in this case the calcitonin gene, to individual DNA prepared as described above. Each lane represents the pattern for a given individual depicted in pedigree directly above the autoradiograph. The radioactive probe reveals two polymorphic or varying fragments of sizes. 8.0 and 6.5 kb at the top of the gel. Predictably, inheritance of fragment size, and thus DNA sequence, is consistent with the laws of Mendel throughout the three-generation family. (From ref. 57, with permission.)

are inherited, and they serve as an important basis for linkage studies in that they provide a means of identifying the mutant gene for the genetic disease of interest. Linkage refers to a normal gene closely associated with the mutant gene responsible for the inherited disease under study.

LINKAGE STUDIES

Linkage analyses provide several advantages. First, linkage markers that will segregate in a pedigree for the mutation responsible for a genetic disease can provide a precise means of documenting that a similar clinical phenotype in two separate families is a result of entirely different mutations. In such circumstances one family would show appropriate linkage for the marker, whereas the other family would not. A common phenotype may be associated with entirely different genotypes. This relationship has been seen in patients with Charcot-Marie-Tooth disease or one of the spinocerebellar degenerations in which linkage studies for specific biochemical markers have been positive in only some of the families that clinically seem identical (4). Second, positive linkages between the presence of the genetic disease and a closely located marker locus for a biochemical function provide a means to develop cDNA probes to the marker locus that will segregate for the presence of the genetic disease. The objective is to find a cDNA probe that binds to a marker gene, thus identifying a specific RFLP by producing a hybridization or bonding pattern on a gel that occurs only with those who have the clinical disorder (Fig. 5). Third, linkage studies will be crucial in locating and, ultimately, isolating the mutant gene and determining precisely its altered DNA sequence (5,48,54).

The power that linkage studies using appropriate restriction endonucleases and identification of specific RFLPs have for identifying the linked marker gene is that

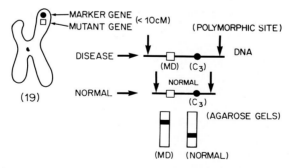

FIG. 5. A cDNA probe for a marker gene linked closely to the mutant gene for a dominantly inherited neurologic disease. DNA fragments (RFLPs) are obtained from patients and controls, and hybridization signals are produced on blots with the cDNA probe for the marker gene that is closely linked to the mutant gene of interest. The mutant gene in this instance is for myotonic dystrophy (MD). The abnormal genotype for the mutant gene can be clearly identified when a hybridization pattern is produced that segregates with affected patients and not with persons not at risk in a pedigree.

in well-characterized family pedigrees the genetic disease under study theoretically could be eliminated if the family cooperated. Such linkage studies have been successfully carried out already with a number of important neurologic diseases. Several important inherited diseases have been mapped to a chromosome (25,46), including the following: chromosome 1, Charcot-Marie-Tooth disease, Gaucher's disease, and phosphofructokinase deficiency; chromosome 3, GM_1 gangliosidosis and Morquio's disease; chromosome 5, Sandhoff's disease; chromosome 6, spino-cerebellar degeneration; chromosome 11, acute porphyria; chromosome 15, Tay-Sachs disease and Prader-Willi syndrome; chromosome 17, Pompe's disease; chromosome 19, myotonic dystrophy; chromosome 22, metachromatic leukodystrophy and Hurler-Scheie syndrome; the X chromosome, Duchenne's dystrophy, adreno-leukodystrophy, Lesch-Nyhan syndrome, and the fragile X mental retardation syndrome.

For practical purposes linkage should be less than 2 centimorgans (cM) between the marker and mutant genes. This means that the chance for recombination (separation between mutant and marker genes) is 2% when homologous chromosomes exchange segments during the meiotic phase of gametogenesis. Thus, with tight linkage the marker gene will always segregate with the mutant gene and hence will be a useful clinical genetic marker (Fig. 6). The statistical significance of linkage is measured by lod scores (log value of the odds), and a value greater than 3 is significant. A lod score of 3 is actually a log value (10^3), indicating the two genes are closely linked with a probability of 1,000:1.

cDNA PROBES AND NONNEUROLOGIC DISEASES

Several nonneurologic genetic diseases have been successfully diagnosed *in utero* before the 20th week of gestation at the genomic or DNA chromosomal level by cDNA probes using cells obtained by amniocentesis or by biopsy of chorionic villus tissue (12). Sickle cell disease and non-insulin-dependent diabetes mellitus are two examples. In the case of sickle cell disease, Chang and Kan (7) and Orkin and colleagues (34) used a new restriction endonuclease, Mst II, which cleaves DNA at the sequence CCTNAGG (C, cytosine; T thymine; A, adenine; G, guanine; N, any of these four bases). In the normal β-globin gene this sequence is present in the genomic region that corresponds to amino acids 5, 6, and 7 (CCT-GAG-GAG: proline, glutamate, glutamate). The cloned normal human β-globin gene was digested by Mst II into two fragments that were 1.15 and 0.2 kb long, respectively. The sickle mutation at B^6 (glutamate to valine) changed the sequence of DNA to CCT-GTG-GAG, abolishing the Mst II recognition site to produce a single 1.35-kb fragment instead of the two normal ones. Using a 1.15-kb 5′ Mst II fragment as the radioactive cDNA probe for hybridization, Orkin and colleagues (34) found a 1.15-kb fragment only in the *AA* normal genotype, the 1.35-kb fragment only in the *SS* homozygote, and both 1.15-kb and 1.35-kb fragments in the *AS* heterozygote. As little as 1 μg of genomic DNA gave a detectable hybridization signal, indicating that the test can be done prenatally on cells obtained by amniocentesis (19) or chorionic villus biopsy (12).

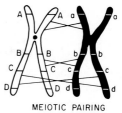

MEIOTIC PAIRING

FIG. 6. Illustration of segmental nature of inherited chromosomes. Products of meiosis are single recombinant chromosomes that represent a mosaic of segments, here shown in black and white, from both parental chromosomes. (From ref. 57, with permission.)

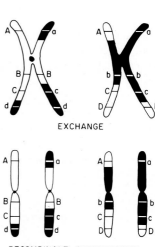

EXCHANGE

RECOMBINANT CHROMOSOMES

Polymorphisms in the 5′ flanking region (the region of DNA occurring just before the start of the insulin gene) of the human insulin gene on chromosome 11 have been identified and represent a molecular genetic marker for non-insulin-dependent diabetes (45). A DNA RFLP using two different restriction endonucleases produced a cDNA probe that identified a fragment 7.8 kb in length upstream on the 5′ side (initial segment) of the insulin gene in normal subjects. Individuals having non-insulin-dependent diabetes mellitus were found to have a unique DNA fragment (polymorphism) in this region resulting from a 1.6-kb insert, resulting in a new, longer fragment identified with the same probe that is 9.5 kb rather than the normal 7.6 kb long. One theoretical explanation for the presence of diabetes mellitus is that as a result of this 1.6-kb insert, transcription or synthesis of RNA from DNA becomes less efficient, producing a less stable available message and, as a result, the synthesis of less insulin.

cDNA PROBES AND INHERITED NEUROLOGIC DISEASES

The greatest achievements thus far have been in finding a cDNA probe for two X-linked neurologic disorders: Lesch-Nyhan syndrome and Duchenne's muscular dystrophy. Brennand and colleagues in 1982 (6) and Jolly and colleagues in 1982

(18) reported cloned cDNA sequences for the mouse and human hypoxanthine-guanine phosphoribosyltransferase (HGPRT) genes, respectively. HGPRT is the enzyme deficient in patients with Lesch-Nyhan syndrome. HGPRT enzyme mutants from unrelated patients with Lesch-Nyhan syndrome were identified, and each exhibited a unique structural and functional abnormality (58). HGPRT$_{Kinston}$ was identified from a patient with Lesch-Nyhan syndrome; the mutation was a result of a codon change incorporating asparagine instead of aspartate into position 193. The change resulted in a K_m mutant enzyme, with K_m values being increased 200-fold, indicating very low affinity of the substrate for the enzyme. Nussbaum and colleagues (33) recently described an indirect DNA hybridization method for detecting HGPRT deficiency by using the endonuclease Bam HI, which mapped specific RFLPs at several sites in the HGPRT gene. Wilson and associates (58) isolated DNA from several members of a family with the mutant HGPRT$_{Toronto}$ allele, associated clinically with hyperuricemia and gout. Patient DNA was restricted with another enzyme (Taq I) and analyzed by methods already described (52) using a nearly full-length HGPRT cDNA as the probe. The normal 2.0-kb RFLP was replaced by a 4.0-kb fragment in the HGPRT$_{Toronto}$ gene and provided a definitive assignment of the genotype of several family members with this variant allele (58). The stage is now set to make a definitive genomic diagnosis using these probes for the HGPRT$_{Kinston}$ allele from a patient with Lesch-Nyhan syndrome, and this event is likely to occur in the immediate future (33).

A cDNA probe for Duchenne's dystrophy was developed in Williamson's laboratory by Murray and colleagues (31) at St. Mary's Hospital, London, by generating random DNA fragments of X chromosomes. A probe, λRC8, was hybridized to the terminal tip of the short arm of the X chromosome, as determined by cell hybridization studies. Through use of this probe and its application to a family pedigree with Duchenne's dystrophy, an obligate female carrier was found to express two hybridization signals, one at 5.3 and the other at 3.2 kb. An affected son expressed only one hybridization signal, at 5.3 kb, and this was the distinguishing feature. These researchers posit that the probe identifies a genetic locus close to the locus for Duchenne's dystrophy but not entirely identical to it. It segregates with the presence of the Duchenne locus with 85% concordance (11,15,31).

The fragile X mental retardation syndrome on the long arm of the X chromosome at the q27 site is very near the Lesch-Nyhan syndrome and the glucose-6 phosphate dehydrogenase (G6PD) loci (24,49,53). cDNA probes now available in several laboratories for the HGPRT (Lesch-Nyhan syndrome) and G6PD genes are being applied to genomic DNA fragments from patients with the fragile X syndrome to provide a molecular means of identifying the presence of fragile X disease.

The use of unique sequence derived cDNA probes described by Wyman and White (59) will be a powerful tool in predicting the occurrence of dominantly inherited diseases. We have initiated hybridization studies using genomic DNA obtained from brain and lymphocyte samples of patients with Joseph disease, using cDNA probes obtained for several genes as well as probes generated from random

DNA fragments. Preliminary data indicate a primary gene mutation on chromosome 1 near the amylase locus and a modifier gene on chromosome 2 at p23 near the erythrocyte acid phosphatase locus. Gusella and colleagues (14), using the same approach and techniques, have undertaken a systematic study of two families with Huntington's disease to obtain a definitive restriction fragment pattern that identifies the genotype for the mutant gene. They recently reported that the Huntington's disease gene in both families is linked to a DNA marker fragment that maps to the short arm of human chromosome 4 near its terminus. They propose to extend these data to other families, isolate the specific DNA fragment with the Huntington's disease mutant gene, and determine the primary genetic defect and thus the altered gene product.

Progress in the investigation of the spinocerebellar degenerations might be readily achieved by using probes developed for the immune response genes on chromosome 6. At least one form of olivopontocerebellar degeneration links to human lymphocyte antigens (HLA).

The myotonic muscular dystrophy mutation has been mapped to chromosome 19 by means of linkage studies associating disease with the third component of complement (C_3). Roses and co-workers (44) are currently moving down, or "walking," the chromosome, beginning with C_3 cDNA probe as a primer and adding flanking (adjacent) segments of DNA to it in both the 3′ (end of the molecule) and 5′ (initial segment of the molecule) directions from the C_3 locus. It is not known whether the myotonic dystrophy locus is on the 5′ or the 3′ side of the C_3 locus, and "walking" will continue until the randomly generated probes identify a hybridization signal on a blot that correlates with the presence of disease.

The abnormal locus in some patients with Charcot-Marie-Tooth disease has been assigned to chromosome 1 by virtue of linkage studies showing association to the Duffy blood group (4) and to the antithrombin 3 locus (37). A cDNA probe to the antithrombin 3 gene is available and should provide the means to develop a precise Charcot-Marie-Tooth disease probe. Using a similar approach, the abnormal gene locus in a family with dominantly inherited antithrombin deficiency recently was identified (37). Affected individuals did not have associated neurologic disease, but the study was important in that it showed major deletions of segments of the antithrombin gene, making it one of the first studies to show that dominantly inherited disease can be associated with major gene deletions. Perhaps families will be described in which both antithrombin 3 deficiency of varying severity and various expressions of Charcot-Marie-Tooth disease exist because of the presence of variable degrees of gene deletion in this region.

In situ hybridization is a powerful new technique to visualize molecular differentiation. It can indicate the degree of mRNA levels in a specific cell or tissue, as developed by W. S. T. Griffin in the developing mouse cerebellum and seen in Fig. 7. Specific cDNA probes will hybridize to complementary mRNAs, and diseases with a similar neuropathology will be separable on the basis of different specific message levels.

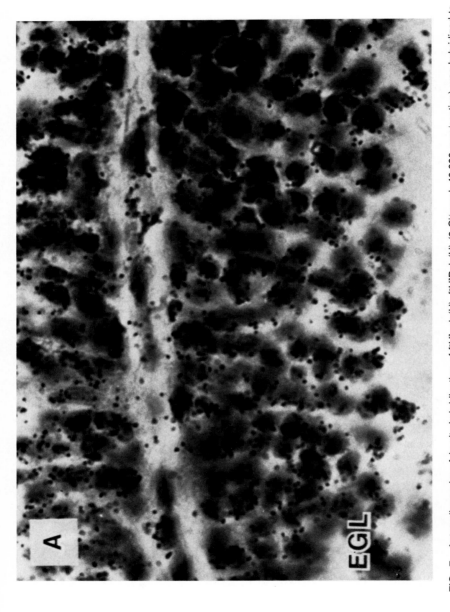

FIG. 7. Autoradiographs of *in situ* hybridization of [³H]poly(U). [³H]Poly(U) (3 Ci/mmol; 40,000 cpm/section) was hybridized to cerebellar sections from 14-day-old rats. Autoradiographic exposure was for 5 days. (Courtesy Dr. W. Sue T. Griffin, University of Texas Health Science Center at Dallas.) **A:** Grain density over granule cells in the external granule layer. *(Continued.)*

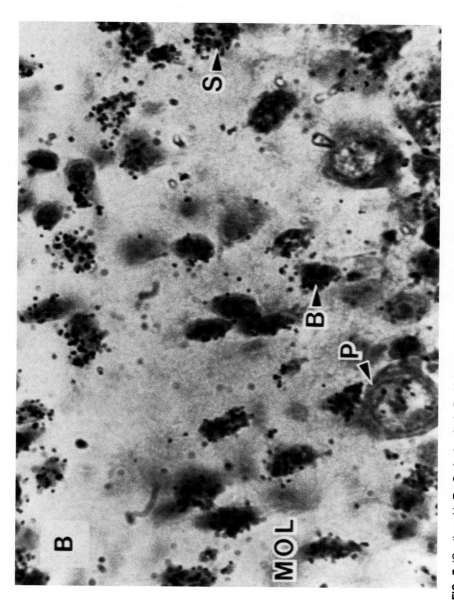

FIG. 7. *(Continued.)* **B:** Grain density in Purkinje cells (P) as well as in migrating cells, stellate cells (S), and basket cells (B) in the molecular layer (MOL).

GENE THERAPY

The correction of genetic defects by gene therapy is not new. Cells deficient in HGPRT, galactose-1-phosphate uridyltransferase, or β-galactosidase have been described in culture in which a low rate of correction of the enzyme defect was made possible by cellular incorporation of the deficient gene with a viral vector. This approach is inappropriate for patient treatment. A more practical approach was taken by Ley and colleagues (23), who utilized 5-azacytidine as a means for selectively increasing fetal globin synthesis in a patient with severe thalassemia. They treated a patient for 14 days, during which time there was considerable synthesis of fetal globin and suppression of the thalassemic β-globin gene product. Incorporation of 5-azacytidine into the patient's genomic DNA (DNA at the chromosomal level) prevented DNA methylation and allowed gene transcription to take place. The approach suggests that diseases such as Huntington's disease, spinocerebellar degeneration, tuberous sclerosis, and neurofibromatosis are the result of the normal inhibition of one isogene and the induction of a mutant isogene at any of several stages of life. Such genetic chronobiological findings would imply that a whole series of isogenes could become induced throughout life, a process analogous to the changes that occur in fetal and adult hemoglobin genes or in fetal and adult creatine phosphokinase genes. Brain isoenzymes, receptor isoproteins, or structural isoproteins may be expressed in a series of isogene inhibitions and inductions occurring regularly throughout life. Reinduction of the repressed normal fetal gene to compensate for an adult mutant isogene may become a research strategy in the future (41).

The introduction of a desired gene into somatic cells has been successfully carried out by Palmiter and associates (35). These workers fused the mouse metallothionein I gene with the rat growth hormone gene and injected the recombinant gene into fertilized pronuclei of mouse embryos so as to generate mice twice the size and weight of normal littermates. This approach suggests both a means of investigating the regulation of the growth hormone gene and a theoretical method of correcting gene mutations in the future.

Comings predicted in 1980 (9) that recombinant DNA techniques would have a major impact on clinical medicine and basic research: "Since the degree of departure from our previous approaches and the potential of this procedure are so great, one will not be guilty of hyperbole in calling it the 'new genetics.'" Recombinant DNA techniques and the "new genetics" have entered the arenas of clinical neurology and neurobiology and are providing a precise means of examining inherited neurologic diseases. More generally, the techniques will provide a profound new approach for understanding the regulatory events responsible for the development of the human brain.

GLOSSARY

Autosome   Any of the chromosomes 1 to 22; not the X or Y chromosome.

Blot   An identified fragment of DNA on a filter produced by the hybridization of a radiolabeled cDNA probe to it.

5

Neurooncogenes

RETROVIRAL ONCOGENES

A potentially deep immediate insight into the molecular mechanisms involved in carcinogenesis occurred with the discovery of the oncogene. An oncogene is a gene that encodes for a protein that eventually leads to the transformation of a normal cell into a malignant one. It was in 1969 that Huebner and Todero proposed the "oncogene hypothesis" in their paper "Oncogenes of RNA Tumor Viruses as Determinants of Cancer" (6). It was their view that retroviruses, viruses that contain RNA as their genetic material rather than DNA, inserted their genetic material into the germ line of eukaryotic animal cells early in evolution, and that these viral oncogenes have been carried through the germ line to all animals, even humans, since that early event. They believed that these acquired oncogenes remained quiescent but that activation of them by radiation or carcinogens would result in clinical cancer. Their concept of inherited oncogenes is a correct one but the origin of these genes is opposite to the view they proposed. It is now known that oncogenes are normal cellular genes that are required for development and differentiation and that span the evolutionary spectrum from yeast to man. The normal oncogene form is referred to as a c-oncogene (c for cellular) or protooncogene and has a close DNA sequence homology to retroviruses. During evolution it is hypothesized that normal oncogenes became associated with retroviruses and converted into cancer-causing genes. Evidence for the sequence homology similarity between retroviruses and c-oncogenes was provided by Bishop and Varmus (3), who prepared radio-labeled complementary DNA (cDNA) probes against RNA from the Rous sarcoma virus. These probes were then used to hybridize with DNA obtained from normal chicken cells. A segment of the RNA from the tumorigenic Rous sarcoma virus referred to as the *src* gene hybridized specifically to a complementary segment of chicken DNA. Thus genomic DNA of normal chickens contains a copy of the Rous *src* gene.

ORIGIN OF ONCOGENES

It was then possible to ask the question, Which came first, the retroviral *src* gene or the normal cellular oncogene? Are cellular oncogenes captured retroviral

DNA segments, or did cellular oncogenes precede evolutionarily their retroviral cousins? They are obviously closely allied, with similar sequences.

The answer to this important riddle came from the pivotal observation that the normal cellular oncogene contains introns or intervening sequences and the retroviral *src* gene does not. In the normal processing of primary transcript RNA into mRNA, the introns are spliced out at specific splice sites by endogenous restriction endonucleases. Thus the *src* gene must have originated first in the cell's genomic DNA and subsequently in evolution become devoid of its introns. If the virus had been the source of the c-oncogene and then became incorporated into the cell's genome, it is clear that it could not have acquired introns subsequently. It is now believed that the oncogene is a normal cellular gene that was parasitized by the Rous sarcoma virus through recombination (5). To date 17 cellular protooncogenes have been identified, and each of them is known from its association as an active oncogene with a specific retrovirus (16).

What is the origin of the oncogene in the human? Weinberg points out that the answer came from several laboratories, including Michael Wigler's group at the Cold Spring Harbor Laboratory, Mariano Barbacid's laboratory at the National Cancer Institute, and his own. These groups isolated a human bladder oncogene. This human bladder oncogene served as a probe for exploring the normal human genome, and it indeed hybridized with a homologous DNA sequence in the normal genome. More complete characterization of the normal human gene and the bladder oncogene showed almost identical sequences. They could not be absolutely identical, as they functioned *in situ* obviously in a different manner. Cloned oncogene DNA transformed cells and cloned DNA of the related normal gene did not. The oncogene DNA obtained from tumor cells was transfected into NIH 3T3 cells, transforming them into tumor cells. The cells did not form a normal monolayer in culture but overgrew into several layers and caused tumors when injected into animals. Normal DNA transfected into NIH 3T3 cells did not result in tumor cell formation. Thus in the normal human genome there exists a protooncogene closely related to the cancer-causing gene, an oncogene.

ONCOGENE ACTIVATION

The mechanisms involved in the conversion of a normal cellular protooncogene into a tumorigenic oncogene are several. The first was elucidated in Weinberg's laboratory as a pont mutation found in the EJ human bladder carcinoma cell line. A segment of 350 DNA nucleotides from the human bladder cell line, when introduced into the protooncogene to produce a hybrid molecule, converted it into a transforming molecule. As Weinberg points out, the critical difference between the oncogene and the corresponding segment of the protooncogene consists of only one base: a guanine in the protooncogene is replaced by a thymine in the oncogene. Thus a single base change in a 5,000-nucleotide normal human gene could convert it into a tumorigenic oncogene.

More recently another mechanism of oncogene activation has been found to be due to chromosomal rearrangement. The human protooncogene *myc* is activated to cause human Burkitt's lymphoma by a chromosomal abnormality resulting in a reciprocal translocation or exchange of DNA between chromosomes 8 and 14. Sometimes a segment from chromosome 8 is transferred to the short arm of chromosome 2 or to the long arm of chromosome 22. The common feature of all of these translocations is that all of the chromosomes that receive translocated material from chromosome 8 contain genes for immunoglobulin chains. The translocated piece of chromosome 8 is the precise site for the c-*myc* gene and thus it is abnormally introduced into sites of active transcription, which results in its own active transcription. Thus the association of the protooncogene with these sites of immunoglobulin gene transcription results in protooncogene deregulation and its conversion into a tumorigenic oncogene (16).

Protooncogene amplification resulting in large numbers of copies of the gene per cell and thus gene expression has an oncogenic effect as well. Thus critical point mutations in protooncogenes, chromosomal rearrangements, and gene amplification of protooncogenes all can result in cellular transformation and cancer.

ONCOGENE PRODUCT

The oncogene product is frequently a protein kinase that phosphorylates tyrosine residues of protein molecules located on plasma membranes of cells. It forms a unique class of kinases, as most normal phosphorylation occurs at serine and threonine residues. This oncogene-determined kinase is located on the cell membrane exactly at points where cells join and on adhesion plaques where cells adhere to a fixed surface. It is interesting to note that one target of the oncogene-determined kinase is vinculin, which when phosphorylated causes the cells to lose attachment and round up typically of tumor cells. The *src* kinase must also be involved in the phosphorylation of other proteins, several of which are probably involved in cellular division (5).

Recently Michael Wigler of the Cold Spring Harbor Laboratory reported that the transforming protein encoded by the *ras* gene is an activator of the enzyme adenylate cyclase of yeast (9). This enzyme converts ATP (adenosine triphosphate) into cyclic AMP (adenosine monophosphate), which is an important second messenger transmitting hormonal signals from the membrane into the cell interior. This observation is an extension of the previous work by Deborah Defeo-Jones and Edward Scolnick that yeast contains the *ras* gene. It is now known that in addition to humans and yeast, many living species, including rodents and fruit flies, contain the *ras* gene, whose normal function is to regulate growth and differentiation of normal cells.

The Wigler and Scolnick groups have found that yeast contains two *ras* genes, designated *ras* 1 and 2. They found that the proteins encoded by the yeast genes are about 90% homologous to the mammalian proteins for the first 80 amino acids and 50% homologous for the next 80. In addition, inactivation of one *ras* gene in yeast still allows growth, but inactivation of both is not compatible with growth. This is a finding again consistent with the view that cellular oncogenes regulate cell growth. Of considerable importance is the finding that a human *ras* gene can substitute for the inactivated endogenous yeast gene and sustain yeast growth. Thus these genes have been tightly conserved throughout evolution for 600 million years.

The linking of the *ras* gene to the adenylate cyclase system is a major step forward but does not solve the problem of how the transforming or the normal protooncogene functions. Much research will be required to resolve both points. There is some speculation that oncogenes may be related to growth factors, as they are known to activate protein kinases in the cell membrane. Oncogenes *sis* and *erb B* have been linked to growth factors already, and the association of the *ras* oncogene with an important cell regulatory system, the adenylate cyclase system, indicates that oncogenes must be necessary for maintenance of cell growth and differentiation (9).

Neurooncogenes

Neuroblastoma and retinoblastoma are two tumors of neural origin in which specific genetic defects have been described as the basis for malignant transformation. Both tumors have been associated with specific chromosomal deletions. Consistent with the hypothesis that protooncogenes are activated to transforming oncogenes is the view that these chromosomal deletions result in the loss of a suppressor element whose normal function is to turn off embryonic genes, the protooncogenes, which allow cells to become mature, postmitotic neurons or retinal cells. Thus in the absence of suppression, these undifferentiated cells remain embryonic and eventually become malignant.

Neuroblastoma

Neuroblastoma was found to be associated with amplification by 20- to 140-fold of a domain of DNA designated N-*myc* in 24 of 63 untreated patients (38%). It is important to note that amplification was found in 0 of 15 patients with stage 1 or 2 disease and in 24 of 48 patients with advanced disease and thus is a marker of a poor prognosis (4,13). An additional karyotypic finding has been identified that is characteristic of human neuroblastoma, a deletion of the distal short arm of chromosome 1. This deletion has been identified in about 70% of both primary neuroblastomas and tumor-derived cell lines. Perhaps this deletion on chromosome 1 results in the loss of the postulated suppressor gene and subsequent activation and amplification of the N-*myc* oncogene on chromosome 2, locus p23 (11).

Further *in situ* hybridization localizes amplified N-*myc* genes in neuroblastoma cells to homogeneously staining regions on different chromosomes (12). Experimentally, neuroblastoma gene amplification can be induced with chemotherapeutic agents, as we showed in 1981, with the formation of double minute chromosomes and homogeneously staining regions on chromosomes associated with increased dihydrofolate reductase activity because of the selective inductive pressure of methotrexate (1).

Retinoblastoma

Familial autosomal dominantly inherited retinoblastoma has been described in the genetic literature for many years (15). On the average 50% of the children of an affected parent will develop disease, and when it occurs the tumors involve both eyes and occur in the first few years of life. Nonfamilial sporadic cases are unilateral and occur later in life.

The Knudson (7) model of cancer, which requires two specific mutations to occur to express disease, has been suggested as an explanation of familial bilateral retinoblastoma. Thus two specific, different mutations must occur in a single cell in the retina to result in cancerous change. In inherited disease one mutation has already occurred in each cell of the patient by virtue of a germ line mutation from the patient's parent, and thus a second, new somatic retinal cell mutation is necessary to result in tumor production. There is a statistical probability that a second somatic mutation will occur, because new mutation occurs once in every million cell divisions and there are about two million cells in the developing retina. This hypothesis implies that familial retinoblastoma will produce a mendelian pattern that is autosomal dominant, but that the genotypic defect is autosomal recessive, i.e., allelic loci on both chromosomes are mutant.

In 1983 Sparkes et al. (14) found in three families with hereditary retinoblastoma close linkage of the gene for this tumor with the genetic locus for esterase D. They assigned the gene for the hereditary form of retinoblastoma by deletion mapping to band q14 on chromosome 13, which is exactly where the chromosome deletion form of the eye tumor exists. They argued that in the nondeletion form of hereditary retinoblastoma, a "submicroscopic change" (mutation) occurred at the same site in both alleles, rendering the retinoblastoma cell hymozygously affected.

Benedict et al. (2) extended the initial observation of esterase D linkage in the chromosomal deletion form of hereditary retinoblastoma and showed that 11 patients had esterase D activity that was 50% of normal in nontumor cells because of a systemic mutation. They described one female patient who had 50% esterase D activity in all normal cells but no deletion of 13q14 at the 550 band level. Two stem lines were obtained from a retinoblastoma of this patient; each had a missing chromosome 13 and no detectable esterase D activity was found in the tumor, indicating that the normal nondeleted chromosome 13 was lost in both lines. They showed that there is a total loss of genetic material at the 13q14 locus including the retinoblastoma gene within the tumor and that a homozygous, recessive genotype exists to express the malignancy. The retinoblastoma cancer gene is recessive, and both alleles must be lost for tumors to develop. One 13q14 allele is deleted by a germ line mutation from the affected parent with hereditary retinoblastoma, and this mutation is carried in all the somatic cells of the affected patient. The second acquired genetic defect in these two lines from the female patient of Benedict was a loss of chromosome 13 from the tumor cells. It may be that all hereditary retinoblastomas are caused by mutations at locus 13q14 of both alleles within the tumor cell. Where the nature of the mutations is known, it proves to be a deletion

(10). Murphree and Benedict do distinguish between their hypothesis that the production of the tumor is caused by loss of a suppressor element at 13q14 and the oncogene mechanism of carcinogenesis (8). Actually they are closely related, as the loss of the suppressor does result in activation of an oncogene.

Lee et al. examined 10 retinoblastoma samples from separate patients for evidence of oncogene activation and found the N-*myc* oncogene transcriptionally active in all and amplified in two. Schwab et al. also found that N-*myc* is amplified in retinoblastoma in the late stages of tumor development and may portend a poor prognosis (12).

Oncogenes activated by mutation, amplification, translocation, or suppressor deletion transform cells into cancer cells. Abnormal tyrosine residue phosphorylation of cell surface, plasma membrane proteins and increased levels of intracellular cyclic AMP as well as other mechanisms may also be involved. In a rather short period of time the molecular basis of carcinogenesis has been elucidated and applied to tumors of neural origin. Similar molecular alterations must be operative to explain familial astrocytomas, meningiomas, and the multiple tumor forms of neurofibromatosis. Research opportunities in neurooncology have never looked brighter. Perhaps a combination of chemotherapeutic agents can be devised exploiting the knowledge of oncogene cellular transformation by inactivating oncogene transcription or its specific protein kinase gene product.

REFERENCES

1. Baskin, F., Rosenberg, R. N., and Dev, V. (1981): Correlation of double minute chromosomes with unstable multi-drug cross-resistance in neuroblastoma transport mutants. *Proc. Natl. Acad. Sci. USA*, 78:3654–3658.
2. Benedict, W. F., Murphree, A. L., Bainerjee, A., Spina, C. A., Sparkes, M. C., and Sparkes, R. S. (1983): Patient with 13 chromosome deletion: Evidence that the retino-blastoma gene is a recessive cancer gene. *Science*, 219:973–975.
3. Bishop, J. M., and Varmus, H. (1982): Functions and origins of retroviral transforming genes. In: *RNA Tumor Viruses*, 2nd. ed., edited by R. Weiss et al., pp. 999–1108.
4. Brodeur, G. M., Seeger, R. C., Schwab, M., Varmus, H. E., and Bishop, J. M. (1984): Amplification of N-myc in untreated human neuroblastoma correlates with advanced disease stage. *Science*, 224:1121–1124.
5. Brown, M. S. (1983): Oncogenes: The wrong genes in the wrong place at the wrong time. Medical Grand Rounds, March 24, 1983.
6. Huebner, R. J., and Todero, G. J. (1969): Oncogenes of RNA tumor viruses as determinants of cancer. *Proc. Natl. Acad. Sci. USA*, 64:1087–1094.
7. Knudson, A. G. (1971): Mutation and cancer: Statistical study of retinoblastoma. *Proc. Natl. Acad. Sci. USA*, 68:820–823.
8. Lee, W. H., Murphree, A. L., and Benedict, W. F. (1984): Expression and amplification of the n-myc gene in primary retinoblastoma. *Nature*, 309:458–460.
9. Marx, J. L. (1984): Oncogene linked to cell regulatory system. *Science*, 226:527–528.
10. Murphree, A. L., and Benedict, W. F. (1984): Retinoblastoma: Clues to human oncogenesis. *Science*, 223:1028–1033.
11. Schwab, M., and Alitalo, K. (1983): Amplified DNA with limited homology to myc cellular oncogene is shared by human neuroblastoma cell lines and a neuroblastoma tumour. *Nature*, 305:245–250.
12. Schwab, M., Varmus, H. E., Bishop, J. M., Grzeschik, K.-H., Naylor, S. L., Sakaguchi, A. Y., Brodeur, G., and Trent, J. (1984): Chromosome localization in normal cells and neuroblastomas of a gene related to C-myc. *Nature*, 308:288–291.

13. Shiloh, Y., Shipley, J., Brodeur, G., Bruns, G., Korf, B., Donlon, T., Schreek, R., Seeger, R., Sakai, K., Latt, S. (1985): Differential ampliciation, assembly, and relocation of multiple DNA sequences in human neuroblastomas and neuroblastoma cell lines. *Proc. Natl. Acad. Sci. USA*, 82:3761–3765.
14. Sparkes, R. S., Murphree, A. L., Lingua, R. W., Sparkes, M. C., Field, L. L., Funderburk, S. J., and Benedict, W. F. (1983): Gene for hereditary retinoblastoma assigned to human chromosome 13 by linkage to esterase D. *Science*, 219:971–973.
15. Vogel, F. (1979): Genetics of retinoblastoma. *Hum. Genet.*, 52:1–54.
16. Weinberg, R. A. (1983): A molecular basis of cancer. *Sci. Am.*, 249(5):126–142.

6

Clinical Neurogenetics

The classic eponymic neurologic diseases discussed in this section produce characteristic pathologic changes in specific nuclei and fiber tracts in brain, spinal cord, and peripheral nerve. The disorders are usually progressive and symmetrical in their pathologic and clinical expression, and they often have a clear genetic basis of inheritance or suggestion of familial involvement. The disorders involve specific regions or systems of the nervous system, such as cerebellar nuclei and fiber tracts or the corticospinal or extrapyramidal motor systems, resulting in specific neurologic symptoms and signs referred to as system degenerations.

Gowers in 1902 referred to these inherited degenerative diseases as *abiotrophies* or inborn errors of metabolism. This term implies the occurrence of neurologic disease as a result of an impairment in the metabolic state of the brain, spinal cord, or peripheral nerve. Recently, as will be discussed, enzyme deficiencies, chromosomal breaks, specific immunologic defects, and slow latent viral-like infections of the brain have been identified as specific etiologic bases for some of these abiotrophies.

It is of great interest and importance that in most of the inherited degenerative disorders to be discussed the primary emphasis of disease involves the neuron, with changes produced in astrocytes and oligodendrocytes being presumably of a reactive and secondary nature. Intensive research is currently underway in many laboratories concerning most of the disorders mentioned here, and it is anticipated that, with a better understanding of the program of molecular genetic differentiation of the neuron, obtained by recombinant DNA techniques and by study of the altered gene products present or defects in the regulation of their synthesis in these various disorders, the mechanisms of the pathogenesis of these diseases will become clearer and specific therapy will become available.

We have witnessed in the past decade an exponential increase in our knowledge of the basic enzyme defects and metabolic consequences of many autosomal recessive disorders in the categories of the gangliosidoses, leukodystrophies, mucopoly-

Portions of this chapter are modified, expanded, and updated from chapters published previously by R. N. Rosenberg and J. W. Pettegrew in *Neurology, Vol. 5; Science and Practice of Clinical Medicine*, edited by J. Dietschy, Grune and Stratton, New York, and in *The Clinical Neurosciences, Vol. 1, Neurology*, edited by R. N. Rosenberg, Churchill-Livingstone, New York, with permission.

saccharidoses, glycogenoses, and heavy metal storage disorders. When these autosomal recessive diseases are used as models, it is hoped that the basic molecular defect in several autosomal dominant system degenerations discussed here, such as Huntington's disease, olivopontocerebellar atrophy, Joseph disease, myotonic dystrophy, tuberous sclerosis, and neurofibromatosis, will become clarified (64).

Progressive Dementias

ALZHEIMER'S DISEASE

This disorder was originally described in 1910 by Alois Alzheimer (7), and it refers to the occurrence of a presenile dementia with an associated diffuse atrophy and resultant reduction in mass and weight of the brain. The occurrence of the presenile dementia is insidious and progressive over many years, and it is usually not associated with other significant neurologic abnormalities. It is important to distinguish this disorder from a senile dementia that similarly produces an insidious and progressive impairment in intellectual functioning but in an older population. A convenient arbitrary division between a senile and a presenile dementia might be age 60 years, when the first symptom of impairment occurs. The presenile dementia of Alzheimer's type and senile dementia represent similar disorders both neuropathologically and clinically, with the Alzheimer form merely occurring earlier in age and progressing more rapidly.

Pathology

The characteristic gross appearance of the brain is a severe, symmetrical, and diffuse atrophy with associated flattening of gyri and widening of the sulci. The entire ventricular system is uniformly enlarged. The histologic findings in general are a diffuse loss of neurons in the cerebral and cerebellar cortices, the basal ganglia, the brainstem, and the spinal cord. In particular, there is prominent neuronal loss in the basal nucleus of Meynert (substantia innominata), the septal nuclei, and the diagonal band of Broca. These basal forebrain nuclei normally provide a cholinergic input into the cerebral cortex diffusely, and their loss is the basis for the significant reduction in acetylcholine throughout the cortex (108,635). Comparison of cell counts in the basal nucleus of Meynert by immunohistochemistry and choline acetylase enzyme activity suggests that enzyme loss is greater than loss of cholinergic cells *per se* (411). However, it is not simply a cholinergic disorder, as norepinephrine is reduced in the cerebral cortex due to impairment and loss of adrenergic neurons that project to the cortex from the locus ceruleus (601), and serotonin is reduced in cortex as well because of raphe neuronal loss. Cortical levels of somatostatin, γ-aminobutyric acid (GABA), and substance P are reduced, but cholecystokinin and vasoactive intestinal polypeptide are normal, as is the density of cholinergic receptors.

At the molecular level, compared with age-matched controls, total cellular RNA and polyadenylated RNA are significantly reduced in Alzheimer's disease cortex, which has numerous plaques and neurofibrillary tangles. These RNA changes were associated with an increase in ribonuclease activity caused by an abnormality in the ribonuclease inhibitor complex. The marked reduction in rates and levels of protein synthesis in Alzheimer's disease brain as described in translation systems *in vitro* with patient cortical messenger RNA (mRNA) may be related to high levels of ribonuclease, which severely reduce mRNA concentrations (517).

This neuronal loss is replaced by astrocytic gliosis without inflammatory cells. Several important additional features that characterize Alzheimer's disease include neurofibrillary tangles and senile plaques. The occurrence of Alzheimer neurofibrillary inclusions in nerve cells is demonstrated using the Golgi silver stain impregnation method. Dense tangles of material occur within the cytoplasm of neurons, often displacing the nucleus to the side. At the electron microscopic level, these tangles are in actuality twisted neurofilaments, also called paired helical filaments, showing the characteristic 240 Å diameter with a central canal. The structure of neurofilaments is composed of polymerized globular subunits, the subunits having molecular weights of 53,000 and 55,000 daltons. Recently Roberts et al. (487) reported that the tangle-bearing neurons were those that also contained somatostatin. This proliferation of neurofilaments resembles that seen in experimental aluminum poisoning in animal studies, but those in the human disease appear more twisted. It is of interest that there are several scholarly reports indicating significant elevations in brain aluminum content in the Alzheimer brain, but a precise relationship of the pathogenesis of disease to aluminum or other toxins is unclear. So-called senile plaques, which appear as deposits of granular amorphous material at the light microscopic level, look like nonspecific globules at the electron microscopic level.

Plaques represent transected terminal axons of degenerating neurons in the basal forebrain nuclei and become associated with amyloid, as shown by birefringence using polarized light and typical amyloid fibrils in electron micrographs. The strategic location of plaques is important to explain memory deficits in patients, as it appears their placement disconnects the hippocampus from other brain structures. Plaques are located in the subiculum of the hippocampal formation and in layers 2 and 4 of the entorhinal cortex and thus effectively disconnect the hippocampal formation from the association cerebral cortex, basal forebrain, thalamus, and hypothalamus (294). Biochemically, the senile plaque also contains immunoglobulin-like material.

The precise cause of nonfamilial Alzheimer's disease is not known. However, genetic factors may be involved, as there are several reports indicating familial Alzheimer's disease (185) and affected twins (102), and another set of identical twins with Alzheimer's disease has been described in a family with an autosomal dominant inheritance (321).

In 1983 Kuzuhara et al. (337) reported a Japanese family with a chronic progressive disease characterized by dementia, cerebellar dysfunction, and pyramidal and extrapyramidal abnormalities. Of note on neuropathologic examination were massive multiform plaques of Kuru type as well as multicentric senile (Alzheimer) types. There were no spongiform changes. These clinical and neuropathologic features were consistent, according to Kuzuhara et al., with autosomal dominant Gerstmann-Sträussler-Scheinker disease (GSS disease). It is of considerable importance, however, to point out that several cases of GSS disease have been reported that did have a spongiform encephalopathy, and Masters et al. have reported a slow, latent viral-like agent that was isolated from GSS disease brain. Thus at least some atypical inherited multisystem involvement forms of presenile dementia resembling Alzheimer's disease may be due to the Creutzfeldt-Jakob agent (377,378).

This infectious agent has been recently characterized as a proteinaceous infective particle or prion (53,473). Prion rod-like particles have been associated with amyloid ultrastructurally and even show green birefringence by polarization microscopy after staining with Congo red dye. Prusiner (473) concludes that amyloid plaques observed in transmissible degenerative neurologic diseases, such as GSS disease, might consist of prions.

Prusiner's data strongly suggest that for a protein to be infectious and transmissible, it must be able to replicate. They imply that a prion protein may be an inducer of the gene, allowing RNA polymerase II access to transcribe the gene into mRNA, which is translated to make more prion protein. Such a view is surely against current dogma of the stream of information flow from DNA to RNA to protein, or, with reverse transcriptase, from RNA to DNA to RNA to protein. Recently, the gene for the prion protein, PrP 27-30, was cloned from a scrapie infected hamster brain cDNA library. Using this probe, PrP-related mRNA was found at similar levels in normal and scrapie infected hamster brain and other normal tissue. No PrP-related nucleic acids were found in purified preparations of scrapie prions indicating that PrP 27-30 is not encoded by a nucleic acid carried within the infectious particles (441). This discussion, it must be emphasized, only applies to these unusual inherited forms of GSS disease in which Alzheimer-like presenile dementia is associated with a rare unique spinocerebellar-like degeneration inherited as an autosomal dominant (89). Routine Alzheimer's disease brain has been inoculated into many animal hosts, but no disease-like state clinically or pathologically has yet been produced in the host animals. These observations do not rule out a prion infectious agent as the cause of Alzheimer's disease, since the animal hosts selected may not be appropriate for expression of the prion or the incubation period may be well beyond the laboratory experiment time or even the life-span of the animal. To date there is no evidence that nonfamilial or familial Alzheimer's disease is caused by a transmissible, infectious agent.

Of considerable interest is the recent report of Weinreb (626) showing an altered fingerprint pattern in Alzheimer patients. If this preliminary finding can be reproduced by others, it would provide strong genetic evidence for the causation or predisposition for this disorder. Alzheimer patients are reported to have an increased frequency of ulnar loops on their fingertips and an associated decrease in the frequency of whorls and arches compared with age-matched controls. These same features have also been reported by Schaumann and Alter (524) to be increased in patients with Down's syndrome, offering another linkage between these two disorders that produce a similar neuropathology.

Recently Robison et al. (489) reported that DNA repair mechanisms are defective in Alzheimer patient fibroblasts grown in culture and exposed to methylmethane sulfonate. This observation, if confirmed, would suggest that a primary gene defect underlies Alzheimer's disease and is incorporated universally in all cells in genomic DNA.

According to Morrison's (411) recent review, there are no chromosome defects in the disease but there is circumstantial evidence of involvement of chromosome 21. Patients with Down's syndrome having trisomy 21 who live into the fourth decade of life have senile plaques and neurofibrillary tangle neuropathologic features like Alzheimer's disease. There is also an increased frequency of Down's syndrome in families with Alzheimer's disease. The region of chromosome 21 responsible for Down's phenotype is 21q22. One gene in that region is for superoxide dismutase, which is now being cloned and used as a DNA probe to find linkage between it and a postulated Alzheimer gene locus.

Clinical Manifestations

The disease is characterized by the progressive and insidious development of intellectual impairment, going on to a profound dementia over several years' time. The disease usually begins in the fifth or sixth decade of life and is usually sporadic in its occurrence in a family. Familial involvement is recorded in 25 to 40% of cases, and an autosomal dominant mode of inheritance in 10% of families has been documented. The patient is usually aware of problems in memory or judgment in the early stages of the disorder, and as it becomes more advanced, he loses insight and appreciation of his deficits. Marked swings in mood may occur, including difficulty in controlling manic behavior alternating with depression. Judgment, insight, introspection, and memory gradually become impaired, producing a total dementia with dissociation from the environment and virtual mutism after 10 years of disease. Appearing in the late stage of the disease, aphasic syndromes and, rarely, signs of extrapyramidal involvement, including bradykinesia and rigidity, may occur. Seizures and myoclonus may also occur.

The neurologic examination may indicate, in addition to the dementia, the presence of primitive reflexes, including the snout reflex, the palmomental reflex, and symmetrical mild hyperreflexia. The cerebrospinal fluid (CSF) and routine blood chemistry studies are negative. The electroencephalogram (EEG) during the advanced stages of the disease shows diffuse and symmetrical slowing. A computerized axial tomographic (CT) brain scan shows both ventricular enlargement and gyral atrophy, with increased sulcal markings. This diffuse atrophy can be confirmed by pneumoencephalography showing both ventricular enlargement and cortical atrophy.

Terminally the patient appears dissociated, demented, mute, and decorticate. Death is usually from pulmonary or urinary tract infection. Unfortunately, no specific treatment is available. Oral treatment of patients with lecithin, choline, or physostigmine has not been useful. A preliminary report of intrathecal or intraventricular infusion of bethanechol, a cholimimetic, suggested some mental improvement.

Diagnosis

Alzheimer's disease is diagnosed in the young to middle-aged adult who shows progressive signs of intellectual deterioration without significant associated neurologic signs or symptoms. The neurologic examination is normal except for the emergence late in the course of primitive reflexes. Diffuse cerebral atrophy is confirmed by a CT scan and pneumoencephalogram. The CSF is unremarkable.

Differential Diagnosis

Alzheimer's disease must be differentiated from other disorders that similarly produce progressive intellectual deterioration. The presence of a space-occupying mass lesion in the frontal lobe, such as a chronic subdural hematoma, metastatic tumor, primary astrocytoma, or brain abscess, must be considered. In general, mass lesions in the frontal lobe of the types mentioned often produce dementia and associated focal neurologic signs, including deficits of the corticospinal pathway producing asymmetrical hyperreflexia, clonus, Babinski's sign, and sometimes evidence of increased intracranial pressure. There may be an early loss of social graces and amenities with an early disheveled appearance and urinary bladder incontinence in the patient with a frontal lobe mass lesion, unlike the patient with Alzheimer's disease, who presents a neater and cleaner manner and retains most social graces. Other entities to be considered are low-pressure hydrocephalus or exogenous intoxications such as bromides, drugs, and heavy metals. Hypothyroidism, myxedema, vitamin B_{12} deficiency with associated subacute combined degeneration, and neurosyphilis must be considered.

PICK'S DISEASE

Pick's disease refers to a circumscribed brain atrophy with predilection for the frontal and temporal lobes. It spares the more posteriorly located structures. In 1984 Morris et al. (409) described an autosomal dominant disorder that could be considered as part of a Pick-Alzheimer spectrum of cortical neuronal degenerations. They referred to their class of disorders as hereditary dysphasic dementia and the Pick-Alzheimer spectrum. Clinical manifestations include in late adulthood the occurrence of progressive dementia and severe dysphasia. Neuropathologic examination shows typical Pick's disease or asymmetrical focal cerebral atrophy, Alzheimer's disease with typical plaques, and neuronal loss in the substantia nigra indicative of Parkinson's disease. The disorder needs to be included in the spectrum of the inherited dementias, and the precise classification will require further cases to be studied.

Pathology

The neuropathologic changes are clear from examination of the gross brain, which shows prominent atrophy involving the frontal and temporal lobes, with preservation of the posterior regions of the brain. The frontal and temporal horns of the lateral ventricles are similarly focally enlarged. The hippocampal formation in the medial ventral portion of the temporal lobes is preserved, but there may be atrophic changes in basal ganglia, thalamus, and brainstem. Neurons contain a large amorphous cytoplasmic basophilic structure referred to as a "Pick body."

Clinical Manifestations

It is difficult to differentiate Alzheimer's disease from Pick's disease by neurologic examination. Alzheimer and Pick patients both show a dementia, but the Pick patient usually has a better preservation of memory and insight into his defective thinking problem early in the disorder. The neurologic examination is otherwise unremarkable.

FAMILIAL AMYOTROPHIC LATERAL SCLEROSIS, PARKINSONISM, AND DEMENTIA

Families have been described in which there occur progressive dementia, parkinsonism, and amyotrophic lateral sclerosis inherited in an autosomal recessive manner. Neuropathologic examination has found Alzheimer-type neurofibrillary tangles in the substantia nigra, innominata, locus ceruleus, parahippocampal gyrus, and also in the hippocampus and cerebral cortex. Complex forms of dementia including these other neurologic features have been reported in natives of Guam, the Kii Peninsula of Japan, New Guinea, and Europe (533).

Treatment

There is no effective therapy available for Alzheimer patients. Most important is to be sure that the diagnosis is correct and that a treatable condition resembling Alzheimer's disease is not present such as metabolic encephalopathy, benign or malignant brain tumor, chronic meningitis, cerebral vasculitis, or depression. Recently Harbaugh et al. (257) have reported that a few patients with Alzheimer's disease have been treated by bethanechol administered into the CSF by an intracranial catheter. The preliminary results of this cholimimetic form of therapy were encouraging and they plan additional studies.

Basal Ganglia Diseases

HUNTINGTON'S DISEASE

In 1872 George Huntington, a physician living on Long Island in New York, noted a family that expressed a disorder that included progressive dementia and

Clinical Neurogenetics 101

chorea. Much has been learned about this disorder in the past 113 years, but the precise molecular defect remains unknown, although a DNA polymorphism associated with the disease has now been described and the mutant gene has been mapped to chromosome 4 (244). It is characterized by an autosomal dominant mode of inheritance with almost uniform clinical expression.

Pathology

Examination of the gross brain demonstrates a symmetrical and severe atrophy involving predominantly the frontal and temporal lobes. The atrophy is symmetrical and extends into the parietal and occipital lobes as well. The lateral ventricles are uniformly enlarged, with an emphasis in the frontal horns. The caudate nucleus is severely atrophied and in fact may be concave where it projects to the surface of the lateral ventricle. Histologically there is diffuse neuronal loss in the cerebral cortex, basal ganglia, thalamus, inferior olives, and anterior horn motor neurons of the spinal cord.

A significant reduction in the activity of the enzyme glutamic acid decarboxylase (GAD) and its reaction product (GABA), an important neurotransmitter, has been reported in the neostriatum of Huntington's disease brain as compared with control brain. Further, there was a 50% reduction in the activity of the acetylcholine-synthesizing enzyme choline acetylase (CAT) in the frontal lobe and neostriatum in some Huntington brains. The concentration of dopamine, however, was normal in these regions, although the dopamine to GABA ratio was increased. The binding affinities of the serotonergic and muscarinic cholinergic receptors were also defective in the neostriatum in the Huntington brain when quantitative binding measurements with analogs were carried out (174). Patients also had low basal and impaired prolactin responses to both chlorpromazine and thyrotropin-releasing hormone (TRH). These findings are compatible with enhanced hypothalamic dopaminergic activity in this disease. Neurotensin, somatostatin, and TRH were significantly elevated in concentration in the caudate nucleus in patients compared with control brain (428). Substance P, enkephalin, and cholecystokinin were reduced in concentration in patient brain (374). These changes are probably the result of the primary gene defect and not causal of disease. It is clear that the neurons in the frontal lobe and in the corpus striatum are most vulnerable to this dominant gene mutation and its altered gene product with resultant neuronal demise. The biochemical findings of a reduced GAD activity, CAT activity, reduced GABA levels, and an increased dopamine to GABA ratio are probably biochemical markers of the morphologic changes. Use of nonneural tissue such as erythrocytes, fibroblasts, and lymphocytes and applications of ^{31}P nuclear magnetic resonance, electron spin resonance, and membrane fluorescent probes to find a molecular defect have not been of diagnostic value. Growth characteristics of patient fibroblasts in culture are also normal, despite earlier claims to the contrary (97).

Clinical Manifestations

The clinical manifestations are those of progressive dementia, including impaired judgment and insight, bizarre behavior, and a personality change that is also present in other affected family members with an autosomal dominant mode of expression. Associated with the mental changes are involuntary choreiform movements described as quick, random, jerking movements. At times there may be more rhythmic, twisting, and slow movements that are characteristic of athetosis. If the disorder occurs in childhood, it may present with progressive rigidity, and especially so if it is the paternal gene that expresses the disease. As mentioned, the disorder begins in the fourth, fifth, or sixth decades of life and runs a progressive and relentless course of dementia and chorea. Late in the course the occurrence of corticospinal deficits, including hyperreflexia, clonus, Babinski's sign, and decortication may result. The children of affected women have significantly older mean ages of onset than offspring of affected men. The absence of increased father-daughter similarity indicates that modification is not X-linked (422).

Differential Diagnosis

Huntington's disease is easily diagnosed when a family history of an autosomal dominant disorder producing dementia and chorea can be obtained. Other entities that must be considered in the absence of a clear family history of Huntington's disease would include Alzheimer's disease in its late stage, in which extrapyramidal signs have occurred. The symptoms of patients who may have chorea because of prolonged or excessive phenothiazine administration, perhaps for a primary psychiatric disorder, may be difficult to differentiate from those of patients with Huntington's disease, in which there are similar psychiatric symptoms and chorea. Wilson's disease, with associated personality change and choreoathetosis, can be easily identified by the determination of a Kayser-Fleischer ring, low serum ceruloplasmin, increased hepatic levels of copper, and elevated 24-hr urinary excretion of copper.

A dramatic advance was achieved recently by Gusella et al. (244), who found a DNA polymorphism associated with the disease. It was achieved by testing their eighth unique sequence cDNA probe with the restriction endonuclease Hind III on genomic DNA obtained from large informative kindreds from Indiana and Venezuela. A specific genetic haplotype cosegregated with the presence of disease in these two families and offers a means to identify the presence of disease in at risk persons. It is a precise and powerful approach and one that offers the means to eliminate this disorder in families who utilize it along with careful genetic counseling (244). Careful screening of additional families is now underway to see if all families can be ascribed to the same polymorphism or if other allelic or nonallelic forms of the disease exist. The probe used would not be useful if nonallelic forms exist and great care must be taken to avoid false negative determinations. By somatic cell hybrid studies and *in situ* hybridization, Gusella has been able to map the Huntington's disease gene to the subterminus of the short arm of chromosome 4 (243,244). Of considerable interest is the recent report of Folstein et al. (195a) who found linkage of the HD locus to the G8 probe, provided by Gusella, in two families with differing clinical features.

Treatment

There is no specific treatment to stop the progression of the disease process, but the use of haloperidol (1–5 mg three or four times daily) or chlorpromazine (20–100 mg two or three times daily) may be very effective in reducing the involuntary movement and calming the patient. Perry et al. (458) reported several patients in whom choreoathetosis resolved after treatment with INH (isonicotinic acid hydrazide).

WILSON'S DISEASE (HEPATOLENTICULAR DEGENERATION)

Von Frericks in 1861 probably described the first case of Wilson's disease when he reported on a young boy who had severe liver disease, violent tremors and convulsions, and, at autopsy, cirrhosis of the liver (38). Kayser in 1902 (316) described a greenish ring at the limbus of the cornea in a patient who was diagnosed as having multiple sclerosis. In 1903 Fleischer (193) reported the corneal ring as an integral part of a neurologic disease associated with cirrhosis of the liver. In a series of papers between 1903 and 1912, Fleischer proposed that the changes in the eye, brain, and liver were all caused by a common metabolic factor. Wilson in 1912 (640) published his monograph "Progressive Lenticular Degeneration: A Familial Nervous Disease Associated with Cirrhosis of the Liver." Rumpel in 1913 (514) was the first to demonstrate the increased copper and silver content in a patient with "pseudosclerosis," and in 1922 Siemerling and Oloff (556) suggested that the pseudosclerosis of Westphal-Strumpell was caused by copper deposition in liver, eyes, and brain. Glazebrook in 1945 (221) firmly established the role of copper in the pathogenesis of Wilson's disease. Cummings in 1948 (112) first recommended the use of the copper chelating agent dimercaprol (BAL) to remove excess copper from tissues. In 1952 Scheinberg and Gitlen (530) and Bearn and Kunkel (39) independently reported a deficiency of circulating ceruloplasmin in Wilson's disease. Penicillamine was discovered by Walshe in 1956 (624), and in 1968 Sternlieb and Scheinberg (579) suggested that presymptomatic diagnosis was possible leading to early therapy to prevent organ damage (see ref. 38).

Genetics

This is an autosomal recessively inherited disorder. It has been linked to the esterase D locus on chromosome 13 (204).

Clinical Features

Wilson's disease presents with the triad of neurologic deterioration (movement disorder and psychiatric symptoms), cirrhosis of the liver, and Kayser-Fleischer rings of the cornea. The age of onset is variable, most patients exhibiting signs and symptoms in adolescence or early in adulthood. The onset may be as early as 4 years or as late as the fifth decade. It has an incidence of 1 in 10,000 and is inherited as an autosomal recessive disorder.

There are two neurologic forms of the disease, with clinical intermediates. In one form the major manifestations are spasticity, rigidity, dysarthria, and dysphagia with drooling of saliva. This form occurs predominantly in young adults. The other neurologic form has flapping tremors of the wrists and shoulders as the major feature, with rigidity and spasticity much less marked. This form occurs at any age in either sex.

Psychiatric manifestations are common but variable in type and degree. Behavioral changes include aggressiveness, childishness, and euphoria. In spite of these changes, the intellect remains quite intact. Patients may present with frank schizophrenia.

The earliest sign of liver involvement is an enlarged, firm liver with splenomegaly. The earliest abnormality of liver function is increased serum transaminase (580). It has recently been documented that the earlier the onset of the disease, the more likely it is that the presentation consists of hepatic disease alone. The neurologic symptoms may develop at any time, and sometimes they are misinterpreted as portal-systemic encephalopathy.

Kayser-Fleischer rings are still considered the single most diagnostic sign of the disease. They are golden-brown or greenish rings at the margin of the cornea near the limbus. Sometimes the rings can be detected with the unaided eye, but usually a slit-lamp examination is required. Slit-lamp examination reveals granules deposited on the inner surface of the cornea in Descemet's membrane. The rings are always bilateral, and because of the vertical flow of the aqueous fluid in the anterior chamber, the deposition may be more marked superiorly and inferiorly. Kayser-Fleischer rings are rarely seen in a child under the age of 7 years and are invariably present in patients with overt neurologic disease. They fade and eventually disappear with penicillamine therapy.

Clinical laboratory evidence of diffuse renal involvement is frequently present. This may consist of hematuria, proteinuria, glycosuria, aminoaciduria, hyperphosphaturia, reduced concentrating ability, or reduced acidification of the urine. Penicillamine therapy reverses these findings. Before starting penicillamine therapy, however, the renal status should be characterized, as penicillamine can have renal toxicity.

A low blood ceruloplasmin is one of the most constant biochemical findings in Wilson's disease, although the degree of depression is variable and some patients with normal values have been reported. Evidence has been presented that there is a reduced rate of hepatic synthesis of ceruloplasmin and that the deficit is not in synthesis of the apoenzyme but in the incorporation of copper into newly synthesized ceruloplasmin.

The non-ceruloplasmin-bound serum copper is elevated in Wilson's disease, but the total serum copper concentration is lower than normal. The elevated non-ceruloplasmin-bound copper is thought to give rise to increased urinary excretion of copper.

The diagnosis of Wilson's disease can be accurately made on clinical findings. Confirmatory laboratory findings include lowered serum ceruloplasmin levels, lowered total serum copper, elevated urinary copper excretion, and elevated liver copper content by needle per cutaneous biopsy.

Families that include a patient with Wilson's disease should be screened for ceruloplasmin levels in order to identify asymptomatic patients. The identification of asymptomatic patients is very important so that therapy can be started to prevent organ damage.

Pathology

The liver is the earliest site of copper deposition. Early in the disease the copper deposition is diffusely distributed in the hepatocyte cytoplasm. The copper deposition precedes the cirrhosis.

Copper is widely distributed in the brains of patients, but the basal ganglia are the most severely affected. The excess copper is nonspecifically associated with a number of proteins. The copper deposition appears to be more in glial cells than in neurons.

Therapy

Untreated Wilson's disease is invariably fatal. Treatment is aimed at restricting dietary copper and chelating the excess copper from tissues (454).

Dietary copper is reduced to 1.0 to 1.5 mg/day by the avoidance of foods with high copper content, such as liver, nuts, cocoa, mushrooms, shellfish, and chocolate.

The recommended dose of penicillamine is 1 g/day in two divided doses for children over 10 years and adults and 0.5 to 0.75 g/day for children under 10 years. The clinical improvement with penicillamine therapy is slow, and during the first 6 to 8 weeks the clinical condition may worsen. With early diagnosis and treatment, the development of the disease can be prevented. Patients with early organ involvement can usually be restored to a normal state with therapy.

PARKINSON'S SYNDROME

Parkinson's syndrome is usually thought of as a sporadic disorder, but familial clustering of components of parkinsonism has been reported. It has been estimated that parkinsonism occurs as a familial disorder in 5 to 15% of patients. An autosomal dominant form of disease has been reported in some of these families (375,574). Rarely, familial parkinsonism has been reported as an autosomal recessive or X-linked recessive disorder. Martin et al. (375) reported a multifactorial polygenic model of inheritance for familial parkinsonism and suggested a genetic defect in tyrosine hydroxylase, the rate-limiting enzyme in the pathway for dopamine synthesis. The risk for an individual to develop familial parkinsonism increases with the number of affected individuals in the at risk person's family. The occurrence of dementia may be part of the parkinson syndrome, and in these families an increased risk of developing parkinsonism will occur when the onset of the illness occurs earlier in life (273).

HALLERVORDEN-SPATZ DISEASE

Clinical Findings

Hallervorden-Spatz disease (HSD) includes the development of childhood rigidity and hypertonia resembling parkinsonism associated with dysarthria and dysphagia. Late in the course of disease, dementia and corticospinal degeneration with spasticity and decerebrate posturing occur. Pigmentary retinal degeneration, optic atrophy, and visual loss also occur.

Pathology

There is a pigmentary degeneration of the pallidum and nigra due to the excessive deposition of iron. Neuronal loss and demyelination in these regions also occur, associated with axonal swellings referred to as spheroid bodies.

Genetics

The disease is inherited as an autosomal recessive disorder (141,636). In 1985 Jankovic et al. (302) described a family with autosomal recessive HSD disease in which four of five siblings developed the syndrome presenting as familial parkinsonism. This family presented with late onset disease, with the propositus dying at 68 years after 13 years of dementia and parkinson features rather than a dyskinesia. The disorder thus does not have to present in young adulthood. The cause of the disorder is not known.

NEUROAXONAL DYSTROPHY OF SEITELBERGER

This syndrome overlaps with HSD and some consider them as variants of a common disorder. In general this disorder occurs earlier in life and is more aggressive than HSD. Early dementia with extrapyramidal type of rigidity and dystonia are typical features. The main difference from HSD is the paucity of pigment accumulation. Axonal spheroid bodies and demyelination occur throughout the brain (not limited to the basal ganglia as in HSD) and peripheral nervous system. It is inherited as an autosomal recessive disorder. The cause of the disease is not known (107).

GILLES DE LA TOURETTE SYNDROME

Clinical Findings

This syndrome is characterized by the onset in childhood of motor tics of the face, head, and extremities that resemble blinking, facial grimacing, and other muscle twitching. These tics are accompanied by vocal grunting, clearing of the throat, and even spitting movements. Uncontrolled vocal expletives without cause are a cardinal feature of the syndrome but not necessary for the diagnosis. Other findings include sleep problems, echolalia, tremor, and depression. Stress exacerbates the syndrome (99).

Genetics

The syndrome is probably inherited as an autosomal dominant disorder with variable penetrance, but the precise type of inheritance is not clear (85).

Pathogenesis

The cause of the syndrome and its precise pathogenesis are not known. A beneficial response to dopamine receptor blockers such as haloperidol strongly suggests that a hypersensitivity state of the dopamine system may be of primary concern in this syndrome (161).

Therapy

Clonidine was helpful in reducing motor and phonic tics (346). Haloperidol has been used for many years and has been found to be effective in reducing tics and abnormal behaviors.

FAMILIAL CHOREOATHETOSIS

A variety of familial syndromes involving progressive choreoathetosis inherited as autosomal dominant traits have been described. They are all essentially benign disorders with late childhood onset of the involuntary movement disorder and with preservation of intellect. Distinctions have been made within this group according to whether the syndrome is associated with (a) progressive or nonprogressive choreoathetosis, (b) involuntary movement induced with a voluntary act, (c) dystonia, (d) acanthocytosis, or (e) the presence of basal ganglia calcifications. Familial Syndenham's chorea associated with acute rheumatic fever must be included in this spectrum as a familial entity that requires antibiotic therapy for streptococcal disease. Syndenham's chorea can be the sole manifestation of an acute rheumatic fever attack, and it may appear in a familial setting (426).

BENIGN ESSENTIAL TREMOR

The occurrence of tremor without other neurologic deficits has been reported as an autosomal dominant disorder. There is wide variation in the age of onset in a family and in the degree of severity of the tremor (109). The tremor may be focal, involving only the head as a head-nod, the arms and hands, the legs, or the muscles of speech and swallowing, or it may become generalized, involving the trunk and impairing walking.

TORSION DYSTONIC SYNDROMES

This group of disorders is characterized by slow involuntary twisting movements due to forceful muscle contractions. The resultant dystonic postures are the cardinal feature of the torsion dystonia. These dystonic postures or muscle spasms may be local, as in writer's cramp, or may involve the neck muscles to produce torticollis on the pelvis and hence tortipelvis. Oromandibular dystonia (Meige's syndrome), in which spasms of jaw muscles, tongue protrusion, and blinking occur, may also be a familial disorder. The distribution may be generalized and is known then as dystonia musculorum deformans (DMD). An autosomal recessive form of DMD is found among Ashkenazic Jews, and an autosomal dominant is also reported (158). Paroxysmal dystonic choreoathetosis or the Mount-Reback syndrome may be an epileptiform discharge from the basal ganglia resulting in severe muscle spasms and may be inherited as an autosomal dominant disorder (281).

DYSTONIA MUSCULORUM DEFORMANS

This disorder is inherited as an autosomal dominant trait with marked variation in clinical expression. Four generations of a family of 121 persons of whom 16 were affected as autosomal dominants have been reported. It has been described as concordant in twins as an autosomal recessive, with onset in the twins being years apart (156). Clinical manifestations include dystonia of cervical musculature (torticollis) and dystonia of the trunk (tortipelvis). The disorder may be severe, producing marked deformity of the neck, extremities, and trunk (309). Minor changes, including neuronal loss and reactive gliosis, have been described, involving the striatum, globus pallidus, and dentate nucleus of the cerebellum. Larsen et al. (342) have described a family with dominantly inherited dystonia and intracranial calcifications in the basal ganglia, dentate nucleus of the cerebellum, and frontal lobes.

Differential Diagnosis

This disorder must be separated from HSD disease, which is an autosomal recessive genetic disorder beginning in the first decade of life and producing progressive dystonia and athetosis. The basal ganglia, which are pigmented by a brownish pigment, especially in the globus pallidus, contain iron. HSD thus is a heavy metal storage disease because of iron deposition, and it can resemble dystonia musculorum deformans (657). Fahr's disease is a disorder involving abnormal deposition of calcium within the basal ganglia; it produces dystonia, athetosis, and tremors. It is most likely inherited as an autosomal recessive trait. Finally, Parkinson's disease, with rigidity and tremor at rest, has been reported to occur in several families (375,474,574). Recently Romanul et al. (493) reported a family of Portuguese ancestry with autosomal dominant Parkinson's disease in association with cerebellar findings and peripheral neuropathy.

Spinocerebellar Degenerations

The spinocerebellar degenerations represent a series of clinical deficits including ataxia and dysmetria resulting from the predominant involvement of the cerebellum and its afferent and efferent pathways. These disorders are system degenerations, and many of them are specific entities clearly inherited as genetic disease or as familial entities in an autosomal dominant or autosomal recessive manner. Although the clinical manifestations and neuropathologic findings of cerebellar disease are the most predominant in the spinocerebellar degeneration, there may also develop characteristic changes in the basal ganglia, optic atrophy, retinitis pigmentosa, and peripheral nerve disease (554). There are many gradations in the spectrum from pure cerebellar involvement to mixed cerebellar and brainstem involvement, cerebellar and basal ganglia involvement, or spinal syndromes including associated peripheral nerve disease. The clinical picture may be rather consistent in one family, but examples occur in which the disease assumes a characteristic form in the majority of family members and is entirely different in one or several members.

The typical clinical picture and the age of onset of symptoms and signs are used to classify these inherited spinocerebellar diseases. Major categories of disease are included in this designation, but it should be pointed out that these divisions are arbitrary and that gradations between the various entities are encountered. The important and common inherited spinocerebellar degenerations include (a) Friedreich's syndrome, the spinal form of spinocerebellar degeneration, (b) Roussy-Levy syndrome, (c) Refsum's syndrome, (d) Bassen-Kornzweig syndrome, (e) olivopontocerebellar degeneration, (f) Joseph disease, (g) dyssynergia cerebellaris myoclonica, (h) ataxia telangiectasia, (i) Marinesco-Sjögren syndrome, (j) hereditary spastic paraplegia, and (k) Charcot-Marie-Tooth disease (Table 1).

These entities, as classified by Greenfield (232), can be grouped into predominantly spinal forms, spinocerebellar forms, and pure cerebellar forms. The olivopontocerebellar degenerations (OPCD) were subclassified by Konigsmark and Weiner (327) into at least five subgroups with both autosomal dominant and autosomal recessive forms of inheritance. The many minor variants of OPCD described, for example, by Brown in 1892 (76), Marie in 1893 (371), Dejerine and Thomas in 1900 (125), Holmes in 1907 (279), and Schut in 1950 (538), as listed by Konigsmark and Weiner (327), might represent examples of genetic disease in which all the phenotypic variability could theoretically be explained by a single gene mutation transmitted as an autosomal recessive trait and another single gene mutation transmitted as an autosomal dominant trait in which many other host genes modify expression and penetrance of the mutant gene.

Insights into the molecular causes of these diseases are beginning to be described in some of the spinocerebellar diseases, including Friedreich's syndrome, Refsum's disease, and Bassen-Kornzweig syndrome (Table 2). In the remaining spinocerebellar degenerations, although the disorders are well described both clinically and pathologically, the specific cause of disease remains elusive. The spinocerebellar

TABLE 1. *Summary of the spinocerebellar degenerations*

Type	Age of onset	Development	Reflexes	Sensory change	Cerebellar	Other important features
Spinal syndromes Friedreich's syndrome	1st decade	Slowly progressive	Absent myotatic deep tendon reflexes; extensor plantar response	Moderate loss	Severe	Dysarthria; nystagmus; moderate mental retardation; skeletal defects; defect in pyruvate dehydrogenase; defect in mitochondrial malic enzyme; autosomal dominant or recessive or sporadic; cardiomegaly with fibrosis
Hereditary spastic paraplegia	1st or 2nd decade	Slowly progressive	Hyperreflexia; clonus; extensor plantar response	Minimal loss	None	Paraplegia; impaired bowel and bladder function; autosomal dominant or recessive or may occur in families with typical Friedreich's syndrome or olivopontocerebellar degeneration
Roussy-Levy syndrome (included in types I and II hereditary motor sensory neuropathy of Dyck)	1st or 2nd decade	Slowly progressive	Absent myotatic deep tendon reflexes; extensor plantar response	Moderate loss	Moderate	Absence of dysarthria with peroneal muscular atrophy; intermediate between Friedreich's and Charcot-Marie-Tooth diseases
Polyneuropathy (Charcot-Marie-Tooth disease (types I and II hereditary motor sensory neuropathy of Dyck)	1st or 2nd decade	Slowly progressive	Absent	Moderate loss	None	Predominant peroneal muscle atrophy; nerves may be hypertrophic; usually autosomal dominant; can be autosomal recessive or X-linked; optic-acoustic nerve involvement occurs
Dejerine-Sottas (type III hereditary motor sensory neuropathy of Dyck)	1st or 2nd decade	Slowly progressive	Absent	Moderate loss	None	Tremor; nystagmus; dysarthria; scoliosis; hypertrophic nerves; usually sporadic or autosomal recessive; elevated CSF protein

Disease	Age of onset	Course	Reflexes	Sensation	Ataxia	Features
Ataxia telangiectasia	1st or 2nd decade	Slowly progressive	Reduced	Minimal loss	Severe	Telangiectatic lesions involving sclerae, face, pinna, and neck; pulmonary infections; increased incidence of lymphoma; hypo-γ-IgA; autosomal recessive
Bassen-Kornzweig syndrome	1st decade	Slowly progressive	Absent	Moderate loss	Severe	May have mental retardation; acanthocytosis; steatorrhea; pigmentary retinal degeneration; a-β-lipoproteinemia; autosomal recessive
Tangier disease	1st decade	Slowly progressive	Reduced	Moderate loss	None	Enlarged yellowish-appearing tonsils; defect in high density lipoproteins; autosomal recessive
Refsum's disease	1st decade	Slowly progressive	Absent	Severe loss	Severe	Nyctalopia; pigmentary retinal degeneration; ichthyosis; cardiac conduction defects; deafness; elevated serum phytanate; defect in lipid α-oxidase activity; autosomal recessive
Cerebellar syndrome, olivoponto-cerebellar degeneration	1st or 2nd decade	Slowly progressive	Hyperreflexia; clonus; extensor plantar response	Moderate loss	Severe	Late development of optic atrophy and muscle atrophy; may develop a moderate dementia; seizures are rare; may be autosomal dominant or recessive; contrast studies including CT scan show pontine and cerebellar atrophy
Carcinomatosis cerebellar degeneration	Adult	Less than 10 progressive	Reduced	Moderate loss	Truncal	Truncal greater than extremity ataxia; dysarthria and nystagmus minimal; lung carcinoma most common association
Alcoholic cerebellar degeneration	Adult	Slowly progressive	Reduced	Moderate loss	Truncal severe	Truncal greater than extremity ataxia; dysarthria and nystagmus minimal; peripheral neuropathy present
Dyssynergia cerebellaris of Ramsay Hunt	Adult	Slowly progressive	Reduced	Normal	Moderate	Diffuse myoclonic jerks; generalized seizures; sporadic or recessive; mitochondrial defects
Marinesco-Sjögren syndrome	1st decade	Slowly progressive	Reduced	Normal	Moderate truncal	Associated with mental retardation and cataracts in early childhood

TABLE 2. *Biochemical disorders in the inherited ataxias*

Biochemical disorder	Clinical type	Age of onset	Clinical features
Lipid disorders (see Fig. 27 for review of biochemical pathways)			
Autosomal recessive			
Storage of phytanate due to defect in α-oxidase	Refsum's disease	20–30 yr	Ataxia; retinitis pigmentosa; deafness; ichthyosis; cardiac arrhythmia; polyneuropathy
a-β-Lipoproteinemia	Bassen-Kornzweig syndrome	5–10 yr	Ataxia; acanthocytosis; retinitis pigmentosa; polyneuropathy; malabsorption of fat
Arylsulfatase A deficiency	Juvenile onset metachromatic leukodystrophy	5–20 yr	Ataxia; mild mental retardation; polyneuropathy
Storage of GM₂ ganglioside due to hexosaminidase A deficiency, α-locus type	Juvenile onset atypical spinocerebellar ataxia	3 yr	Progressive ataxia; spasticity; dysarthria; muscle atrophy; pes cavus; normal intelligence
Storage of GM₂ ganglioside due to hexosaminidase A deficiency, β-locus type	Juvenile onset atypical ataxia with cherry-red spots	2 yr	Progressive ataxia and intention tremor; macular cherry-red spots
Partial deficiency of hexosaminidase A and B	Adult onset spinocerebellar degeneration	20 yr	Gait and limb ataxia; head titubation; dysarthria; tremor grimacing; chorea
Galactosylceramide lipidosis	Late infantile to adult progressive cerebellar deficits	Late infantile	Multiple periventricular hypodense lesions suggestive of leukodystrophy; sural nerve shows demyelination; reduced leukocyte galactocerebrosidase activity (597)
X-Linked recessive			
Storage of long-chain (C24–30) fatty acids	Adrenoleukomyeloneuropathy (Nixon-Blaw disease)	5–20 yr	Cortical blindness and spasticity; skin pigmentation; childhood onset of adrenal cortical insufficiency; adult onset with ataxia and polyneuropathy

Carbohydrate disorders (see Fig. 25 for review of biochemical pathways)

Autosomal recessive

Pyruvate carboxylase or pyruvate dehydrogenase deficiencies (inhibitor of thiamine triphosphate formation in brain; inhibitor of thiamine pyrophosphate-ATP phosphotransferase)	Leigh's disease (subacute necrotizing encephalopathy)	birth–5 yr	Acute episodic extraocular muscle palsies; optic atrophy; hypotonia; ataxia; mental retardation; somnolence; hyperreflexia; extensor plantar responses; elevated serum pyruvate and lactate
Biotin-responsive multiple carboxylase deficiency	Neonatal or infantile intermittent ataxia	birth–1 yr	Intermittent ataxia responsive to biotin; ketosis; lactic acidosis; infections; hyperammonemia; hypotonia
Lipoamide dehydrogenase deficiency; mitochondrial malic enzyme	Friedreich's ataxia	5–15 yr	Progressive gait and limb ataxia; dysarthria; nystagmus; areflexia; extensor plantar reflex; distal sensory loss
Oxidative metabolism with elevated serum lactate and pyruvate	Adult onset neuromyopathy with ataxia, Kearns-Sayre syndrome	20–50 yr	Retinitis pigmentosa; neuromyopathy; ophthalmoplegia; ataxia; cardiac arrhythmias; muscle biopsy shows ragged red fibers

Disorders of amino acid metabolism

Autosomal recessive

Deficiency in branched-chain keto acid decarboxylase	Maple syrup urine disease and variants	birth-5 yr	Mental retardation; seizures; failure to thrive; irritability; anorexia; ataxia; maple syrup odor to urine; excretion of branched-chain amino acids and keto acids
Hyperglycinemia	Spastic paraparesis with muscular atrophy and arm dysmetria	2–10 yr	Spastic paraparesis; peroneal muscle atrophy; distal sensory loss; pes cavus; optic atrophy; arm dysmetria
5-Oxoprolinuria due to deficiency of glutathione synthetase	Ataxia and defect in the γ-glutamyl cycle (I) (reduced glutathione synthesis)	10 yr	Progressive mental retardation; spasticity; limb and gait ataxia; tremor; hemolytic anemia with intermittent jaundice
Generalized amino aciduria due to deficiency of γ-glutamylcysteine synthetase	Ataxia and defect in the γ-glutamyl cycle (II) (reduced glutathione synthesis)	20 yr	Hemolytic anemia; areflexia; gait and limb ataxia; distal sensory loss; staccato speech; acute psychosis

(Table continues on next page)

TABLE 2. (continued)

Biochemical disorder	Clinical type	Age of onset	Clinical features
Defect in tryptophan absorption from gut; aminoaciduria	Hartnup disease	5–25 yr	Intermittent ataxia; episodic pellagra-like skin rash; progressive mental retardation; spasticity; choreoathetosis
Deficiency in glutamate dehydrogenase	Olivopontocerebellar degeneration	20–40 yr	Progressive gait and limb ataxia; spasticity; mild extrapyramidal features; late distal amyotrophy and sensory loss; rare mental changes
Disorder or urea cycle metabolism			
Autosomal recessive (see Fig. 24 for review of urea cycle pathway)			
Argininosuccinate synthetase deficiency	Citrullinemia	Infancy	Vomiting; somnolence; tremor; ataxia; seizures; delay in mental and physical development; hyperammonemia
Disorder of immunologic function			
Autosomal recessive			
Reduced serum immunoglobulins (IgA, IgG, and IgM); lymphopenia	Ataxia telangiectasia (Louis-Barr syndrome)	5–12 yr	Telangiectasia of face and sclerae; Friedreich's phenotype with ataxia; dysarthria; areflexia; extensor plantar responses; oculomotor apraxia
Disorder of protein metabolism (Increased amount of glial proteins)			
Autosomal dominant			
Increased glial acidic filamentous protein and a complex of 40,000 MW proteins in cerebellum and basal ganglia seen on 2-D gels	Joseph disease	20–65 yr	Gait ataxia often with either corticospinal and extrapyramidal findings or late onset polyneuropathy
Disorder of endorphin enkephalin metabolism			
Increased endorphin and enkephalin levels in brain and CSF	Necrotizing encephalopathy (Leigh's syndrome)	1–2 yr	Attacks of coma; miosis; ptosis; clumsiness; pallor; hyperhydrosis; may respond to naloxone; 20 × increase in brain enkephalins and CSF endorphins (67)

system is highly vulnerable to a series of molecular abnormalities, as evidenced by very different molecular defects such as Bassen-Kornzweig syndrome and Friedreich's syndrome, yet the system can respond only in a limited manner and without a great deal of pathologic variation, as evidenced by the similarity of neuropathologic findings in these various disorders. Common neuropathologic features, from the peripheral nerve through the spinal cord and up to the cerebellum with its associated connections, are seen in the broad spectrum of these spinocerebellar degenerations, and the interesting aspect of these generalized and nonspecific changes is that they represent specific clinical syndromes caused by separate molecular defects inherited in a characteristic autosomal recessive or autosomal dominant manner.

HEREDITARY SPINAL AND CEREBELLAR ATAXIA OF FRIEDREICH (FRIEDREICH'S SYNDROME)

Friedreich's syndrome is a collection of spinocerebellar degenerations that occur in childhood as a familial disorder or that may be clearly transmitted as a genetic autosomal recessive or dominant disorder. Sporadic or isolated examples of the syndrome are reported (576). Friedreich's syndrome represents a series of several specific entities that share common clinical features and pathologic changes. The syndrome includes a variety of inborn errors of metabolism, including several disorders of lipids (phytanic acid storage disease, a-β-lipoproteinemia, moderate β-galactosidase deficiencies, and juvenile arylsulfatase deficiencies), diseases of oxidative metabolism (deficiencies of the pyruvate dehydrogenase complex, defect of mitochondrial malic enzyme, neuromuscular disorders with "ragged red" fibers, and abnormalities of cytochrome *b* or of nicotinamide adenine dinucleotide (NADH) oxidation), aminoacidurias (intermittent maple syrup urine disease, γ-glutamyl-cysteinyl transferase deficiencies, and Hartnup disease), and the partial deficiency of hypoxanthine guanine phosphoribosyl transferase (HGPRT) deficiency. The clinical expression of these inborn errors of metabolism includes involvement of cerebellar functions and corticospinal functions that are progressive and symmetrical, compatible with Friedreich's syndrome.

In addition to those inborn errors producing spinocerebellar degeneration, already mentioned, deficiencies of enzymes of the pyruvate dehydrogenase complex that catalyze the conversion of pyruvate to acetyl-CoA and carbon dioxide have also been identified in patients having ataxia and peripheral neuropathy. Pyruvate oxidation defects have also been described in patients with ataxia and peripheral neuropathy caused by nongenetic acquired conditions such as thiamine deficiency, alkylmercury poisoning, and elemental mercury poisoning.

Friedreich's syndrome in which pyruvate oxidation was low in muscles has been described in children. Muscle from four of seven Friedreich's syndrome patients was used, as well as muscle from four of 12 patients with other ataxias and from eight of 19 patients with familial or idiopathic neuropathies. Fibroblast cultures from patients with a deficiency in pyruvate oxidation have also been described. Further, the activities of several enzymes of oxidative metabolism in cell-free extracts of fibroblasts from four patients with Friedreich's ataxia and from a fifth patient with a variant of this syndrome were assayed by Blass and co-workers (49,50) for (a) the total pyruvate dehydrogenase complex, (b) the thiamine-dependent first enzyme of the complex (pyruvate decarboxylase), and (c) the 2-oxoglutarate dehydrogenase complex and mitochondrial marker enzyme cytochrome *c* oxidase. There is one enzyme common to the pyruvate and 2-oxoglutarate dehydrogenase, i.e., lipoamide dehydrogenase (reduced NAD-lipoamide oxidore-ductase). The pyruvate dehydrogenase complex from disrupted fibroblasts was assayed from four patients with this syndrome and was found to be 43% of that in 16 controls. There was a 50% reduction in the activity of the 2-oxoglutarate dehydrogenase complex in the patient's cells compared with that of controls. The activity of cytochrome *c* oxidase was normal in patient cells. Patients with less than 15% of normal pyruvate dehydrogenase activity but with normal oxoglutarate dehydrogenase generally have had severe neurologic disease and lactic acidosis beginning in infancy. Several deficiencies of both complexes have been described in one infant with severe disease. Several patients with 20 to 30% of normal pyruvate dehydrogenase activity had a milder illness in which ataxia was the predominant sign. The patients with Friedreich's syndrome having 40 to 50% of normal pyruvate dehydrogenase activity together with 50% of normal oxoglutarate dehydrogenase activity may be associated with ataxia beginning at puberty and progressing slowly, typical of Friedreich's syndrome. Several patients have been reported by Stumpf et al. (583) in whom mitochondrial malic enzyme of fibroblast cultures has been reduced by at least 50%, but other patients reported by Chamberlain and Lewis (92) and Gray and Kumar (231) had normal levels in fibroblast cultures. Patients in whom a defect in oxidative metabolism can be documented might be referred to as having Friedreich's disease, and those patients sharing the same phenotype but not having the oxidative defect might be referred to by the nonspecific designation, Friedreich's syndrome.

Pathology

The primary area of pathology is the spinal cord and the peripheral nerves. The spinocerebellar tracts, lateral corticospinal tracts, and posterior columns are specifically and selectively involved. The peripheral nerves may also undergo degenerative changes, including demyelination. The primary sensory neurons undergo neuronal loss, with secondary demyelination occurring in the posterior columns of the spinal cord. Neuronal loss also occurs in Clarke's column, which is the cell nucleus of origin for the spinocerebellar tracts. Anterior horn neurons of the spinal cord may also be lost, as well as neurons of the cerebellar cortex and deep cerebellar nuclei.

The spinal cord and cerebellum usually appear normal on gross inspection, but in some instances the cord and cerebellum may be atrophied. The cerebral cortex is histologically normal, and demyelination and secondary gliosis in the corticospinal tracts usually do not extend above the level of the medulla.

Incidence

Friedreich's ataxia and the spinocerebellar degenerations are uncommon disorders. They may be inherited in a sporadic or isolated manner as a familial disorder without a clear genetic pattern or as an autosomal recessive or autosomal dominant trait. They usually begin in the first decade of life but occasionally in the second decade, presenting with gait ataxia as the earliest and predominant feature (610). Deformed feet, including pes cavus and pes equinovarus (clubfoot), with scoliosis, minor ataxia, and absent deep tendon reflexes may be encountered as an incomplete form of the disease.

Clinical Manifestations

Truncal ataxia as manifested by a discoordination of gait, frequent falling, and titubation may be the earliest and most severe aspect of this syndrome. Gait instability may be the only manifestation of the disease for many years, but eventually dysarthria of speech and incoordination of arm and hand movements develop. By the second decade of life, the progression in gait ataxia usually develops to the point where assistance in walking becomes necessary (274,576).

The neurologic examination indicates the presence of nystagmus, loss of fast saccadic eye movements, truncal titubation, dysarthria of speech, and dysmetria and ataxia of extremity and truncal movement. Important findings in the motor examination include extensor plantar responses with normal tone in trunk and extremities and absent deep tendon reflexes (609). Weakness and extremity atrophy with fasciculations may be noted. Cardiac disease may develop that includes cardiomegaly, murmurs, bundle-branch block, T-wave inversions, and complete heart block as recorded on the electrocardiogram (EKG) (56,596). Congestive heart failure requiring diuretics and digitalis may develop. Cardiomegaly with subsequent cardiopulmonary arrest has been reported. Moderate mental retardation or psychiatric syndromes may be present in a small percentage of patients (121,264).

Diagnosis

The occurrence in childhood of truncal and extremity ataxia with dysarthria followed by nystagmus, extensor plantar responses, and areflexia is compatible with Friedreich's syndrome. The subsequent development of fasciculations, muscle atrophy, and mild mental retardation may be encountered. Two forms with associated neuropathy can be separated on the basis of a determination of motor and sensory nerve conduction velocities as well as the pattern seen on electromyography. The more common neurogenic form of neuropathy appears to be a result of loss of motor anterior horn cells without attendant demyelination. Thus the motor nerve conduction velocities are normal, but fasciculations and an impaired interference pattern are seen on electromyography, indicative of denervation. In the hypertrophic form of associated neuropathy, motor nerve conduction velocities are slowed, and the peripheral nerves may be somewhat enlarged on palpation because of recurrent demyelination and remyelination. The latter hypertrophic form of peripheral nerve disease associated with Friedreich's syndrome is quite rare and is more often encountered in Charcot-Marie-Tooth syndrome. The CSF protein is normal. A neurogenic type of group atrophy may be seen in the muscle biopsies from some patients. Kyphoscoliosis and pes cavus foot deformities are also typical findings. Finally, cardiac conduction defects as recorded by the EKG and cardiomegaly on the chest X-ray may be of diagnostic value.

A determination of pyruvate dehydrogenase or mitochondrial malic enzyme specific activities utilizing fibroblast cultures from Friedreich's syndrome patients may demonstrate at least a 50% reduction in enzyme activity. Thus, the term *Friedreich's disease* as distinct from the syndrome should be restricted to those patients who appear to have an abnormality in carbohydrate metabolism as reflected by these enzyme defects.

Differential Diagnosis

Included as differential diagnostic entities are multiple sclerosis, Roussy-Levy syndrome, and subacute combined degeneration of the spinal cord resulting from vitamin B_{12} deficiency. Roussy-Levy syndrome is separated from Friedreich's syndrome because of the relative absence of nystagmus and dysarthria associated with the childhood onset of ataxia, areflexia, and skeletal changes. Refsum's disease, which results from a defect in lipid α-oxidase, produces a clinical syndrome similar to Friedreich's syndrome, but these patients in addition have elevated serum phytanate levels along with optic atrophy, pigmentary retinal degeneration, ichthyosis, and deafness. Friedreich's syndrome associated with a-β-lipoproteinemia, steatorrhea, and acanthocytosis indicates the presence of Bassen-Kornzweig syndrome. Patients with hereditary spastic paraplegia are distinguished from Friedreich's syndrome patients by the presence of hyperreflexia, extensor plantar responses, and progressive paraparesis that may be associated with peroneal muscular atrophy, skeletal deformities, and nystagmus. Early in the course these patients present with findings that may be similar to the spinocerebellar degenerations, or they have family members with more typical cerebellar deficits and thus are nosologically included.

Treatment

Blass in 1979 (49) reviewed specific pharmacologic treatment for patients with pyruvate dehydrogenase complex deficiency and the Friedreich phenotype. A high fat diet is suggested to provide substrate and bypass the error in sugar metabolism. Thiamine, steroids, physostigmine, choline, and lecithin may also benefit selected patients. Infants with intermittent ataxia, immunodeficiency, and multiple carboxylase deficiencies may have improvement in ataxia with high doses of dietary biotin, as reviewed by Sander et al. in 1980 (518). It is of note that Griggs et al. in 1978 (238) found a subset of ataxia patients with paroxysmal ataxia and a positive family history that promptly and completely responded to acetazolamide.

HEREDITARY ATAXIA WITH MUSCULAR ATROPHY (ROUSSY-LEVY SYNDROME)

Roussy-Levy syndrome, originally described in 1926 (508), is an example of an intermediate form between Friedreich's syndrome and Charcot-Marie-Tooth syndrome. It is placed in the intermediate category because it represents a combination of minor cerebellar deficits with atrophy of the muscles of the legs, especially in a peroneal distribution. Harding and Thomas (259) include it as a form of hereditary motor and sensory neuropathy types 1 (slow conduction velocities) and 2 (normal conduction velocities). It is fair to state that this syndrome represents a variation of Friedreich's syndrome in which there develops a prominent amount of muscle wasting with a relative absence of cerebellar findings. In reports of Friedreich's syndrome in large families, the presence of the Roussy-Levy variant is seen in some family members (440).

OLIVOPONTOCEREBELLAR DEGENERATIONS

The olivopontocerebellar syndromes represent a collection of disorders that produce progressive involvement of cerebellar functions and that share a common impairment or reduction in neurons in the inferior olivary nuclei of the medulla, in the basis pontis, in the cerebellar cortex, and in the deep cerebellar nuclei (217).

Pathology

Gross atrophy of the cerebellum, cerebellar peduncles, and basis pontis clearly develops. There is a severe impairment of Purkinje cells at the light microscopic level, reduction in the number of granule cells of the cerebellar cortex, and marked neuronal loss in the deep cerebellar nuclei, including the dentate nucleus (197,571). According to Landis et al. (341) an increased number of stacked cisternae, curvilinear densities, pleomorphic membranous tubules, and crystalloid inclusions are found as early lesions in Purkinje cells by electron microscopy (Figs. 1 and 2). Although these ultrastructural alterations in the cerebellar cortex obtained from live patients at various stages of disease do disclose a variety of abnormalities, these changes nevertheless do not reveal anything of unequivocal pathogenetic significance. The possibility that infectious agents may participate in the pathogenesis of some autosomal dominant olivopontocerebellar degenerations is raised by the finding of paramyxovirus-like tubular structures and crystalloid inclusions in the degenerating cerebellar neurons (Figs. 1 and 2).

Clinical Manifestations

Progressive ataxia, dysarthria, dysmetria, dysadiodochokinesia, nystagmus, loss of fast saccadic eye movements, and subsequent development of spasticity, optic nerve atrophy, distal sensory involvement, and late intellectual dysfunction represent the essential clinical features of the olivopontocerebellar degenerations (268,327). As previously mentioned, there may be modifications and new clinical phenomena in different families expressing either an autosomal recessive or a dominant disease

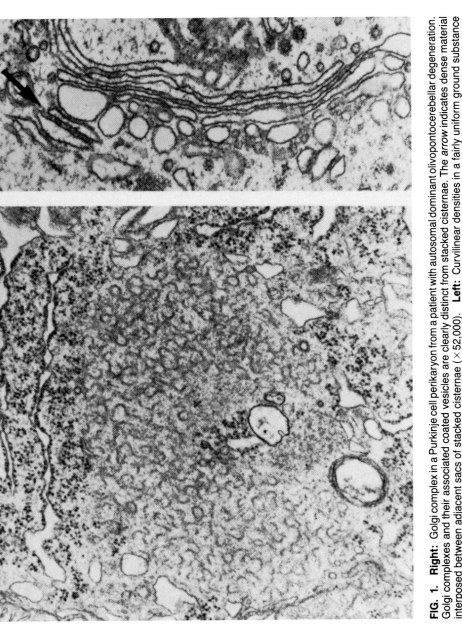

FIG. 1. Right: Golgi complex in a Purkinje cell perikaryon from a patient with autosomal dominant olivopontocerebellar degeneration. Golgi complexes and their associated coated vesicles are clearly distinct from stacked cisternae. The *arrow* indicates dense material interposed between adjacent sacs of stacked cisternae (×52,000). **Left:** Curvilinear densities in a fairly uniform ground substance in a Purkinje cell perikaryon. At high magnification the "curlicues" appear to have faint cross-striations (×42,000). (From ref. 341, with permission.)

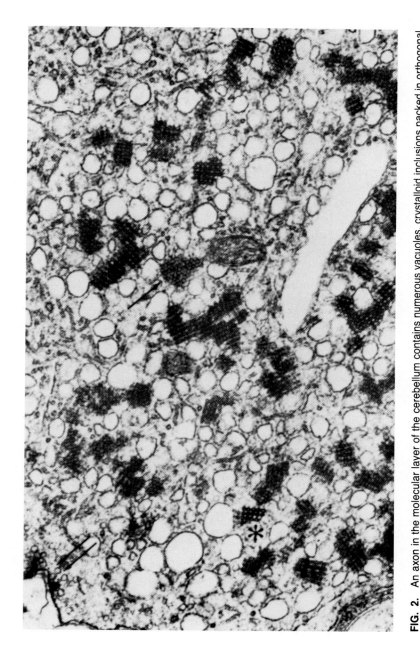

FIG. 2. An axon in the molecular layer of the cerebellum contains numerous vacuoles, crystalloid inclusions packed in orthogonal array in some instances (above *asterisk*) and packed hexagonally elsewhere *(single arrow)*, and numerous vermiform tubules 30 to 35 nm in external diameter in longitudinal and cross-section. A synaptic junction with an unidentified process is indicated by *double arrows* (×48,000). This is from a patient with autosomal dominant olivopontocerebellar atrophy. (From ref. 341, with permission.)

as classified by Konigsmark and Weiner (327). It is important to note that the variants previously described by Holmes, Sanger-Brown, and Marie, among others, cited by Konigsmark and Weiner (327) are quite similar as clinical entities and are separated by arbitrary minor differences in clinical features (647). It can be argued that the olivopontocerebellar degenerations inherited as autosomal dominant (327) (Fig. 3) or autosomal recessive (258) genetic disorders represent a very small number of unique clinical diseases and that the primary gene mutation has its penetrance and expression altered clinically by other modifying genes.

In the second or third decade of life, extremity and truncal ataxia with dysmetria and dysarthria progressively develops. Spasticity associated with clonus, hyperreflexia, and extensor plantar responses subsequently develops. Nystagmus, optic nerve atrophy, and loss of fast saccadic eye movements may occur. A late occurrence of muscle atrophy with fasciculations involving the facial muscle, the muscles of mastication, and the lingual muscles is encountered owing to the involvement of lower motor neurons in this system degeneration. Sensory involvement in a distal

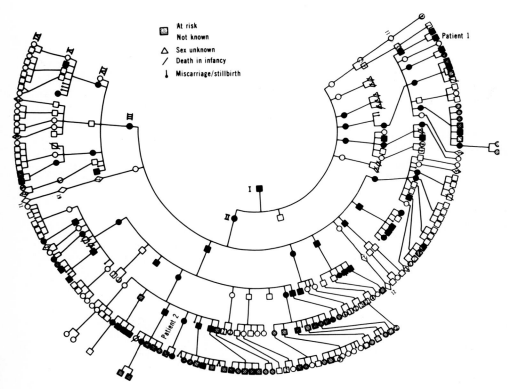

FIG. 3. Pedigree of the Schut-Swier kindred correct to 1970. Certain sets of siblings not at risk are represented by *diamonds*; the numbers within the diamonds indicate the number of siblings so represented. This illustrates the autosomal dominant form of inheritance in this family with olivopontocerebellar atrophy. (From ref. 341, with permission.)

distribution may also occur. Intellectual deterioration and the eventual development of a dementia may occur in some patients late in the disease process (88). Ophthalmoplegia, extrapyramidal signs, and optic atrophy with visual loss may be encountered. Conry et al. (101) reported a family in which this syndrome complex was dominantly inherited, but it was not clear if it was autosomal or X-linked dominant. The family was unique in that two distinct presentations were noted. Patients either began at 1 to 4 years of age with a rapidly progressive disorder or had a later onset at 9 to 40 years, with a slowly decreasing visual acuity that preceded the onset of a spastic ataxia by several years. This kind of wide variation is most unusual for typical olivopontocerebellar syndrome and more in keeping with several Joseph disease pedigrees.

The syndrome of dyssynergia cerebellaris myoclonica of Ramsay-Hunt (291) is another rare variant beginning in childhood or early adulthood, and it includes myoclonus, seizures, and progressive ataxia inherited in an autosomal dominant manner (562).

Diagnosis

The development early in life of progressive symmetrical involvement of cerebellar functions followed by progressive and symmetrical development of spasticity is characteristic of the olivopontocerebellar degenerations. Abnormalities of eye movement, intellectual impairment, and muscle atrophy with sensory distal loss may complete the clinical picture. Cerebellar atrophy, pontine atrophy with minor cerebral atrophy, and large lateral ventricles may be visualized by CT brain scans or, if necessary, pneumoencephalography. There may be slowing of motor nerve conduction velocities with denervation as demonstrated on electromyography. The CSF protein and cell counts are normal. Jackson et al. (300) and Haines et al. (254) in 1984, studying the Schut-Swier kindred, have presented convincing evidence recently of linkage between the gene for ataxia and the human lymphocyte antigen (HLA) complex situated on chromosome 6. These data may become most useful as a marker of disease for purposes of genetic counseling.

In general, the spinocerebellar degenerations represent syndromes producing progressive and symmetrical involvement in their pathologic and clinical expression and often have a clear genetic basis of inheritance or suggestion of familial involvement. Rosenberg et al. (505a) reported an abnormal organic acid composition in urine from affected patients. An increased incidence of echinocytes (649) and an abnormally low aspartate concentration in the CSF from patients (456) are also reported. Plaitakis et al. (464,466) and Duvoisin et al. (147) reported a 50% reduction in glutamate dehydrogenase (GDH) activity in nonneural tissues from recessively inherited and dominantly inherited with incomplete penetrance patients, respectively, which could result in toxic levels of glutamate in the cerebellum, producing potential excitotoxic degeneration of cerebellar neurons. Recently, dominantly inherited patients have been reported having low GDH activities in leukocyte homogenates (189). This is an important observation, but it is not clear if this enzyme defect is a primary or secondary change. Progress is being made in research on this disorder, and perhaps the recent glutamate dehydrogenase data will lead to a better understanding of pathogenesis and therapy.

Therapy

No specific therapy is available. It is important to be sure the patient does not have a malabsorption of vitamins A and E secondary to gastric surgery resulting in a blind loop syndrome and a spinocerebellar syndrome as a secondary event. Treatment with antibiotics and supplemental vitamins will often result in some improvement (71).

JOSEPH DISEASE

A nongenetic form of striatonigral degeneration was described initially by van der Eecken et al. in 1960 (612). The patients involved were diagnosed clinically as having Parkinson's disease, but their symptoms differed neuropathologically in that they had bilateral degeneration of the corpus striatum and substantia nigra, particularly the zona compacta portion. No cause has been found in any of these cases.

In 1976 Rosenberg et al. (502) described a family of Portuguese ancestry with autosomal dominant spinocerebellar and striatonigral degeneration. This family numbered 329 persons in eight generations (Fig. 4). Romanul et al. (493) described another family of Portuguese-Azorean ancestry with striatonigral degeneration (patient 2) in a clinical setting of parkinsonism and polyneuropathy. The two families are not related and, in fact, are descended from persons from separate and distant Azorean Islands. Joseph disease has also recently been described in two families that have no known relationship to any family in the Azores by Lima and Coutinho (355) in Portugal and by Healton et al. (270) in the United States. The first reports of similar disease were by Nakano et al. (423) and by Woods and Schaumburg (646). It was originally thought that the disorders described by Nakano et al., Woods and Schaumburg, and Rosenberg et al. were separate and distinct. After careful epidemiologic studies and case analyses in the United States, Portugal, the Azores, India, and Japan by Rosenberg et al. (503), Coutinho and Andrade (105) and Barbeau et al. (30), it is concluded these clinical types represent variation in the expressivity and penetrance of the same mutant gene. The presence of a modifier gene is also postulated to be responsible for this clinical variation rather than normal background diffuse genetic heterogeneity. The finding of absence of disease in one large family was statistically correlated with the presence of the BA isoenzyme form of the erythrocyte enzyme acid phosphatase, which maps to chromosome 2p23. It may be that the postulated modifier gene is linked to this locus, and DNA polymorphism studies are underway with cDNA probes for this locus for possible diagnostic presence of this modifier in selected families. Studies of a similar nature are also in progress to find a DNA polymorphism that is

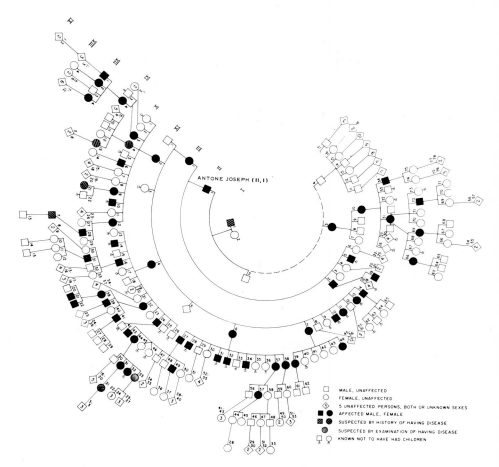

FIG. 4. Pedigree of the Joseph family of California composed in 1975 showing 329 persons in eight generations. In 1978, with further research, the pedigree included 600 persons, with more than 50 persons who have been or are now affected with autosomal dominant striatonigral degeneration (Joseph disease). (From refs. 504 and 505, with permission.)

associated with the primary gene mutation. Preliminary data suggest that Joseph disease gene is on chromosome 1 near the amylase locus.

Pathology

The major pathologic findings in several deceased family members were a severe loss of neurons and glial replacement in the corpus striatum and a severe loss of neurons in the zona compacta portion of the substantia nigra. There was also a moderate loss of neurons in the dentate nucleus of the cerebellum and the nucleus ruber of the midbrain. The cerebellum, cerebellar peduncles, inferior olives, corticospinal tracts in the brainstem, and basis pontis did not show gross atrophy. The cerebellar cortex showed Purkinje cell loss and granule cell loss. The dentate nucleus had cell loss and pyknotic changes. Purkinje cell torpedos and Bergmann cell gliosis were also present histologically. Also the frontal cerebral cortex appeared entirely normal histologically. There was no evidence of demyelination in the cerebellum, its peduncles, or the brainstem.

These findings indicate a spinocerebellar degeneration with a striatonigral degeneration caused principally by neuronal loss and glial replacement. Although the putamen showed significant neuronal loss, there was no increased pigmentation characteristic of the nongenetic forms of the striatonigral degenerations (106,503).

Clinical Manifestations

Type 1

The main neurologic findings beginning in the first two decades include extremity weakness and spasticity of all extremities, especially the legs, often with associated dystonia of the face, neck, trunk, and extremities (Fig. 5). Patellar and ankle clonus are common, as are extensor plantar responses. The gait is slow and stiff with a slight increase in base and lurching from side to side; this results from spasticity, not true ataxia. Affected persons have no truncal titubation. Pharyngeal weakness and spasticity cause difficulty with speech and swallowing. Of note is the prominence of horizontal and vertical nystagmus, loss of fast saccadic eye movements, hypermetric and hypometric saccades, and impairment of vertical gaze upwards. Facial fasciculations, facial myokymia, lingual fasciculations without atrophy, ophthalmoparesis, and ocular prominence are common and early manifestations (Figs. 6 and 7).

Type 2

The hallmarks are the additional presence of true cerebellar deficits including dysarthria, gait, and extremity ataxia beginning in the second to fourth decades, along with corticospinal and extrapyramidal deficits of spasticity, rigidity, and dystonia. Type 2 is the most common form of the disease. Ophthalmoparesis, upward vertical gaze deficits, and facial and lingual fasciculations are also present, as they are in type 1 disease. It must be separated from olivopontocerebellar degeneration.

Type 3

The onset of disease occurs in the fifth to the seventh decades of life with a pancerebellar disorder including dysarthria, gait, and extremity ataxia. Distal sensory loss to pain, touch, vibration, and position senses and distal atrophy are prominent. The deep tendon reflexes are depressed to absent, and no corticospinal or extrapyramidal findings occur. In all instances the intelligence of patients is preserved (30,503) (Fig. 8).

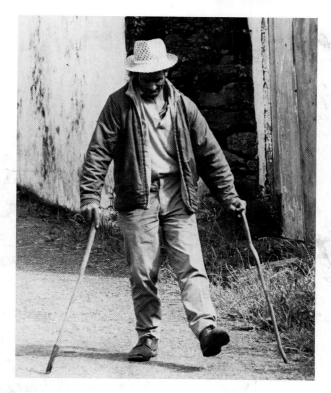

FIG. 5. A 36-year-old patient with Joseph disease is shown with obvious impairment of gait due to lurching from side to side when walking because of spasticity. The presence of facial dystonia is also visible. He is patient NS (V,32) in our original paper in 1976 (494). (From refs. 504 and 505, with permission.)

The disorder is inherited in an autosomal dominant manner, with the mean age of onset of symptoms in affected family members examined being 25 years. Neurologic deficits invariably increased progressively and resulted in death from debilitation within 15 years of onset, especially in types 1 and 2 patients. Patients retained full intellectual function, and the only significant involuntary movement was tremor at rest or dystonia in some affected members.

Diagnosis

Autosomal dominant Joseph disease should be considered in persons with an appropriate family history who develop progressive dystonia, rigidity, and spasticity of pharynx, trunk, and extremities with associated hyperreflexia, clonus, and extensor plantar responses during the first or second decade (type 1). This entity is distinguished from Huntington's disease by the preservation of intellect and the absence of choreoathetosis. Dystonia musculorum deformans can be distinguished

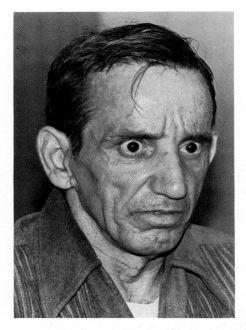

FIG. 6. Patient JL, age 36 years, who has a family history of autosomal dominant striatonigral degeneration. He has Joseph disease but is not a Joseph family member, originating from a family that emerged from the island of St. Miguel, Azores. He has marked Parkinson's disease and a distal sensory polyneuropathy. The ocular prominence without proptosis is shown and is present in several other patients with Joseph disease. (From refs. 504 and 505, with permission.)

FIG. 7. A patient with Joseph disease is illustrated to show the presence of extraocular muscle involvement. He is a 40-year-old man examined on the island of Flores, Azores (June 1977), who has generalized ophthalmoparesis, facial fasciculations, extensor plantar responses, hyperreflexia, spasticity, and truncal ataxia. (From refs. 504 and 505, with permission.)

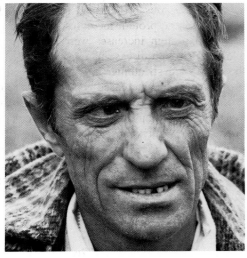

because of the prominence of spasticity and the characteristic eye findings present in Joseph disease (types 1 and 2). These findings, along with typical cerebellar deficits of dysarthria, gait, and extremity ataxias in the second to fourth decades, indicate type 2 disease. Some patients in large families develop distal extremity atrophy, areflexia, distal sensory loss, hypotonia, and definite cerebellar truncal

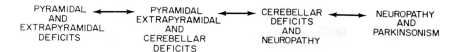

FIG. 8. Spectrum of clinical manifestations in Joseph disease. Type I refers to prominent pyramidal and extrapyramidal deficits. Type II disease is present when pyramidal and extrapyramidal findings include definite cerebellar deficits. Type III disease is present when cerebellar deficits occur with distal, sensory, and motor neuropathy. One family has been described with autosomal dominant parkinsonism and distal sensory neuropathy. (From refs. 504 and 505, with permission.)

and extremity ataxia (type 3). Assays of the CSF for homovanillic acid are of value, as the mean concentration of this metabolite of dopamine in the CSF of five affected persons was 15.3 ng/ml, compared with a control value of 43.4 ng/ml (502).

More recently the brain from an affected 73-year-old woman was autopsied, and neuropathologic findings included atrophy of the pons and cerebellum with extreme degeneration of the thoracic spinal cord. Axonal terminal swellings were noted. Bergmann glia were increased in cerebellum. Two-dimensional Coomassie-stained gels were used by Rosenberg et al. (501,506), Comings (98), and Morrison and Rosenberg (412) to analyze proteins from cerebellar cortex, putamen, and cerebellar cortex from this patient and five adult controls. Two classes of proteins were significantly increased in putamen and cerebellum, including the 50,000 MW glial acidic filamentous protein and two 40,000 MW proteins that migrate near actin (Fig. 9). These protein increases most likely represent secondary gliosis. In 1980 the same protein increases were found in cerebellum and basal ganglia of five additional Joseph disease patients. These protein increases in the putamen support the view of a striatonigral degeneration in this patient in addition to cerebellar involvement. The increased glial proteins represent gliosis, the result of the disease process. DNA polymorphism associations will be necessary to determine the primary altered gene product. Such a molecular marker will be a constant, irrespective of the clinical variations. Dawson et al. (123) have described electrooculographic findings in patients, including defects in caloric response, sinusoidal tracking, opticokinetic nystagmus, refixation saccades, and gaze paretic nystagmus, that can be diagnostic and extremely useful for an early diagnosis of disease in subjects at risk because of an affected parent.

ATAXIA TELANGIECTASIA

Syllaba and Henner in 1926 (588) and Louis-Barr in 1941 (358) described a neurocutaneous disorder that begins in the first decade of life with permanent telangiectatic lesions involving the conjunctivae (Fig. 10A), malar eminences, ear lobes, and occasionally the upper neck regions (Fig. 10B); it is associated with cerebellar deficits and nystagmus (261). Although the disorder usually is sporadic in occurrence and isolated in families, it may present in families with a pattern consistent with an autosomal recessive genetic disorder. A chromosome transloca-

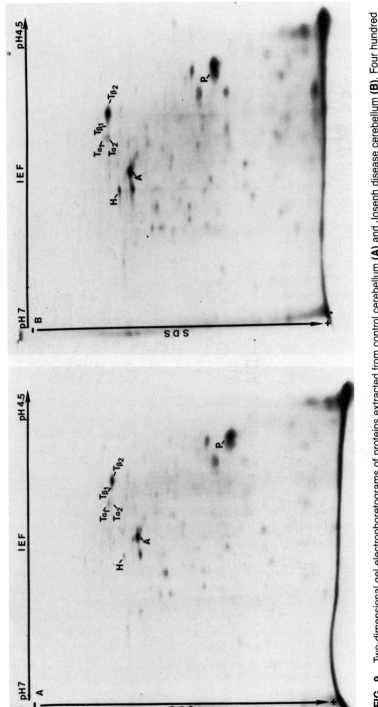

FIG. 9. Two-dimensional gel electrophoretograms of proteins extracted from control cerebellum (**A**) and Joseph disease cerebellum (**B**). Four hundred micrograms of protein was loaded on each gel. A, Actin; H, glial fibrillary acidic protein complex; J, J protein complex; L, L protein complex; SDS, sodium dodecyl sulfate; IEF, isoelectric focusing gel; P, protein P; T, tubulin. (From ref. 412, with permission.)

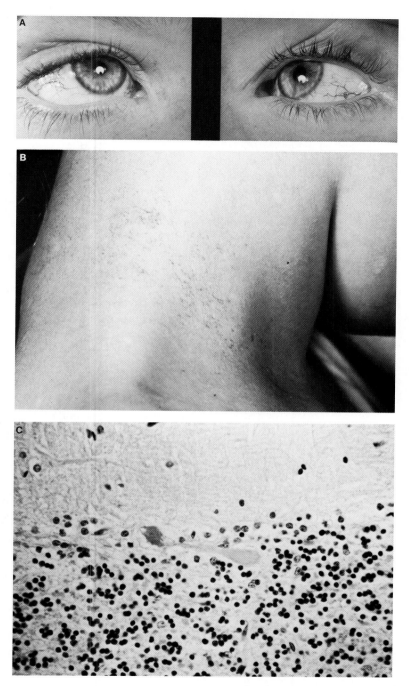

FIG. 10. Ataxia telangiectasia is a neurocutaneous disorder that produces characteristic capillary lesions **(A)** in the sclerae, **(B)** on the side of the neck, and **(C)** associated with cerebellar histologic abnormalities such as Purkinje cell torpedos and granule cell loss. (Courtesy of Dr. M. E. Blaw, University of Texas Health Science Center at Dallas.)

tion involving chromosome 7 and 14, a marked reduction in lymphocyte response to phytohemagglutinin, and increased chromosome breakage have been noted in some patients (271).

Fiorilli et al. (190) have indicated that spontaneous breakages at chromosome bands 7p14 and 14q32 in patient lymphocytes are caused by faulty rearrangements of the T and B cell receptor genes, which also map there (190), thus explaining the immunologic defects in this disorder. Increased sensitivity of patient G_1 chromosomes in stationary fibroblast cultures to X-irradiation has been quantitated. There is a fivefold increase in breaks that do not rejoin in patient cultures compared with control cultures (104).

Pathology

The most striking neuropathologic changes include loss of Purkinje, granule, and basket cells in the cerebellar cortex as well as of neurons in the deep nuclei of the cerebellum (Fig. 10C). The inferior olives of the medulla also may have neuronal loss. There is a loss of anterior horn neurons in the spinal cord and of ganglion cells in spinal ganglia associated with posterior column demyelination in the spinal cord. A poorly developed or absent thymus gland is the most consistent defect of the lymphoid system (3).

Biochemistry

Perry et al. (457) recently reported biochemical abnormalities in autopsied brain of a patient. Glutamic acid content was markedly reduced and taurine content was somewhat reduced in the cerebellar cortex, while GABA content was greatly reduced in the dentate nucleus. GABA receptor binding was reduced by 70% in cerebellar cortex. Phosphoethanol amine content was greatly reduced in the cerebellar cortex and inferior olivary nucleus. Perry et al. indicated that this same compound was also deficient in 10 other brain areas and was the only noncerebellar neurochemical abnormality found.

Clinical Manifestations

In the first decade of life there is the onset of progressive telangiectatic lesions associated with progressive deficits in cerebellar function and early nystagmus. The neurologic manifestations correspond to those seen in Friedreich's syndrome, and this entity should be included in that differential diagnostic category. Truncal ataxia, extremity ataxia, dysarthria of speech, extensor plantar responses, myoclonic jerks, areflexia, and distal sensory deficits may develop. There is a high incidence of recurrent pulmonary infections and neoplasms of the lymphatic-reticuloendothelial system in these patients, as reviewed by McFarlin et al. in 1972 (383).

Diagnosis

The combination of Friedreich's syndrome, including prominent and progressive symmetrical truncal ataxia and other cerebellar deficits, and apractic eye movements associated with characteristic telangiectatic lesions indicates the presence of this syndrome. Serum protein electrophoresis is helpful in documenting the common occurrence of the deficiency of γ-globulins, especially IgA and IgE (8). Lymphocytopenia, a reduced response to skin test antigens, and a lack of sensitization to dinitrochlorobenzene (DNCB) are characteristic findings indicating cellular immune abnormalities. The progression of the disease usually results in death during the first or second decade of life, usually as a result of lymphatic or reticuloendothelial tumors or pulmonary infection.

PARENCHYMAL CEREBELLAR DEGENERATION

The syndrome of intrinsic cerebellar degeneration begins with symmetrical cerebellar deficits primarily involving truncal and leg functions in the fifth to seventh decades of life, males being more frequently involved than females; it is slowly progressive. It may be inherited in a recessive pattern (260), but usually it is sporadic. Impaired coordination is most severe in the legs and may extend to the upper extremities and also be associated with dysarthria and nystagmus. The gait is ataxic and wide-based. The cerebellar cortex is primarily involved, with a partial loss of Purkinje cells and some involvement of granule, stellate, and basket cells (448). The syndrome has been associated with chronic and severe alcoholism (492,561,617) and the occurrence of carcinoma of the lung (66) and other tumors (382). The precise mechanism of disease and a specific form of therapy have not been determined (164). Removal of the malignant neoplasm and cessation of the excessive use of alcohol may result in improvement.

ACUTE CEREBELLAR ATAXIA OF CHILDHOOD

This is usually a benign syndrome occurring in children less than 6 years of age (628). It develops abruptly, with prominent truncal and extremity ataxia, nystagmus, apractic eye movements, intention tremor of extremities, and irritability. It may begin after a viral-type upper respiratory tract or gastrointestinal (GI) infection. There is no evidence on clinical examination and by lumbar puncture of increased intracranial pressure; the CSF is normal; the EEG is also normal; and the course is benign, with complete recovery within 1 year. A similar acute cerebellar syndrome may occur as the remote effect of focal or systemic neuroblastoma. This diagnosis is confirmed by bone marrow aspiration demonstrating neuroblastoma tumor cells, X-rays of long bones showing lesions, and the presence of an elevated vanillylmandelic acid excretion level in urine.

BASSEN-KORNZWEIG SYNDROME

This syndrome, described in 1950 (35), was the first entity with specific diagnostic features associated with the typical picture of Friedreich's syndrome (540). Acanthocytosis, steatorrhea, impaired chylomicron formation, and retinitis pigmentosa are the diagnostic features (35,252,391). Further, the electrophoretic pattern of the serum proteins is grossly abnormal because of the absence of β-lipoproteins. Children with this syndrome develop progressive truncal and extremity ataxia, dysarthria, nystagmus, and muscle atrophy and weakness in a peroneal distribution with distal sensory involvement. Mental retardation is rare and usually mild when present. Cardiomegaly and progressive cardiac failure may develop. The disease is a rare one and must be considered in a child presenting with a progressive cerebellar deficit (329). An adult onset may be associated with malabsorption of vitamins A and E, resulting in nyctalopia, optic atrophy, and cerebellar deficits, which are improved with vitamin A and E therapy.

MARINESCO-SJÖGREN SYNDROME

This is a rare syndrome in which progressive cerebellar deficits begin in early childhood. It is associated with bilateral cataracts and mental retardation, and is another rare example in which the general Friedreich's syndrome is associated with additional specific features, in this case cataracts and mental retardation (9,600). Walker et al. (623) studied four patients' skin fibroblasts by electron microscopy and found numerous enlarged lysosomes that contained whorled lamellar or amorphous inclusion bodies, indicating that this syndrome is probably a lysosomal storage disorder caused by an enzyme defect.

COCKAYNE'S SYNDROME

This is a most rare autosomal recessive disorder described in 1936 and associated with multiple features. Mental retardation, optic atrophy, dwarfism, neural deafness, cataracts, and retinal pigmentary degeneration are the major findings. Cerebellar, pyramidal, and extrapyramidal deficits and peripheral neuropathy may occur with bird-headed facies and normal pressure hydrocephalus.

Demyelination, perivascular microcalcification, and gliosis are the neuropathologic findings. In 1980 a patient was reported by Kennedy et al. (320) with late onset of disease at the age of 19 years, associated with completion of a successful pregnancy. This syndrome must be considered in the evaluation of mental retardation and syndromes with progressive cerebellar or pyramidal degenerations.

In 1985 Lehmann et al. (348) diagnosed the syndrome prenatally. This was accomplished by examining amniotic cells cultured *in vitro*. RNA synthesis after irradiation with ultraviolet light was abnormal in cells from a fetus with the syndrome but not in cells from a normal fetus.

Motor Neuron Diseases

AMYOTROPHIC LATERAL SCLEROSIS

Amyotrophic lateral sclerosis (ALS) represents a spectrum of motor system degenerations involving the corticospinal and corticobulbar pathways and motor neurons associated with the cranial nerves and anterior horn cells of the spinal cord. It is inherited in about 10% of instances, usually as an autosomal dominant with variable penetrance and expressivity (498). Dysfunctions of motor neurons produce clinical manifestations of spasticity and muscular atrophy, either singly or in combination. The presence of diffuse atrophy, weakness, fasciculations, and reduced myotatic reflexes indicates a variant of the system degeneration known as progressive spinal muscular atrophy. Progressive weakness and atrophy of muscles innervated by cranial nerves indicate the development of another variant referred to as progressive bulbar palsy (498). A pure expression of corticobulbar and corticospinal involvement, i.e., with signs of upper motor neuron deficits including weakness and spasticity with hyperreflexia, clonus, and extensor plantar responses, but without evidence of muscular atrophy, corresponds to another variant known as primary lateral sclerosis (18,34).

Incidence

The syndromes of ALS are common ones encountered on neurology services. The incidence rate of 1.4 per 100,000 population is also recorded in many nations. As many as 10,000 patients may have one form of this syndrome at any one time in the United States. Although the disease may occur at any age, according to a review by Bobowick and Brody in 1973 (52), it develops mainly in the fifth, sixth, and seventh decades of life and runs a progressive course, lasting about 7 years. The median age of death of patients dying of ALS in the United States for the 3-year period 1959 to 1961 was approximately 62 years (335,365). The mean age at onset is about 52 years. There is a familial form of the disease (498,599). An interesting feature of both the sporadic and Guamanian forms of ALS is that in all series the male rate of occurrence is from 1.2 to 2.5 times higher than the female rate. The familial form of disease has a one-to-one male to female ratio. There are no well-documented racial differences for ALS with the exception of foci on Guam and in Japan (55,275).

In the 51 fatal cases reviewed by Vejjajiva et al. in 1967 (615), the clinical groupings according to presenting symptoms were as follows: 53% of patients had ALS in mixed forms, 27% of patients had progressive muscular atrophy, and 20% of patients had a flaccid bulbar palsy. The initial site of involvement was also tabulated, and the figures show 40% beginning in the upper extemity, 25% in the lower extremity, 25% in the head, and about 10% in mixed sites. The sporadic form of motor neuron disease is indistinguishable in clinical expression from the hereditary form of ALS seen in the United States and in the Guamanian and Kii Peninsula forms, but neuropathologic distinguishing features have been reported. Of importance is a recent study of Mulder and Howard (418) demonstrating in a prospective study of 100 patients with this disorder that 20 patients were living at least 5 years after the onset of disease. Those patients having a more benign form of disease did not have any predictive identifying features and were unique only because of their protracted course.

Etiology

Several toxic chemicals such as tricresyl phosphate and organic compounds derived from mercury as well as elemental lead exposure may be responsible for the development of a syndrome similar to ALS, but this represents a small number of patients. It has been suggested but not proved that ALS is the result of a slow latent viral infection. Attempts to isolate a transmissible agent in chimpanzees injected with ALS tissue have not been successful. Further, attempts to rescue virus from neurons fractionated out of ALS spinal cord and fused with carrier-helper cells to form heterokaryons have proved negative. Defects in collagen biosynthesis, an angiopathy, impaired dopamine metabolism, a factor present in serum from patients that results in demyelination of myelinated tissue cultures, a serum factor that blocks neurite outgrowth in culture, and a primary metabolic abnormality of neurometabolism have all been suggested as causes of the disease. In 1976 Horton et al. (283) identified at least three types of familial motor neuron disease based on clinical, pathologic, and genetic studies of 14 families. Most of their families had an inheritance pattern indicative of an autosomal dominant disorder. In a smaller number an autosomal recessive form of inheritance was suggested. In families with autosomal dominant transmission, a spectrum of clinical involvement was recorded, from a rapid progressive loss of motor function to a form that was quite benign, with some individuals living longer than 20 years.

Recently Oldstone and associates have reported finding immune complexes associated with the mesangium of the renal glomerulus and basement membrane in typical patients with motor neuron disease who had a more aggressive form of disease. This finding suggests that motor neuron disease may be the result in part of an autoimmune disorder and raises speculation as to the primary basis for the break in immunologic tolerance in these patients (443). A slow latent viral infection, such as a mutated poliovirus, might be pathogenetic. The precise mechanism and cause of disease in ALS are currently not known.

Motor neuron disease has been well studied on Guam, in the Kepi region of New Guinea, and in the Kii Peninsula of Japan, where it occurs with an unusually high incidence. The incidence has fallen in recent years, however. These endemic forms of the disease may be the result of environmental factors interacting with multifactorial or polygenetic mechanisms. The incidence of ALS in the Chamorro people on the island of Guam is on the order of 50 to 100 times the rates observed in other nations. The Guamanian form of the disease is clinically indistinguishable from sporadic ALS, except that patients are younger than those with the sporadic form of ALS and they survive somewhat longer. A syndrome consisting of the triad of dementia, parkinsonian rigidity, and the findings of ALS has been well documented (162,163).

Pathology

Neuronal loss develops in the motor cranial nuclei and motor neurons in the anterior horns of the spinal cord. Similar degenerative changes with neuronal loss result in motor neurons of the cerebral cortex in Brodmann's areas 4 and 6. The neuronal loss occurs without diagnostic features and results in a secondary atrophy of the musculature that is innervated by motor cranial nuclei and motor anterior horn cells because of denervation (93,94). In the autosomal dominantly inherited form of ALS, in addition to the typical pathologic findings of sporadic ALS, there occurs a degeneration in Clarke's column with demyelination of the posterior columns and spinocerebellar tracts of the spinal cord (572). Bundles of neurofilaments are present in the remaining anterior horn motor neurons of the spinal cord (420). In the Guamanian form of ALS, there are similar widespread neurofibrillary tangles present in remaining cortical motor neurons and subcortical areas (72).

Clinical Manifestations

A slowly progressive impairment of motor function, as evidenced by muscle atrophy of the intrinsic muscles of the hand, develops over a period of a year, spreading to produce a symmetrical picture of muscle atrophy involving the forearms and shoulder girdle musculature. Prominent and early is the occurrence of fasciculations as a result of diffuse denervation of entire motor units (196). Mild distal paresthesias and muscle cramps may occur. Rarely a cervical rib might coincidentally coexist with an ALS presentation (36). The deep tendon reflexes are maintained or slightly impaired during the early phase of disease. Clear signs of upper motor neuron involvement may become manifest within the first year of the illness, producing spasticity in the lower extremities with associated hyperreflexia, clonus, and bilateral extensor plantar responses (203). The cremasteric and abdominal reflexes, as well as the bladder and anal sphincters, remain intact. A combination of fasciculations and muscle atrophy may occur associated with exaggerated reflexes. A characteristic of ALS is the presence of this combination of both upper and lower motor neuron deficits. The clinical variant of ALS known as primary lateral sclerosis is suggested when the clinical picture is that of spasticity involving the pharynx, larnyx, and extremities without evidence of lower motor neuron involvement, including atrophy and fasciculations. Bulbar ALS or the progressive spinomuscular atrophy form of ALS is suggested by the loss of the gag reflex, pharyngeal paralysis, lingual atrophy, and fasciculations, as well as diffuse atrophy and fasciculations of the extremities and impaired myotatic reflexes. It is rare for musculature innervated by the 3rd, 4th, and 6th cranial motor nuclei to be involved. Rather, musculature innervated by the 5th, 7th, 11th, and 12th cranial motor nuclei is involved in the bulbar form of disease (367). Minor sensory involvement including paresthesias may be present (625). Emotional lability may be present, but formal mental testing indicates absolute preservation of intellectual functions. The CSF cell count, glucose, and protein values are normal. Fasciculations, positive waves, and fibrillations of acute denervation are identified by electromyography with normal motor nerve conduction velocities even in the presence of severe atrophy, which is a helpful feature in distinguishing this disorder from the peripheral motor neuropathies, in which conduction velocities are reduced early in disease.

Differential Diagnosis

ALS must be clinically differentiated from spinal cord tumors, cervical spondylosis, syringomyelia, arachnoiditis, or chronic myelomeningitis. The presence of a cervical level spinal cord tumor and the necessity for myelography would be suggested by atrophy and fasciculations in musculature innervated by motor neurons in the cervical cord region associated with a clear sensory level in the cervical regions. Similarly, significant skeletal changes on cervical spine roentgenograms suggestive of spondylosis indicate the need for myelography to document a spinal nerve root or spinal cord compression. Arachnoiditis or chronic meningitis is suggested by the finding of a CSF pleocytosis and an elevated protein. Polymyositis, an acquired myopathy, or polyneuropathy may present in a similar clinical manner as ALS, but these can be identified by nerve or muscle biopsy in combination with electromyography, measurement of peripheral nerve conduction velocities, and measurement of serum levels of creatine phosphokinase or aldolase.

There is no specific form of therapy at the present time for patients with ALS.

CONGENITAL ARTHROGRYPOSIS

Congenital arthrogryposis is a syndrome associated with fixation of joints at birth; there are other malformations as well (478). This is a rare syndrome resulting from a diverse etiology including multifactorial genetic factors. Drachman and Banker (145) have described a spinal form that results from anterior horn motor neuron injury and loss that presumably has developed in fetal life. In some patients fibrillations with normal nerve conduction velocities have been described by electromyography, indicating the presence of denervation caused by neuronal disease (616). In other patients the disease assumes a myopathic form. It is presumed that the joint fixations result from lack of proper movement *in utero* because of either neuronal or primary muscle disease. This syndrome probably is not etiologically related to Werdnig-Hoffman syndrome, which may also begin *in utero* and may be associated with fixed joints, as the syndrome of spinal arthrogryposis is nonprogressive, static, and without familial involvement (453).

INFANTILE PROGRESSIVE SPINAL MUSCULAR ATROPHY (WERDNIG-HOFFMAN SYNDROME)

This syndrome refers to a generalized neurogenic muscular atrophy beginning in the first year of life and progressing to death within the first 2 years of life. The syndrome with onset in the first year of life with a slower progression and prolonged survival into adolescence or early adulthood is known as Wohlfart-Kugelberg-Welander syndrome and probably represents a benign form of Werdnig-Hoffman syndrome. Epidemiologic studies have suggested an autosomal recessive mode of inheritance (655). Neuropathologic findings include loss of anterior horn cell motor neurons and bundles of focal glial hyperplasia in relation to the anterior spinal roots (84,234,433). There is also a predilection for involvement of type 1 muscle fibers (Fig. 11). The cause of disease and effective therapy are not known (57).

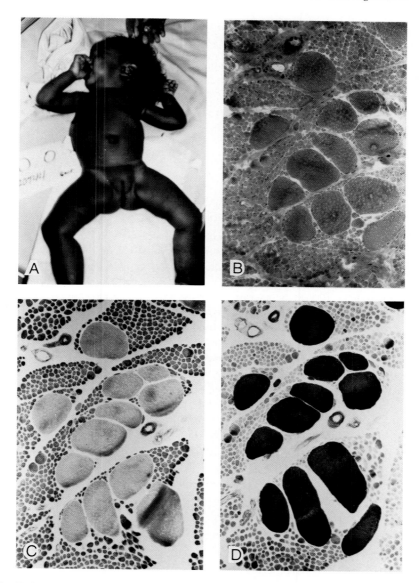

FIG. 11. A: A girl age 11 months with Wernig-Hoffman disease. She is diffusely hypotonic and severely weak. There are obvious muscle atrophy and fasciculations. **B:** Trichrome stain showing the alternation of normal-sized fibers and areas of group neurogenic atrophy (×40). **C:** ATPase stain at pH 9.4, indicating that the large fibers are type 1 and the atrophied fibers are type 2 (×40). **D:** ATPase stain at pH 4.3, showing staining of the type 1 muscle fibers. (Courtesy of Dr. Jay Cook, University of Texas Southwestern Medical School at Dallas, and Grune & Stratton, Inc., New York; from ref. 505, with permission.)

JUVENILE PROGRESSIVE SPINAL MUSCULAR ATROPHY
(WOHLFART-KUGELBERG-WELANDER SYNDROME)

This syndrome has its onset in childhood or adolescence and develops as a progressive, usually proximal neurogenic muscular atrophy that may be confused with Werdnig-Hoffman disease or limb girdle muscular dystrophy (208). Since the original descriptions by Wohlfart et al. (643) and Kugelberg and Welander (334), over 200 case reports have been published; these reports describe approximately 100 cases with infantile onset of disease beginning at less than 2 years of age and about 133 cases with onset in the juvenile years between 3 and 18 years of age (212). A family history is positive in most cases, and the disease is inherited in an autosomal recessive manner, but several families have been reported as having an autosomal dominant mode of inheritance. Namba et al. in 1970 (424) reported a sex ratio of about one to one with infantile onset of disease. The disease produces weakness and muscular wasting in the proximal muscles of the extremities, usually sparing ocular, facial, and other bulbar musculature. Corticospinal and sensory pathways of the spinal cord are not involved. Fasciculations may be prominent in weak or atrophied muscles. This syndrome is distinguished from Werdnig-Hoffman disease by the later onset and benign course; it is also distinguished from ALS similarly because of the slow progression of disease and the absence of any involvement of corticospinal tracts. The limb girdle form of muscular dystrophy can be distinguished from this syndrome by findings on electromyography and muscle biopsy. The Charcot-Marie-Tooth form of neuropathy is distinguished by its production of a predominantly distal muscular atrophy and sensory loss, which is not characteristic of Wohlfart-Kugelberg-Welander disease.

FAZIO-LONDE DISEASE

Progressive bulbar paralysis in childhood is the hallmark of Fazio-Londe disease, as emphasized by Gomez et al. in 1962 (226). It is a rare syndrome beginning in childhood and resulting in progressive bulbar palsies; there is minimum involvement of extremity musculature, however. It may be inherited in an autosomal recessive manner, and it results in progressive paralysis of the muscles of mastication, facial muscles, and pharyngeal and lingual muscles.

FAMILIAL SPASTIC PARAPLEGIA

This syndrome is characterized by the occurrence, in the first two decades of life, of progressive spastic paraparesis leading to paraplegia. The syndrome is inherited as an autosomal recessive, sex-linked recessive, or familial trait (140). It occurs more frequently in males than in females, and its onset may rarely be delayed so that it occurs in adult life (47). It may be related to the spinocerebellar degenerations, as this familial syndrome may be encountered in large families with other forms of spinocerebellar disease (16,213,340,369,490,542,558).

SYRINGOMYELIA

Syringomyelia, or cavitation of the spinal cord, as it was first known, was described by Esteinne in 1546 in his description "La Dissection du Corps Humain." The precise term syringomyelia, referring to a cavitation of the spinal cord, is attributed to Charles P. Ollivier D'Angers, who in 1827 attributed the abnormal dilation of the central canal to a developmental anomaly. Syringomyelia since that time has referred to a chronic and progressive disorder with amyotrophy, pain and temperature sense loss (although position and stereognostic functions are relatively well preserved), paraparesis, skeletal defects including scoliosis, and associated neurogenic arthropathies (269). Syringomyelia occurs more frequently in males than in females, and the first sign of disease begins in the second or third decade of life; it rarely begins in childhood or late adulthood (44). Predisposing genetic factors may be involved in the cause of this disorder because of the developmental abnormalities in the cord and its predominance in males.

Clinical Manifestations

The presentation and progression of disease depend primarily on the location of the cavitary enlargement of the central canal of the spinal cord. The most common location of the syringomyelic cavity is in the midcervical region of the spinal cord, with resultant involvement of anterior horn motor neurons progressing to amyotrophy beginning in the intrinsic muscles of the hands and ascending to the forearms and musculature of the shoulder girdle. Progressive involvement of the lumbrical and interosseus muscles of the hand leads to progressive impairment of terminal extension of the fingers and the development of a claw hand or main en griffe. Weakness and atrophy with fasciculations develop in the forearms and shoulder girdle muscles and are associated with an early loss of the deep tendon myotatic reflexes. Scoliosis and kyphosis may occur early as a result of denervation and atrophy of the dorsomedial and ventrolateral spinal nuclei. The syringomyelic cavity may dissect anteriorly and interrupt the decussating spinothalamic fibers mediating pain and temperature, and this may result in the loss of these sensations with the relative preservation of light touch and posterior column conscious proprioceptive and stereognostic functions. The dissociated impairment of pain and temperature sensations, with other sensations remaining intact, occurs in a shawl distribution across the anterior and posterior upper thorax. Extension of the syringomyelic cavity into the lateral columns of the cord bilaterally results in a rather symmetrical paraparesis with spasticity and associated clonus, hyperreflexia, and extensor plantar responses (384,429). Impairment of bowel and bladder sphincter functions occurs as a late manifestation. The involvement of the second-order sensory neurons in the spinal cord is associated with deep and severe pain, often of a causalgic quality. A Horner's syndrome may be seen as a result of descending central sympathetic fiber involvement. Papilledema may occur as a rare event (6). The presence of dysphagia, pharyngeal weakness and paralysis, weakness and atrophy of the tongue, and loss of pain and thermal sensibility in a trigeminal distribution indicates ascent of the syringomyelic process into the medulla, producing the syndrome of syringobulbia. Analgesic shoulder and knee joints (Charcot's joints of syringomyelia) may occur. Morvan's syndrome, or terminal phalangeal absorption, may be a later occurrence. As reemphasized recently by Sackellares and Swift (516), shoulder enlargement that is painful and associated with complete destruction of the humoral head may develop acutely with cervical syringomyelia early in the course of disease. Angiograms of the shoulder in two adult patients showed hypervascular lesions. Thus the first clinical manifestation of syringomyelia may be a neuropathic painful shoulder arthropathy. Such arthropathies eventually develop in 25% of patients with syringomyelia, and 80% of them involve the upper extremities.

Pathology

Syringomyelia, as defined by Greenfield (233), is a condition with tubular cavitation of the spinal cord extending over many segments. Greenfield considered hydromyelia to be a nosologically distinct entity and a cystic expansion of the central canal of the cord. The syringomyelic cavity may be lined by a thick layer of glial tissue, and such cavities may be in communication with an enlarged central canal (267,631). Developmental abnormalities in the cervical spine and base of the skull (the platybasias) and the Arnold-Chiari malformation, with displacement of the cerebellar tonsils into the cervical canal and cord compression, are commonly encountered (353). Associated findings with syringomyelia include ectopic cerebellar tonsils, hydrocephalus, cerebellar hypoplasia, astrocytomas and ependymomas of the spinal cord, and syringobulbia (471).

Gardner has stressed the concept of "communicating syringomyelia," which refers to a dilated and tense central canal of the spinal cord being in direct communication with the fourth ventricle (211). This malformation develops because of impaired drainage of CSF from the ventricular system. Impaired drainage from the foramina of Magendie and Luschka resulting in Dandy-Walker syndrome leads to a communicating syringomyelic cavity, which is synonymous in his terms with hydromyelia. The common occurrence of the Arnold-Chiari malformation or ectopic cerebellar tonsils is thus explained on the basis of foraminal herniation of the cerebellar tonsils through the foramen magnum during development. Syringomyelia may also occur as a late sequel to trauma of the spinal cord associated with adhesive arachnoiditis. About 2% of patients with traumatic paraplegia develop a progressive ascending myelopathy reaching the cervical cord with a definite syrinx, as demonstrated by myelography.

LUMBAR SYRINGOMYELIA

A location of the syrinx in the lumbar cord may occur alone but usually it occurs in association with a cervical syrinx (613). A lumbar syrinx results in atrophy in the legs, thigh, and pelvic girdle musculature, with a dissociated sensory loss in lumbar and sacral dermatomes. There is a reduction or absence of the deep tendon reflexes in lower extremities, and usually the plantar response is flexor. Impairment of bowel and bladder sphincters usually occurs.

Laboratory Data

The CSF of 31 patients with syringomyelia was analyzed by Merritt (396) and reviewed by Rosenberg (497), with the following findings: (a) The pressure varied between 95 and 285 mm H_2O; pressure was greater than 200 mm H_2O in 7 of the 31 patients. A complete subarachnoid block was present in two patients and was confirmed at the time of operation. (b) The cell count varied from 0 to 20 cells/ mm^3, but only one patient had more than 10 cells/mm^3. (c) The protein was greater than 45 mg% in 15 patients and greater than 100 mg% in two patients with subarachnoid block. Dilation of the spinal cord in the cervical region during myelography is of diagnostic value. Angiography of the shoulder joint may demonstrate a high degree of vascularity and neuropathic changes.

Clinical Course

The progression of syringomyelia is usually slow, extending over many years. Rarely, it may develop rapidly; this is usually in those instances in which syringobulbia occurs.

Differential Diagnosis

ALS, multiple sclerosis, tumors of the spinal cord, skeletal anomalies of the cervical spine, platybasia, and cervical spondylosis are conditions that must be considered and differentiated from syringomyelia. Myelography is important in determining the presence of a spinal cord tumor and severe spondylosis. If there is evidence of diffuse denervation on electromyography, ALS should be seriously considered if electromyography indicates denervation when motor conduction velocities are normal, and if findings on myelography and on examination of the CSF are negative. The occurrence of syringomyelia with subarachnoid block can be separated from a true spinal cord tumor only at the time of laminectomy and direct inspection.

Cervical ribs may result with progressive weakness and atrophy of the shoulder girdle musculature and loss of sensation in dermatomes of a cervical distribution. It should be noted that cervical ribs may be one of the skeletal anomalies associated with true syringomyelia.

Tabes dorsalis may result in absence of the myotatic reflexes in the legs and the occurrence of Charcot joints, suggesting a lumbar location for syringomyelia.

Treatment

At the present time there is no specific therapy for syringomyelia. Radiation therapy to induce glial tissue formation and prevention of extension of the syringomyelic cavity has been of some benefit. Surgical decompression of a cavity may be helpful in selected patients (359). Decompression of the associated Arnold-Chiari malformation by widening the foramen magnum has been of significant value. Associated hydrocephalus should be treated with ventricular shunting procedures and the related spinal cord glioma with radiation therapy and surgical decompression.

HEREDITARY MYASTHENIC SYNDROMES

A sporadic case of a congenital myasthenic syndrome associated with acetylcholinesterase (AChE) deficiency was described in 1977 by Engel et al. (168). A defect in acetylcholine (ACh) resynthesis or mobilization was reported as an autosomal recessive myasthenic syndrome in 1979 by Hart et al. (265). In 1982 Engel and associates (169) described an autosomal dominant myasthenic syndrome and suggested it was associated with an abnormally prolonged open time in the ACh-induced ion channel. Symptoms occurred in the latter syndrome in infancy or later life. There was involvement of cervical, scapular, and finger extensor muscles with ophthalmoparesis. Although there is atrophy of the neuromuscular junction by electron microscopy, there are no immune complexes at the end plate.

Peripheral Nerve Diseases

PERONEAL MUSCULAR ATROPHY

Charcot-Marie-Tooth disease or peroneal muscular atrophy is a genetic disorder of the peripheral nervous system primarily involving the peroneal musculature and other distal muscles of both the upper and the lower extremities. It is most often inherited as an autosomal dominant disorder and less frequently as an autosomal recessive and X-linked dominant or recessive disease (460,604). The specific molecular defect remains unknown.

Pathology

The peripheral nerves in the lower extremities and later in the upper extremities undergo degenerative changes that include demyelination and dissolution of the axon. The occurrence of recurrent demyelination and remyelination with the formation of so-called onion-bulb changes in the peripheral nerve may result in a hypertrophied nerve as a variant; this nerve may be palpated on physical examination. Examination of biopsied skeletal muscle may indicate the occurrence of group atrophy indicative of neurogenic denervation (248). Pathologic changes have been described in the dorsal root ganglion cells, motor neurons of the spinal cord, and posterior columns of the spinal cord.

Incidence

Peroneal muscular atrophy is a rare disorder most commonly seen as an autosomal dominant inherited genetic disease in large families in which atrophy of the peroneal musculature is the dominant expression. It may also be seen in the spectrum of the spinocerebellar degenerations. It usually begins in the first or second decade of life, but delayed onset has been reported. Dyck and Lambert in 1968 (149,150), Dyck in more detail in 1975 (148), and Harding and Thomas in 1980 (259) described an autosomal dominant variant (type I, dominantly inherited hypertrophic neuropathy) in which slow motor nerve conduction velocities were associated with a hypertrophic form of disease resulting from recurrent demyelination and remyelination. A second form (type II, neuronal form of peroneal muscular atrophy) of autosomal dominant disease was not associated with hypertrophy or with slow conduction velocities but rather with denervation, as evidenced by fasciculations and impaired interference patterns on electromyography (149,150). A minor variant was a form of peroneal atrophy without sensory involvement.

Clinical Manifestations

Peroneal muscular atrophy begins in the first decade of life and is most characteristic, with initial atrophy and weakness of the peroneal musculature of the legs, resulting in a steppage gait and obvious footdrop (Fig. 12). Skeletal deformities, including scoliosis and clubfeet, are common. Subsequently, intrinsic muscle atrophy of the hands and forearms may develop (539). The occurrence of cerebellar

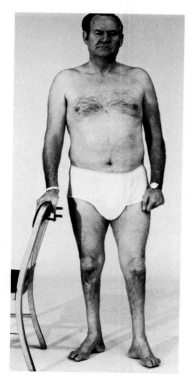

FIG. 12. A 59-year-old man with moderately advanced Charcot-Marie-Tooth disease. He has obvious atrophy of muscles involving the legs distally. (Courtesy of Dr. Jay Cook, University of Texas Southwestern Medical School at Dallas, Grune & Stratton, Inc., New York; from ref. 505, with permission.)

signs and extensor plantar responses indicates a transitional state with Roussy-Levy or Friedreich's syndrome. Harding and Thomas (260) described 25 cases of peroneal muscular atrophy with pyramidal features (extensor plantars) from 15 families. Pyramidal features are rare findings, however. Sensory involvement is frequently present, including conscious proprioceptive, vibratory, pain, temperature, and touch impairment in a distal distribution. The deep tendon reflexes are absent at the ankle and reduced at the knee and in the arms.

Laboratory Data

Motor nerve conduction velocities are slowed in the hypertrophic form of the disease (type I motor sensory neuropathy) (259), and on electromyography denervation of the neurogenic, nonhypertrophied type is found (type II motor sensory neuropathy) (259). Group atrophy is present on examination of biopsied skeletal muscle. The CSF protein is normal in most patients.

Differential Diagnosis

Peroneal muscular atrophy is considered when there is a childhood occurrence of peroneal atrophy with scoliosis and foot deformity and a family history of similar disease. Spinocerebellar disease must be considered with the subsequent development of corticospinal or cerebellar deficits. Hereditary distal myopathy of childhood must also be considered (368). Optic atrophy and acoustic degeneration may be encountered with hereditary peroneal muscular atrophy, as reported by Rosenberg and Chutorian in 1967 (500).

Therapy

Dyck has found a subset of type 1 and 2 patients who respond significantly to prednisone with an improvement in their polyneuropathy.

HYPERTROPHIC INTERSTITIAL NEUROPATHY (DEJERINE-SOTTAS DISEASE)

Dejerine-Sottas disease (124) or hypertrophic interstitial neuropathy (type III hypertrophic neuropathy of Dyck), is a recessively inherited genetic neurologic disorder producing symmetrical and severe involvement of the peripheral nerves; it is associated with impressive hypertrophy beginning in infancy or early childhood (22). It usually begins in the lower extremities but gradually becomes evident in the upper extremities and thoracic musculature, with rare involvement of musculature innervated by motor cranial nerves. There may be impairment of sensory functions, including vibratory and position as well as pain and touch sensations, with spontaneous paresthesia and pain. The deep tendon reflexes are absent and the plantar responses remain flexor. Neuropathologic findings include onion-bulb changes in the peripheral nerve because of redundant numbers of Schwann cells

(598,630). Spinal cord compression has been reported in association with hypertrophic neuropathy (589).

Motor nerve conduction velocities are slowed and the CSF protein may be elevated (220). This syndrome may be related to peroneal muscular atrophy, but this point can only be precisely determined when the molecular defects are defined in both entities. Dyck et al. have reported a great decrease in the peripheral nerve in the amount of cerebrosides in the presence of a normal amount of sphingomyelin and a moderate increase in sulfatides (151).

HEREDITARY SENSORY NEUROPATHY

This disorder is a genetic disease involving the sensory fibers of the peripheral nervous system (127,477). It is inherited as an autosomal dominant trait and it produces progressive sensory deficits beginning in the first or second decade of life (305,536,605). There is a progressive loss of sensations of pain, heat, and light touch, and a loss of proprioceptive functions with associated absence of the deep tendon reflexes and occasional lightning pains. Characteristic painless ulcerations develop in the feet and the digits of the hands. This disorder seems to selectively involve the sensory neurons in the dorsal root ganglion, which undergoes degenerative changes and subsequent neuronal loss. This syndrome must be distinguished from acute sensory-type polyneuritis, in which there is an exclusive and acute impairment of sensory function without motor impairment. An impairment of pain perception in children must raise the question of the Riley-Day syndrome, an autosomal recessive disorder. Riley-Day children also have short stature, recurrent pulmonary infections, absence of circumvallate papillae of the tongue, and vomiting crises (569). Increased homovanillate to vanillylmandelic acid ratios for 24-hr urine excretion of these compounds is a consistent feature of the Riley-Day syndrome. Reduced activity of dopamine-β-hydroxylase in serum has been reported in 25% of Riley-Day patients and may be the primary molecular basis of the disease. With complete absence of cutaneous sensation in children, there may be a complete absence of neurostructures in the skin (356).

FAMILIAL DYSAUTONOMIA (RILEY-DAY SYNDROME)

This syndrome presents in early childhood and is inherited in an autosomal recessive manner (386). It occurs almost entirely in Jewish children. It was originally described by Engel and Aring in 1945 (172) and again in 1949 by Riley et al. (484). Smith et al. in 1963 (570), Dancis and Smith (114), and Smith and Dancis in 1967 (568) suggested that the disorder was caused by a defect in catechol metabolism, since patients demonstrated an increased concentration in urine of homovanillic acid, which is a metabolic product of dopamine metabolism, and an associated decrease in the concentration of vanillylmandelic acid, which is a metabolic product of norepinephrine. These abnormalities in the urinary excretion of these metabolites suggested a defect in the enzyme dopamine-β-hydroxylase. In 1971 Weinshilboum and Axelrod (627) reported a marked reduction in serum dopamine-β-hydroxylase activity in some but not all patients with this syndrome.

Ziegler et al. (659) reported on the norepinephrine concentration in serum and the dopamine-β-hydroxylase plasma activity in dysautonomic patients when reclining or after standing as compared with normal control subjects. Dysautonomic patients, after standing, did not have a normal increase in their levels of norepinephrine and dopamine-β-hydroxylase. Further, they became hypotensive. Their data supported the view that hypotension and hypertension in dysautonomia were related to abnormal rates of norepinephrine release. Siggers et al. (557) found a threefold increase in serum antigen levels of the biologically active β-subunit of nerve growth factor (NGF) in dysautonomic persons as compared with normal subjects. The β-subunit of NGF from dysautonomic persons was functionally abnormal as measured by binding assays and radioimmunoassays. Thus it is suggested that the β-subunit of NGF is qualitatively as well as quantitatively abnormal in dysautonomia. Such abnormalities might provide the molecular explanation of neuropathologic changes in the peripheral nervous system, the autonomic nervous system, and the CNS. Breakefield et al. (69) identified some copies of the β-NGF gene (alleles) in six affected families. Alleles differed in the length of restriction fragments that hybridized to DNA probes for the NGF gene. They found that in two families affected children did not inherit the same two alleles at the β-NGF locus. They point out that since this disease is inherited as an autosomal recessive, the affected children must share the same alleles at the locus causing the disease, and thus their study excludes the β-NGF gene locus as the cause of the disorder.

Degeneration has been reported in neurons of the dorsal root ganglia, thoracic and sacral sympathetic ganglia (573), celiac plexus, and reticular formation of the brainstem, and in preganglionic sympathetic neurons in the lateral horns of the spinal cord, spinothalamic tract, spinocerebellar tract, and posterior columns of the spinal cord (77,650). Several of these neuropathologic changes were also recorded in animals immunosympathectomized by raising antibodies to injected NGF during the neonatal period, thus giving pathogenetic relevance to the altered NGF from patient serum.

Children with this disorder develop symptoms in the first 5 years of life and are usually in the lower 10th percentile for height and weight. Manifestations include irritability, insensitivity to painful stimuli, absence of taste discrimination, attacks of severe vomiting and hyperpyrexia, episodes of hypertension and hypotension, episodes of skin-blotching alternating with pallor, impaired lacrimation, seizures, absent deep tendon reflexes, and dysphagia. Recurrent upper respiratory tract infections with pneumonia may occur. A tetrad of alacrima, corneal hypesthesia, exodeviation, and methacholine-induced miosis may occur (223,452). This syndrome is characterized by the occurrence of periodic attacks, as mentioned above, with death in infancy or early childhood resulting from pneumonia, hyperpyrexia, severe dehydration with electrolyte abnormalities caused by vomiting, upper GI bleeding, or recurrent generalized major motor seizures (223,225).

The important laboratory findings are an increased ratio in the urinary excretion of homovanillic acid to vanillylmandelic acid, low serum dopamine-β-hydroxylase activity, and impaired norepinephrine release. Characteristic findings on physical examination include the absence of fungiform and circumvallate papillae of the tongue, absence of the deep tendon reflexes, and impairment in normal lacrimation. The intravenous administration of edrophonium chloride under carefully controlled circumstances may demonstrate a transient return of taste and lacrimation and a decrease in dysphagia, indicating that the disorder in part is related to an alteration in acetylcholine metabolism (485).

HEREDITARY AMYLOID NEUROPATHY

Peripheral neuropathy may be a component of generalized primary amyloidosis in about one-fifth of patients. There are two major hereditary forms that have been documented where neuropathy is an important clinical feature (513).

Andrade (13) reported several families from northern Portugal with autosomal dominant amyloid neuropathy. The disease process begins in the third or fourth decade, and there develops a progressive and symmetrical impairment in both sensory and motor functions associated with marked autonomic involvement. Typical findings include hyperpathia of the distal lower extremities with an impairment in temperature and pain sensations. A steppage gait caused by a bilateral footdrop subsequently occurs along with areflexia. Evidence for autonomic neuropathy includes distal ulcerations of the lower extremities, sphincter impairment, impotence, pupillary changes, and diarrhea or constipation. The neuropathologic changes include direct deposition of amyloid (a mutant prealbumin glycoprotein) into the peripheral nerves in addition to other organs such as the skin, GI tract, tongue, heart, and kidneys. Several patients with primary hereditary amyloid neuropathy inherited as an autosomal dominant have been treated with colchicine, which has resulted in clinical improvement, reduced amyloid on repeated peripheral nerve biopsies, and an improvement in nerve conduction velocities.

A similar form of autosomal dominant amyloid polyneuropathy has been described in the United States. These patients appear to have a milder form of the disease, with an onset as late as the sixth decade. It begins with a slow progression of motor and sensory deficits in the upper extremities, and it may present initially as a carpal tunnel syndrome.

In the Japanese type of autosomal dominant familial amyloid polyneuropathy, there is also a prealbumin variant with a single amino acid replacement of valine by methionine at position 30, and this mutant protein leads to amyloid fibril formation. Sasaki et al. (523) have cloned and sequence analyzed the cDNA for normal human prealbumin and have detected the mutation in the prealbumin gene for this dominant form of amyloid polyneuropathy. The presymptomatic diagnosis of disease was made in two sons of an affected mother in one family and in a daughter of an affected father in a second family. The demonstration of two abnormal hybridization signals in the first family at 5.0 and 1.4 kb with Nsi I restriction enzyme, indicating unique restriction fragment polymorphism, was sufficient to establish a diagnosis of presymptomatic disease. Similarly, in the second family signals at 5.0 and 1.4 kb indicated a restriction fragment polymorphism pattern associated with the mutant genotype, although presymptomatic. Both families thus had the same mutation, and the probe was highly effective in diagnosing disease in the at risk person. Surely this approach will be a powerful tool to eliminate this disorder not only in Japan, but also in Sweden, Portugal, and the United States, where it is endemic.

TANGIER DISEASE

Inhabitants of Tangier Island in Chesapeake Bay develop a progressive polyneuropathy in the second or third decade of life that involves distal motor and sensory functions of the extremities (173). A deficiency in high density serum lipoproteins (a-α-lipoproteinemia) in the serum of these patients has been a consistent feature associated with lipid deposits within lymphoreticular deposits of the tonsillar fossae of the oropharynx. The primary molecular defect has not been determined, but the disorder is inherited as an autosomal recessive trait.

PORPHYRIC POLYNEUROPATHY

Acute polyneuropathy may be an important component in the acute intermittent Swedish type of porphyria that is inherited as an autosomal dominant trait. The phenotypic neurologic features include episodes of personality change, depression, psychosis, abdominal pain, and severe generalized polyneuropathy. Skin manifestations do not occur in this form of porphyria. Episodes of polyneuropathy may be precipitated by barbiturates or phenytoin. A characteristic syndrome may occur in individual families, and the variation and severity of disease also differ from family to family. Urinary excretion of porphobilinogen is uniformly present. The enzyme uroporphyrinogen synthetase (porphobilinogen deaminase) has been reported to be deficient in liver and erythrocytes from affected patients. Enzyme activities are reduced by 40 to 60% of normal, which apparently is sufficient to alter the rate of metabolism in the porphyrin pathway. Thus porphyria is a most rare example of a dominantly inherited disorder resulting from an enzyme deficiency state. As a result of this enzyme deficiency and the reduced synthesis of its product, uroporphyrin-1, there is a release induction of the activity of the rate-limiting enzyme in the pathway, δ-aminolevulinic acid synthetase. This induction in turn results in an increase in urinary δ-aminolevulinic acid and porphobilinogen. Several patients have been treated with hematin, which corrects the metabolic defects of δ-aminolevulinic acid and porphobilinogen with striking improvement in clinical findings, including polyneuropathy. A high-carbohydrate diet may also prevent attacks and reduce morbidity.

The occurrence of acute polyneuropathy is sudden and often without any apparent cause. Drugs, hormones, or infection may trigger an attack. Severe polyneuropathy may develop with predominantly motor findings in an ascending distribution, with proximal accentuation resembling the Guillain-Barré syndrome. In fact, facial diplegia and bulbar paralysis may also occur in an ascending fashion. Patients may demonstrate an encephalopathy with delirium and seizures as well. Hyponatremia resulting from the inappropriate secretion of the antidiuretic hormone (ADH) has been reported. Rarely, the presentation of a mononeuritis multiplex syndrome occurs, with random, asymmetric involvement of individual nerves resembling a sacral plexus syndrome with severe pain and weakness. Phenothiazines, glucose, and intravenous infusion of hematin are therapeutically effective. Coproporphyria and variegate porphyria are two other autosomal dominant forms of porphyria that result in acute neurologic deficits.

GIANT AXONAL NEUROPATHY

This is a rare autosomal recessive disorder described in 1972 by Asbury et al. (20) and characterized by a symmetrical distal neuropathy, mental retardation, and frizzy, kinky hair (Fig. 13). The peripheral nerve axons are dilated segmentally because of the accumulation of 10-nm neurofilaments as seen on nerve biopsies. Similar axonal pathology is seen in the CNS. 2,5-Hexanedione is a toxin that

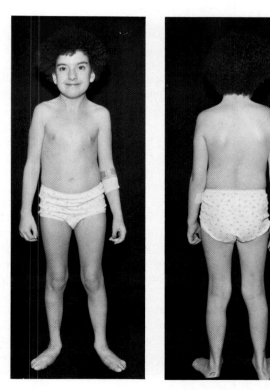

FIG. 13. A 10-year-old girl with giant axonal dystrophy. She has evidence clinically of a peripheral neuropathy with distal weakness and sensory loss in her extremities. Her frizzy curly hair is noted, which is characteristic of the disorder. (Courtesy of R. Tandan, M.D., University of Vermont Medical Center.)

produces an experimental model of giant axonal neuropathy. Monaco et al. (405) reported, using this model system, that the transport of neurofilamentous protein and two other polypeptides was selectively increased. The genetic disorder thus may result from a similar defect.

Phakomatoses or Neurocutaneous Syndromes

NEUROFIBROMATOSIS (VON RECKLINGHAUSEN'S DISEASE)

Neurofibromatosis or von Recklinghausen's disease is a genetic disorder inherited as an autosomal dominant trait and characterized by the occurrence of pigmented skin lesions, multiple tumors of spinal or cranial nerves, tumors of the skin, and associated gliomas and intracranial meningiomas. There is an increased association with pheochromocytomas, cystic lung disease, renal vascular lesions causing hypertension, fibrous dysplasia of bone, GI neurofibromas with chronic blood loss, and medullary thyroid carcinoma and other tumors of the endocrine glands.

Pathology

The characteristic feature of the disease is the occurrence of multiple neurofibromas associated with nerves in their peripheral, intraspinal, or intracranial segments. In the peripheral nervous system these tumors represent the proliferation of neurilemmal sheath cells (Schwann cells) or of fibroblasts of the peripheral nerve, as determined by electron microscopic studies. The tumors may become confluent in the region of the brachial or sacral plexus and produce large plexiform neuromas that can evolve into malignant sarcomas. Intracranial astrocytomas, ependymomas, glioblastomas, and meningiomas are also encountered, as are optic nerve gliomas in childhood. Stenosis of the aqueduct of Sylvius with noncommunicating hydrocephalus is also observed in this disease. The skin manifestations include neurofibromas, pedunculated polyps, lightly colored pigmented lesions with sharp edges referred to as café au lait spots, and depigmented lesions (Figs. 14–16). Neoplasms of endocrine organs, including medullary thyroid carcinomas and pheochromocytomas with associated hypertension, have been reported in a number of patients.

Metabolic bone disease in some patients results in overgrowth of bone with occluding of cranial formina and rarefaction and cyst formation of bone resulting from replacement of normal bone with fibroblasts and fibrocytes similar to fibrous dysplasia. The congenital absence of a portion of the sphenoid bone, resulting in pulsating exophthalmos, congenital vertebral anomalies, bone cysts, pseudoarthrosis of the tibia, local gigantism of an extremity, and scoliosis, are encountered in some patients. Histologic abnormalities of the cerebral cortex, ectopic islands of gray matter, and focal gliosis are described and may be the basis of mental retardation in some patients.

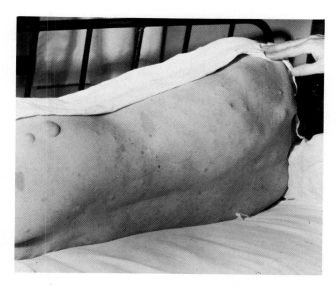

FIG. 14. Neurofibromatosis produces characteristic cutaneous neurofibromas and café au lait spots, as illustrated in this man. (Courtesy Dr. M. E. Blaw, University of Texas Health Science Center at Dallas.)

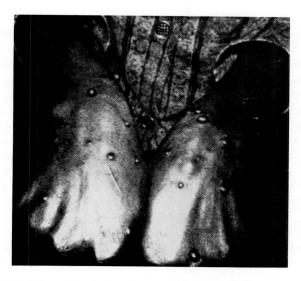

FIG. 15. Pedunculated peripheral nerve tumors typical of neurofibromatosis in a 60-year-old patient. (From ref. 496, with permission.)

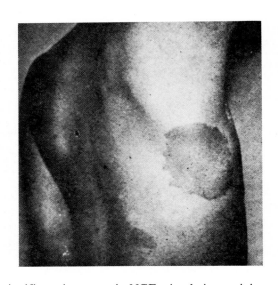

FIG. 16. Typical café au lait lesion of neurofibromatosis. (From ref. 496, with permission.)

Schenkein et al. (531) reported significant increases in NGF-stimulating activity in serum from patients with neurofibromatosis. Nerve growth hormone or factor (NGF) is a protein that stimulates the proliferation and differentiation of spinal and sympathetic ganglia *in vivo* and induces differentiation of neurites from embryonic ganglion cells of the chick, mouse, and human neuroblastoma cells in culture. In patients with disseminated neurofibromatosis, 19 of 24 serums tested (79%) had high titers of serum NGF, as compared with only 3 of 66 control serums (5.6%). In 1979 Fabricant et al. (175) reported on high titers in serum of NGF-antigenically positive material in patients with "central" neurofibromatosis. These were patients with intracranial tumors. It may be, in this autosomal dominant genetic neurologic disorder, that the high titer of NGF during fetal life, when neurilemma sheath cells are most sensitive to NGF, induces a proliferation of sheath cells and transforms them into tumor cells. Clinical manifestations of disease then result from the continued stimulation of these tumor cells that have been transformed by the elevated levels of NGF. These reports of elevated NGF are important, if true, as they represent the first molecular alteration in this disease and may serve as a useful marker in the future for individuals who are at risk. In an excellent review, Riccardi (481) cannot offer strong support to the hypothesis that NGF may be involved in the pathogenesis of disease. Fialkow et al. (187) studied female patients with neurofibromatosis who also were heterozygous for the A and B genes at the X-linked glucose-6-phosphate dehydrogenase locus, and demonstrated both type A and type B isoenzymes from tumor tissue. This interesting fact strongly indicates that hereditary neurofibromas have a multiple rather than a single-cell origin.

Clinical Manifestations

Neurofibromatosis, typical of dominantly inherited disease, can present in a variety of ways, but the presence of multiple cutaneous neurofibromas and café au lait pigmented skin lesions represents the hallmark of this disease. It has been estimated to be more frequent in incidence than Huntington's disease, Duchenne's dystrophy, and myotonic dystrophy combined. Its prevalence in the United States is 60 per 100,000 population. The pigmented lesions are smooth with regular borders and occur most commonly over the trunk and in the axilla. Such lesions can be found in persons not having this disorder; however, lesions greater than 3 cm in diameter and more than six in number are indicative of neurofibromatosis. Individual nerves of the extremities may be involved or the presentation may be multiple and diffuse. The brachial and sacral plexuses can also be affected with en plaque or plexiform neuromas. Multiple cranial nerves are affected as well, resulting in facial weakness, facial numbness, deafness, and visual loss with optic nerve atrophy. Multiple confluent tumors and fibrosis of the affected parts result in elephantiasis neuromatosa. A marked increase in the proliferation and overgrowth of skin and subcutaneous tissues of the skull, neck, and trunk can result in gross asymmetric hypertrophy. Neurofibromatosis may also produce massive leg edema in association with fibrous dysplasia of bone, as seen in Fig. 17. Neurofibromas associated with a nerve root can invade the intervertebral foramen and result in spinal cord compression or brainstem compression. Large neurofibromas of a cranial nerve produce increased intracranial pressure caused by hydrocephalus. Intracranial meningiomas, optic nerve gliomas, and astrocytomas occur in a number of patients. A tumor can present as a cerebellar pontine angle mass lesion with ipsilateral cerebellar signs. The 5th, 7th, 8th, and 10th cranial nerves are commonly involved with neurofibromas, producing facial muscle weakness, facial numbness, weakness of the muscles of mastication with atrophy and also deafness, and vertigo. Rarely, spontaneous fractures of vertebrae or long bones result because of fibro-dysplasia or cystic bone formation. Nodules on the iris, known as Lisch spots, are a common feature of the disorder. The combination of borderline mental retardation, familial pulmonary artery stenosis, and café au lait spots has been reported in a few families (Watson's syndrome).

The CSF protein is elevated in patients having large tumors that result in cord compression. Roentgenograms of the skull and internal auditory meatus show erosion caused by adjacent tumors.

Diagnosis

Neurofibromatosis is diagnosed readily by the occurrence of the characteristic neurofibromas and pigmented lesions of the skin. The tumors are often multiple and vary considerably in size. Most tumors are smooth, multilobulated, and can be palpated along the course of a peripheral nerve. More than six pigmented skin lesions with several greater than 3 cm in diameter indicate strongly the presence of neurofibromatosis. Hypertensive patients must be evaluated with urinary deter-minations of renin and catecholamines for the possiblities of renal artery stenosis, as well as for pheochromocytomas. Cranial nerve palsies, focal neurologic deficits, and hydrocephalus signal the presence of an intracranial neoplasm and the need for

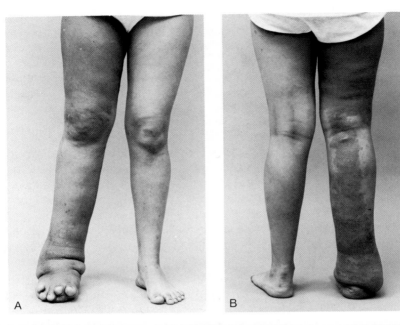

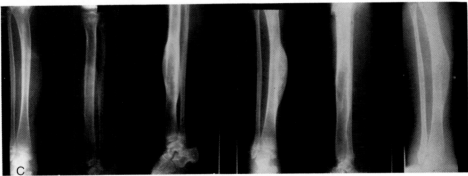

FIG. 17. Neurofibromatosis has produced massive edema of the leg in this 10-year-old child. Note the speckled pigmented lesions over the dorsum of the leg and foot **(A)** and a large café-au-lait spot on the posterior surface of the leg **(B)**. Roentgenograms of the leg are shown in **(C)** for 1978, 1979, and 1980, depicting a front and lateral view taken each year. Note the progressive fibrous dysplasia of bone shown with each year involving the tibia, which is representative of the metabolic bone disease associated with neurofibromatosis. (Courtesy of Dr. Jay Cook, University of Texas Southwestern Medical School at Dallas; from ref. 505, with permission.)

CT brain scans or angiography for precise definition. Cerebellopontine angle meningiomas and cranial nerve or spinal nerve tumors are usually resectable and must be considered in patients manifesting progressive brainstem or spinal cord deficits. There is no treatment for neurofibromatosis other than resection of symptomatic tumors and decompression of hydrocephalus.

TUBEROUS SCLEROSIS (BOURNEVILLE'S DISEASE)

Tuberous sclerosis (Bourneville's disease or epiloia) is a neurocutaneous disorder inherited as an autosomal dominant trait. Its triad of findings includes (a) facial nevi (adenoma sebaceum), (b) epilepsy, and (c) mental retardation. Although the clinical and neuropathologic features are well described, the basic biochemical defect remains unknown.

Pathology

The gross brain may have many firm nodules that are apparent on the surface. These firm nodules are also present in the deep layers of the cortex, the underlying white matter, the basal ganglia, and they line the lateral ventricles as projections; they are referred to as "candle gutterings." These nodules are also encountered in the substance of the spinal cord, brainstem, and cerebellum. The histologic appearance of the nodules shows a proliferation of primitive glia with multinucleated giant cells. Vascular malformations, meningiomas, gliomas, and hamartomas of the brain also occur.

The cutaneous lesions include characteristic facial nevi and areas of fibrosis. These nevi are not true adenomas of the sebaceous glands but rather take their origin from terminal nerves in the subcutaneous regions of the skin, together with a hyperplasia of connective tissue and blood vessels. Fundoscopic examination can disclose similar nodules or phakomas consisting of glial elements, fibroblasts, and ganglion cells arising from the retina. Rarely, an optic nerve glioma develops. Rhabdomyomas of the heart, renal tumors, and neoplasms of endocrine organs including testis, pancreas, ovary, and thyroid may occur. Rarely, an astrocytoma may occur in a child; for example, Fig. 18 shows a CT scan demonstrating an astrocytoma located in the head of the caudate nucleus of a young child.

Clinical Manifestations

The clinical appearance of the patient is characteristic. Patients develop mental retardation and epilepsy during the first decade of life. The first manifestation of disease is usually focal or generalized major motor seizures without other focal neurologic deficits. The occurrence of mental retardation is not evident until age 6 years. Several years after the development of seizures, the characteristic cutaneous facial lesions first develop. The facial nevi or sebaceous adenomas occur in a symmetrical distribution on the malar and nasal regions, and they appear yellow or orange-red in color, varying from several millimeters to a centimeter in size (Figs. 19 and 20). Areas of roughening of the skin (shagreen patches) in the shape of small spheres caused by fibrous hyperplasia, café au lait spots, areas of depigmented nevi, and, rarely, subungual neurofibromas are characteristic of tuberous sclerosis and are evidence for its being genetically related to von Recklinghausen's disease.

Neoplasms of the kidneys are common but usually not clinically evident. Tumors of endocrine organs and the liver occur rarely, and true rhabdomyomas occur in a

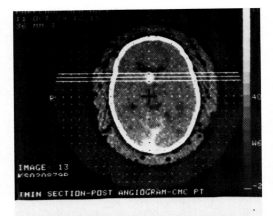

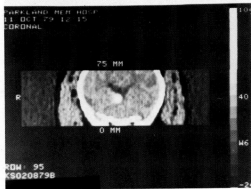

FIG. 18. CT brainscan showing the presence of a contrast-enhancing astrocytoma located in the head of the caudate nucleus of a young child with tuberous sclerosis. (From ref. 505, with permission.)

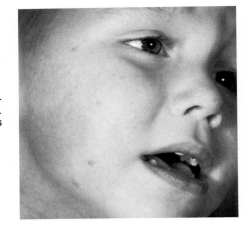

FIG. 19. Child with early skin lesions (adenoma sebaceum) of tuberous sclerosis. (Courtesy of Dr. M. E. Blaw, University of Texas Health Science Center at Dallas.)

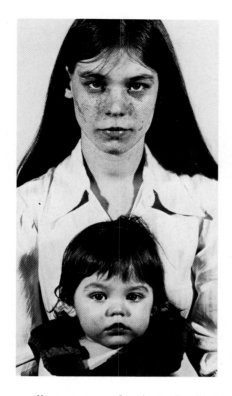

FIG. 20. A 19-year-old female patient with the typical adenoma sebaceous skin lesions of tuberous sclerosis. Her child also has tuberous sclerosis and a right hemiplegia. The mother further had a kidney hamartoma that was surgically removed. The 13-month-old child did have hypsarrhythmia on EEG, which responded to a ketogenic diet. Here is an example of autosomal dominant tuberous sclerosis present in both mother and child. (Courtesy of Dr. Jay Cook, University of Texas Southwestern Medical School at Dallas, Grune & Stratton, Inc., New York; from ref. 505, with permission.)

small percentage of patients. Papilledema and other focal neurologic deficits signal the presence of a large intracranial tumor.

The EEG may show focal slowing and multifocal spikes resulting from associated intracerebral phakomas. Hypsarrhythmia has been reported in a small number of patients. Roentgenograms of the skull may indicate the presence of calcifications in a periventricular distribution.

Diagnosis

This disorder is clearly identified when the triad of facial nevi, epilepsy, and mental retardation occurs. Examination of other family members should be carried out, as this is an autosomal dominant genetic disorder and the infant or child presenting with the onset of generalized seizures may not yet have the characteristic cutaneous lesions that can be clearly seen in older family members. The characteristic periventricular phakomas can be demonstrated with pneumoencephalography or CT brain scans. Large periventricular calcifications seen on skull roentgenograms are diagnostic as well. There is no specific treatment for this disorder, and seizures should be managed by appropriate anticonvulsant medication, while brain tumors or increased intracranial pressure should be managed by surgical intervention and shunting procedures.

STURGE-WEBER DISEASE

This neurocutaneous disease produces a port-wine-colored capillary hemangioma on the face; this is accompanied by a similar vascular malformation of the underlying meninges and cerebral cortex. The etiology is unknown, although the defect has been reported in more than one family member, which indicates a genetic predisposition.

Pathology

The cutaneous hemangioma follows the distribution of one or more divisions of the trigeminal nerve. A neural factor that affects blood vessel proliferation is assumed to be involved but has not yet been identified. The cerebral cortex may undergo atrophy with loss of nerve cells and a proliferation of glia. The capillaries of the cortex may show thickening and calcifications, especially in the second and third cortical layers. The distribution of cortical calcification clearly outlines the cortical mantle in a ribbonlike undulating manner. The atrophy and calcification of the cerebral cortex are presumed to be reactive to the angiomatous malformations of the meninges.

Clinical Manifestations

The diagnosis is easily made by the presence of a port-wine facial nevus following the sensory dermatomal distribution of the first, second, or third portion of the trigeminal nerve (Fig. 21). Generalized or focal motor seizures may also occur and may be associated with mental retardation. The patient may develop hemiplegic atrophy with shortening of the extremities, which occurs contralateral to the atrophic hemisphere with calcification. Exophthalmos, glaucoma, buphthalmos, optic atrophy, and other cutaneous port-wine nevi and retinal angiomas may also be present.

Diagnosis

The characteristic facial port-wine nevus with contralateral hemiparesis and hemiatrophy establishes the diagnosis of Sturge-Weber disease. Seizures and mental retardation are also present. Roentgenograms of the skull often demonstrate a parietooccipital distribution of calcification following the contour of cerebral gyri. There is no specific treatment, and seizures are managed with anticonvulsant drugs.

Differential Diagnosis

In the differential diagnosis, this entity must be distinguished from von Hippel-Lindau disease. The latter disorder is a familial disease inherited without a clear mendelian pattern; it produces hemangioblastomas of the cerebellar hemispheres with associated angiomas of the retina and cystic change in the kidney and pancreas. Sturge-Weber disease presents in early childhood with facial nevi and seizures. von Hippel-Lindau disease, on the other hand, presents in the fourth to sixth

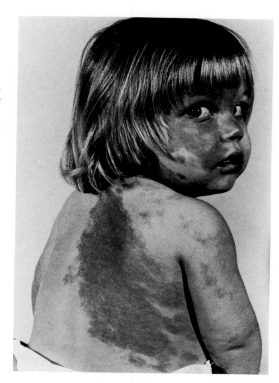

FIG. 21. A 16-month-old girl with Sturge-Weber disease. The capillary vascular lesion follows the distribution of the first and second division of the trigeminal nerve on the right side of her face only. A portion of the third division of the fifth nerve is also incompletely involved. In addition, dermatomal involvement between the first and seventh thoracic dermatomes is shown. It is characteristic for the vascular markings of this disorder to follow discrete dermatomal levels, suggesting a trophic interaction between peripheral nerve and developing capillaries in the fetus and the young child. (Courtesy of Dr. Jay Cook, University of Texas Southwestern Medical School at Dallas; from refs. 504 and 505, with permission.)

decades of life and is usually not associated with cutaneous vascular lesions; it presents with the acute occurrence of a cerebellar hemorrhage resulting in papilledema, impaired level of consciousness, and signs of cerebellar dysfunction. A clinical association with pheochromocytomas and polycythemia has been made in the same patient. The diagnosis of von Hippel-Lindau disease is made on the basis of the patient's presenting with an acute cerebellar lesion and an associated angiomatous tumor of the retina. A cerebellar hemorrhage from an angiomatous tumor requires prompt evaluation by CT scanning or angiography and surgical decompression of the posterior fossa with resection of the cerebellar tumor.

INCONTINENTIA PIGMENTI

This is a rare neurocutaneous disorder inherited in an X-linked dominant manner and recognized as early as 1906 by Garrod (214). It must be differentiated from neurofibromatosis, which is a more common neurocutaneous disorder but one that is inherited as an autosomal dominant. Pigmented skin lesions begin in the first 6 months of life and initially appear as vesicular or bullous eruptions. The skin lesions then become pigmented, forming brown linear patterns or whorls on the face, extremities, and abdomen (Fig. 22). There may be mental retardation, seizures, dystrophy of the fingernails, and alopecia in addition to the skin hyperpigmented lesions. In addition, microcephaly, hydrocephaly, microphthalmia, chorioretinitis,

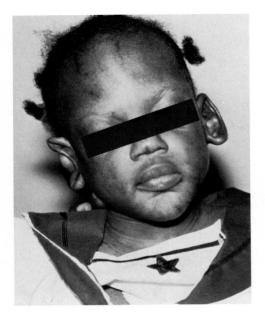

FIG. 22. A child 2 years old showing the characteristic linear hyperpigmented lesions of incontinentia pigmenti. There were three generations of seizures in her family, suggesting a dominant, probably X-linked form of inheritance. Note also the prominent dysmorphic shape of her external ear. (Courtesy of Dr. Jay Cook, University of Texas Southwestern Medical School at Dallas; from ref. 505, with permission.)

and spastic or flaccid quadriparesis may be associated features of the disease. The spectrum of findings was recorded by Sulzberger et al. in 1938 (584) and Carney in 1976 (86). Miller and Parker (401) reported a depigmented form of incontinentia pigmenti achromians (hypomelanosis of Ito) with a chromosome defect. A 6-month-old girl had seizures, the Wolf-Parkinson-White cardiac conduction defect, and a whorled pattern of hypopigmentation over the trunk and limbs. The patient had a balanced translocation between chromosomes 2 and 8. Parental karyotypes were normal. The patient was 46,XX,t(2,8)(q37.2;p21.1).

XERODERMA PIGMENTOSUM

This is a rare but severe disorder of the skin and nervous system. Patients have extreme sensitivity to sunlight or ultraviolet light, resulting in skin freckling, atrophy, and telangiectasia. The nervous system involvement can result in microcephaly, chorea, athetosis, ataxia, deafness, and mental retardation. Patients readily develop skin cancers including basal cell malignancies and melanomas. Medulloblastomas and neuromas also occur. The basic defect involves an impairment in DNA repair. The defect involves the removal of pyrimidine dimers because of deficient endonuclease activity. The patients whose cells in culture show the highest percentage of defect in DNA repair are the ones that develop neurologic disease. The patients with neurologic abnormalities (DeSanctis-Cacchione syndrome) have neuronal death of the pyramidal cells, Purkinje cells, and basal ganglia neurons. It is inherited as an autosomal recessive disorder with an incidence of between 1 per 65,000 and 1 per 250,000 births (218).

Disorders of Purine Metabolism

LESCH-NYHAN SYNDROME

Historical

In 1964 Lesch and Nyhan (352) described a familial disorder of uric acid metabolism with CNS dysfunction, and in 1966 Shapiro et al. (549) reported an X-linked recessive inherited syndrome of mental retardation and hyperuricemia. This was followed in 1967 by a report by Seegmiller et al. (545) of an enzyme defect associated with an X-linked human neurologic disorder (Lesch-Nyhan syndrome) with excessive purine synthesis in erythrocyte lysates and cultured skin fibroblasts. In 1968 the first *in utero* diagnosis of a heterozygous individual was achieved (318).

Incidence and Prevalence

The true incidence and prevalence are not known at this time, but this is a rare entity.

Genetics

This disorder is transmitted in an X-linked recessive fashion.

Clinical

Patients with Lesch-Nyhan syndrome are usually normal for the first 1 to 3 months of life, although some exhibit recurrent vomiting, feeding difficulties, and hypotonia. By 3 to 4 months the infants show signs of slowed motor development, and by 8 to 12 months they develop extrapyramidal signs. The extrapyramidal signs usually consist of combinations of chorea, athetosis, and dystonia of the extremities. These signs, however, are not specific for Lesch-Nyhan syndrome. Around 12 months of age, the patient begins to develop signs of pyramidal tract involvement such as hypertonia, hyperreflexia, and extensor plantar responses. The extrapyramidal and pyramidal signs become more prominent with the passage of time. Between 2 and 6 years of age, many patients develop a striking compulsive, self-destructive type of behavior, consisting of biting their lips, buccal mucosa, and accessible parts of their extremities, such as fingers and toes. These patients also exhibit head-banging and place their extremities in dangerous places. The urge to self-mutilation can be strikingly asymmetrical. Patients also exhibit unusual aggressiveness toward others, and the aggressiveness and self-mutilation can be quite variable from day to day. It has been suggested the aggressiveness is similar to "sham rage." The aggressiveness, agitation, episodes of opisthotonic posturing, and self-mutilation are all increased by placing the patients in stressful situations.

Approximately 50% of patients with Lesch-Nyhan syndrome have been reported to have seizures. Routine IQ testing methods have revealed IQs in the 39 to 65 range. When trying to assess intelligence of these patients, one has to take into consideration their dystonia and movement disorders.

Routine neurologic laboratory studies, including CSF studies, electromyography, and nerve conduction velocities, are normal. EEGs can either be normal or reveal diffuse slowing.

All patients exhibit excessive uric acid production, with excretion ranging from 25 to 143 mg/kg/day, compared with an upper limit of 18 mg/kg/day in normal children. The serum urate concentration ranges from 7 to 18 mg/dl in the absence of renal insufficiency. Because of this variability, determination of serum uric acid concentration is not a reliable screening test. The urine uric acid to creatinine ratio is a nonspecific but valuable screening test. The normal urine uric acid to creatinine ratio is up to 2.8 under 1 year of age and less than 1.0 for ages greater than 10 years. In Lesch-Nyhan syndrome the ratio may be greater than 5.0 for patients less than 10 years old and is usually in the range of 2.0 to 3.0 for patients older than 10 years. Other disorders that are associated with excessive uric acid production include type I glycogen storage disease and lymphoproliferative disorders.

Because of increased urinary uric acid excretion, uric acid cystalluria usually develops at some time in most patients and can lead to the finding of orange crystals on an infant's diaper. The excessive uric acid excretion can also lead to symptomatic uric acid nephrolithiasis and obstructive uropathy. Elevated serum uric acid can lead to gouty arthritis and tophaceous deposits of monosodium urate.

Diagnosis

The diagnosis is considered in a male patient who exhibits choreoathetosis, spasticity, self-mutilation, mental retardation, excessive production of uric acid, and hyperuricemia. The diagnosis is confirmed by finding virtual absence of activity of hypoxanthine-guanine phosphoribosyl transferase (HGPRT) in tissues, erythrocyte lysates, leukocytes, or cultured skin fibroblasts (317,318).

Pathology

In at least eight autopsied patients with Lesch-Nyhan syndrome, the most consistent finding was bilaterally shrunken kidneys with striking deposits of monosodium urate and uric acid. There have been no distinctive pathologic findings in the CNS. Those CNS findings that are present are thought to be either nonspecific or to reflect the severe uremia present prior to death.

Biochemical Findings

There exist two major pathways for purine synthesis in humans. One is a *de novo* pathway from smaller precursors including 5-phosphoribosyl-1-pyrophosphate (PP-ribose-P), glutamine, glycine, aspartate, formate, and bicarbonate through a common intermediate inosinic acid (IMP). The other is a salvage pathway in which free purine bases can be converted directly to their respective ribonucleotides by the appropriate purine phosphoribosyl-transferase in the presence of PP-ribose-P; HGPRT catalyzes the tranfer of the phosphoribosyl moiety of PP-ribose-P to the 9 position of hypoxanthine and guanine to form IMP or guanylic acid (GMP), respectively. The substrate for each HGPRT is $(Mg)_2$-PP-ribose-P.

The highest activity of HGPRT is in brain, and the highest brain activity is in the basal ganglia. There is relatively high activity in leukocytes, fibroblasts, and gonadal tissue, and in general, HGPRT activity is highest in rapidly dividing tissue. The native form of HGPRT is postulated to be a dimer or trimer of subunits of MW 26,000 to 34,500 daltons. Studies have shown a number of electrophoretic forms of the normal enzyme, all of which are immunologically identical, with the same substrate specificity, product inhibition, and degree of substrate inhibition.

In Lesch-Nyhan syndrome, because of decreased synthesis of purine, IMP, and GMP by the HGPRT-mediated salvage pathway, there is an increased *de novo* synthesis. The increased *de novo* synthesis is thought to be secondary to decreased IMP and GMP inhibition of *de novo* synthesis and to increased stimulation of *de novo* synthesis by increased PP-ribose-P. This leads to increased hypoxanthine and xanthine conversion to uric acid by the liver enzyme xanthine oxidase. Since the CNS lacks xanthine oxidase, it cannot convert hypoxanthine and xanthine to uric acid, and therefore hypoxanthine and xanthine levels in the CSF may be three times the plasma levels.

Other associated enzyme abnormalities in Lesch-Nyhan syndrome include increased enzyme activity of adenine phosphoribosyltransferase in erythrocytes; increased inosine 5'-phosphate dehydrogenase in erythrocytes but not in leukocytes or fibroblasts; increased orotate phosphoribosyltransferase and orotidine 5'-phosphate decarboxylase in erythrocytes and increased phosphoribosyl pyrophosphate synthetase in lymphoblasts and fibroblasts but not in erythrocytes. The pyrimidines, uridine diphosphate (UDP), uridine triphosphate (UTP), and cytidine triphosphate (CTP), are also increased in Lesch-Nyhan syndrome, presumably secondarily to increased PP-ribose-P.

Wilson et al. (639) recently reviewed HGPRT mutants of patients and found they are frequently caused by single base mutations that lead to deleterious amino acid substitutions. Major gene deletions or rearrangements in the HGPRT structural gene are rarely present. The majority of patients with the Lesch-Nyhan syndrome retain little if any enzyme protein, as the gene mutations lead to the synthesis of a labile enzyme or disturb the normal processing of HGPRT mRNA. It is suggested that mutations at junctions between coding and intervening sequences may be involved in some patients, as the structural gene contains many intervening sequences and there is a good precedent for such mutation sites in forms of β-thalassemia. It is not at all clear how the HGPRT enzyme defect results in the severe neurologic deficits. A basal ganglia and cortical neurotransmitter disorder involving peptidergic, purinergic, dopaminergic, and serotonergic systems has been implicated.

Yang et al. (648) reported on seven patients who were all found to be genetically distinct on Southern blots, indicating that new mutations occur commonly in this disorder. They predicted that multiple new mutations would be present, as patients fail to reproduce and the heterozygous state does not confer a selective advantage. Thus Haldane's (255) principle would predict that new mutations at the HGPRT locus must occur frequently in order for it to be maintained in the population. In fact, a new HGPRT variant has been described in a child having hyperuricemia and choreoathetosis with no HGPRT activity, but having normal intelligence and no self-mutilation (229).

Somatic gene therapy is becoming feasible for this disorder, since the HGPRT gene was cloned in 1983 by Jolly and associates (311). Recently Miller et al. (400) ligated a human cDNA corresponding to the human gene for HGPRT into a retroviral vector. Transfection of HGPRT-deficient cells with chimeric virus produced HGPRT-positive enzyme in human or rodent cells. These genetically transformed cells contained human HGPRT protein at levels similar to HGPRT in normal cells. The next step is to transfect rodent marrow cells with the hybrid vector and show expression of the human gene insert in the intact animal after marrow transplantation. The stage will then be set, it is hoped, so that sufficient enzyme will cross the blood-brain barrier to achieve therapeutic levels within the brain itself. A nice review of these points has recently appeared by Stein and Morrison (578).

Treatment

Although many specific therapeutic regimens have been tried in this disorder, none has been found to be of long-term benefit. Therefore, supportive measures and drug therapy (tranquilizers, sedatives) (allopurinol) for the disorder appear appropriate. Patients seem less agitated when they are restrained in a manner so that they cannot engage in self-mutilation. For the mutilation of the lips, nothing short of tooth extraction has proved to be of benefit in such patients.

Drugs such as diazepam, haloperidol, and phenobarbital appear to be helpful in treating the movement disorder. Levodopa has also been reported to be of some value. Recently Nyhan et al. (437,438) have treated a series of patients with 5-hydroxytryptophan in combination with the peripheral decarboxylase inhibitor carbidopa and with imipramine. As reported in their article, most patients had a striking alteration in self-mutilative behavior. Within 1 to 3 months, unfortunately, these patients became unresponsive to this therapeutic regimen, and a similar effect could not be reproduced 1 year later. It is important to note that a neuropharmacologic approach did improve patients on a short-term basis, and the behavioral abnormalities these children express may be due in part to CNS neurotransmitter imbalance.

Allopurinol effectively lowers the uric acid content of both serum and urine in patients with Lesch-Nyhan syndrome, and this drug can be used to prevent uric acid stone formation, uric acid and urate nephropathy, gouty arthritis, and the development of tophi. For these reasons patients with the Lesch-Nyhan syndrome should be treated with allopurinol. Uricosuric drug therapy probably should not be used unless allopurinol is also administered, because of the extremely large load of uric acid already being presented to the kidneys. The possibility of xanthine stone formation during allopurinol treatment can be minimized by increasing urine flow.

Prognosis

The prognosis is very poor for these patients at the present time because there is no specific treatment of the CNS aspect of this disorder; however, by minimizing the increased uric acid production by allopurinol and careful management to prevent renal complications of the disorder, the prognosis for life can be somewhat improved.

ADENOSINE DEAMINASE DEFICIENCY

An infantile syndrome caused by a deficiency of the purine salvage enzyme adenosine deaminase (ADA) has been clearly recognized, which includes severe combined immunodeficiency and severe motor and mental retardation. It is inherited as an autosomal recessive disorder. Pendular nystagmus, headlag, increased extensor muscle tone, dystonic and athetoid movements, absent deep tendon reflexes, and mental retardation are some clinical features. Profound lymphopenia, the absence of a thymic shadow, rib concavity, and flattened acetabula are other features. Serum IgA and IgM can be absent and IgG is very low. Peripheral blood lymphocytes do not respond to *in vitro* stimulation with phytohemagglutinin, and T and B cells may be absent. Delayed skin tests for reactivity to dinitrochlorobenzene (DNCB) are nonreactive. ADA deficiency is confirmed by measurement of the enzyme in red blood cells. Neurologic abnormalities have been reported in three of 23 ADA-deficient patients. Importantly, neurologic abnormalities disappeared in one patient during treatment with multiple partial-exchange transfusions of irradiated normal erythrocytes, thus providing enzyme replacement (276).

FAMILIAL PYRIMIDINEMIA AND PYRIMIDINURIA ASSOCIATED WITH FLUOROURACIL TOXICITY

Recently, an autosomal recessive disorder has been described in which patients manifest pyrimidinemia or pyrimidinuria with impairment in level of consciousness progressing to coma and associated with cerebellar deficits when treated with fluorouracil. A 27 year old woman with a breast malignancy was treated with modest doses of fluorouracil and rapidly developed a severe leukopenia, thrombocytopenia, stomatitis, hair loss, diarrhea, fever, weight loss, dysarthria, cerebellar ataxia progressing to confusion, and semicoma. Her neurological symptoms gradually improved when the drug was stopped, but she continued to excrete high amounts of uracil and thymine. Plasma levels of uracil and thymine were also elevated. Her normal brother also had pyrimidinemia indicating that the patient just described had a genetic defect in pyrimidine metabolism which was made clinically manifest when treated with fluorouracil. A defect in the degradation of uracil and thymine is postulated in these individuals and was responsible for an impairment in the degradation of fluorouracil as well. Dihydropyrimidine dehydrogenase, the rate limiting enzyme in pyrimidine metabolism, is postulated as being defective in this patient and her brother as described by Tuchman and associates (606).

Hereditary Cerebral Angiopathy with Cerebral Hemorrhage and Amyloidosis

Hereditary cerebral hemorrhage due to an angiopathy associated with amyloidosis is an uncommon event compared with hypertension-induced cerebral hemorrhage. Arnason in 1935 (17) published a report showing 10 families with a high incidence of cerebral hemorrhage. More recently the fibrillar components of the amyloid deposits in cerebral arteries were isolated and were found to consist of large fragments of the alkaline microprotein γ-trace (240). Patients with hereditary cerebral hemorrhage with amyloidosis had lowest CSF values for γ-trace, and the data are compatible with the hypothesis that the basic defect in this disease is an abnormal metabolism of γ-trace and the abnormality resides in the catabolic processing of the γ-trace. Grubb et al. (240) also point out that the very low concentration of γ-trace in CSF in patients compared with controls can be used as an index in the diagnosis of this serious disorder.

Disorders of Amino Acid Metabolism

PHENYLKETONURIA

This disorder of amino acid metabolism is the most common one in our society, with an incidence of disease in the United States of 1 in 14,000 births, and fortunately it is treatable. It was described originally by Folling (195) in patients who were retarded and excreted urinary phenylpyruvic acid. Based on this excretion product, Penrose and Quastel (455) called it phenylketonuria (PKU). The enzyme defect for this autosomal recessive disorder involves hepatic phenylalanine hydroxylase (304). The therapeutic value of diet restricted in phenylalanine was reported by Bickel et al. (48), and heterozygote identification with a phenylalanine challenge was reported by Hsia et al. (287).

Clinical Features

In general, children at birth are normal, although neonatal disorders, especially vomiting and eczema, have been cited as being increased in incidence. A characteristic odor due to elevated phenylacetic acid in perspiration has been emphasized.

During the first 12 months of life progressive mental retardation and hypopigmentation of hair, skin, and the ocular iris occur. It has been suggested that this hypopigmentation is due to inhibition of tyrosinase by the high titers of phenylalanine in tissues. If patients are not treated early, a very high percentage of them will be severely mentally retarded.

A simple diagnostic test is the ferric chloride test, which produces a vivid green color in the presence of phenylpyruvic acid. A more reliable test is the Guthrie test (246), which gives a more quantitative assessment of blood phenylalanine levels and avoids the false negative assessment of the ferric chloride test in some patients. An abnormal serum phenylalanine is that above 20 mg% in a child older than 1 week and on an average protein and calorie diet.

A major recent advance occurred in 1983 when Woo et al. (645) cloned the gene for phenylalanine hydroxylase and showed its usefulness in diagnosing affected persons, carriers, and noncarriers by showing distinctive patterns of hybridization signals on Southern blots (Fig. 23).

In 1985 DiLella et al. (133) observed two variations of PKU at the mRNA level. The liver from one PKU patient contained abundant phenylalanine hydroxylase mRNA, which was identical in size to normal mRNA. Thus low levels of enzyme activity in this patient are the result of defective or unstable enzyme rather than a transcriptional error from the gene level into its mRNA. Another patient of theirs had barely detectable liver levels of phenylalanine hydroxylase mRNA. Thus this patient had a transcriptional error, and minimal enzyme protein would be synthesized. Thus there is evidence now for molecular variability for the clinical expression of this disorder. In 1985 a full-length cDNA clone of human phenylalanine hydroxylase was inserted into a eukaryotic expression vector and transferred into mouse NIH3T3 cells that usually do not express it. The transformed mouse cells expressed enzyme mRNA. Thus a single gene contains all of the necessary genetic information to code for functional enzyme (347).

Lidsky et al. (354) reported diagnosing classic PKU prenatally in two at risk families by means of a cloned phenylalanine hydroxylase gene probe that was used to analyze DNA isolated from cultured amniotic cells. The diagnoses of a PKU fetus in one family and a heterozygous fetus in another family were confirmed after birth.

Neuropathology

The brain from a PKU patient shows impressive loss of myelin in the cerebral hemispheres and cerebellum. Neuronal loss in the cerebral and cerebellar cortices also occurs associated with gliosis.

Treatment

The use of a diet low in phenylalanine started within a few days after birth provides the best chance for avoiding retardation. A delay in beginning such a dietary regimen can result in severe mental impairment. It is important to have the

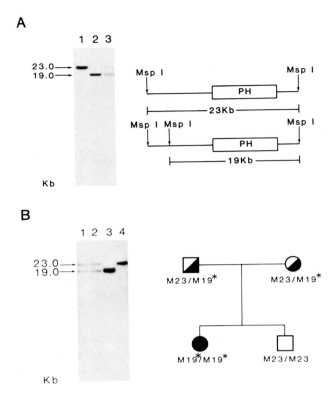

FIG. 23. Msp I restriction fragment length polymorphism in the phenylalanine hydroxylase (PH) gene. **A:** PH gene with polymorphism for a 23-kb and a 19-kb fragment. **B:** Family pedigree in which PKU occurs in a daughter who is homozygous for both alleles for the 19-kb fragment and has clinical PKU. Her parents are heterozygous, and a brother is genotypically normal, having both alleles containing the 23-kb fragment. Thus the mutant PH gene is carried by the 19-kb fragment in this family, and the diagnosis of PKU and carriers can be achieved using a cDNA probe for the PH gene and Msp I as the restriction enzyme. (From ref. 645, with permission.)

serum phenylalanine remain between 3 and 10 mg%, as lower levels will also produce neurologic impairment. It is not absolutely clear how long a child should be maintained on such a diet. It is suggested that it should be strictly enforced until 10 to 12 years of age, tapered yearly with frequent monitoring of mental functioning. Pregnant patients who have PKU also should be placed on the diet to prevent the child who does not genetically have the syndrome from developing a toxic hyperphenylalaninemic encephalopathy due to the placental passage of toxic levels of phenylalanine from the mother (Mabry syndrome) (370).

In addition to classic PKU there have been described at least eight other syndromes with associated hyperphenylalanemia. Various deficiencies of phenylalanine hydroxylase have been reported with mild elevations of serum phenylalanine, which often return to normal with development. A deficiency of dihydropteridine reductase, the cofactor of phenylalanine hydroxylase, has been described in patients with marked mental retardation and seizures in whom there is no clinical response to a diet low in phenylalanine. These patients need to be treated with high doses of folic acid, L-DOPA, and L-tryptophan to provide the developing brain with adequate substrate and cofactor to synthesize dopamine, serotonin, and norepinephrine.

HOMOCYSTINURIA

This is a common aminoacidopathy with an incidence in the United States of 1 in 200,000 births. It was described in patients who were retarded and excreted homocystine (87). Mudd et al. (417) described the enzyme defect to be cystathionine β-synthase for this autosomal recessive disorder. Holowell et al. (280) demonstrated that pyridoxine (vitamin B_6) could increase enzyme activity and lower excretion of homocystine in selected patients.

Clinical Features

Patients develop a characteristic clinical picture that includes mental retardation, ectopia lentis, scoliosis, genu valgum, pectus carinatum or excavatum, a high arched palate, pes cavus, thromboembolism, a malar flush, and prominent livido reticularis. Seizures may be present in a small percentage of patients, and about 10% of patients are mentally normal.

A few patients present in childhood or early adulthood with a schizophrenic-like behavior, homocystinuria, and hypomethioninemia. Their cystathionine β-synthase activity is normal, and they have a methionine regeneration shuttle that is defective because of vitamin B_{12} or folic acid synthesis or reductase enzyme defects.

Neuropathology

Patients may suffer acute infarctions caused by thrombosis of cerebral vessels. Demyelination and neuronal loss of the hippocampus and cerebral cortex have also been reported.

Treatment

A diet low in methionine is the mainstay of therapy. Vitamin B_6 administration may induce the enzyme cystathione β-synthase in selected patients. Patients with a methionine regeneration shuttle defect require vitamin B_{12} and folate therapy to maximize conversion of homocysteine to methionine.

The treatment of homocystinuria that is not responsive to pyridoxine is usually not biochemically or clinically effective, as pointed out by Wilcken et al. (637). They treated 10 patients with cystathionine β-synthase deficiency that was not responsive to pyridoxine and one patient with homocystinuria caused by a defect in cobalamin metabolism with 6 g daily of betaine added to conventional therapy. Betaine therapy was intended to improve homocysteine remethylation. All treated patients had significant decreases in plasma total homocysteine levels and increases in total cysteine levels. In six patients with betaine therapy, there was immediate clinical improvement. Wilcken et al. conclude that treatment of homocystinuria not responsive to pyridoxine and of disorders of homocysteine remethylation should include betaine in doses to ensure maximum lowering of elevated plasma homo-cysteine levels.

Schuh et al. (537) reported a unique case of an inborn error of vitamin B_{12} metabolism in an infant who had severe developmental delay, megaloblastic anemia, and homocystinuria. Treatment with hydroxycobalamin but not with cyanocobalamin and folic acid resulted in rapid clinical and biochemical improvement. The intracellular defect was in methionine synthesis.

METHYLMALONIC ACIDURIA

These patients have a marked motor and mental retardation, often with generalized seizures and ketoacidosis (439,495). Patients may improve biochemically and clinically with high doses of vitamin B_{12} (495). Defects in the enzymes methylmalonyl-CoA racemose and mutase as well as in B_{12} synthetic enzymes have been reported as being associated with this syndrome. It is presumed to be inherited as an autosomal recessive disorder. Another subset of patients consists of those in which methylmalonic aciduria was also present with homocystinuria, cystathioni-nuria, and hypomethioninemia, and these patients were not ketoacidotic.

Treatment consists of a low-protein diet and high doses of vitamin B_{12} for those who respond biochemically with reduced methylmalonic acid excretion and improved mental status. L-Carnitine oral therapy has been advocated in a loading dose of 100 mg/kg, followed by 100 mg/kg/day divided into three or four doses (14,582).

PROPIONIC ACIDEMIA

Patients present in the neonatal period with obtundation, coma, dehydration, and ketoacidosis. Propionic acidemia and aciduria with a deficiency of the enzyme propionyl-CoA carboxylase in fibroblasts or leukocytes are diagnostic of the syndrome. It is inherited as an autosomal recessive. Therapy includes a low-protein diet, vigorous rehydration, and correction of acidosis with bicarbonate. Biotin, a cofactor of propionyl-CoA carboxylase, is given to patients who respond with improvement biochemically and clinically. L-Carnitine oral therapy has been advocated in a loading dose of 100 mg/kg followed by 100 mg/kg/day divided into three or four doses (14,582).

HYPERGLYCINEMIA

This autosomal recessive disorder has as its clinical features neonatal to early childhood onset of episodic ketoacidosis with motor and mental retardation and with hyperglycinemia and hyperglycinuria. During acute episodes urinary excretion of α-methyl-β-hydroxybutyrate, α-methyl acetoacetate, and butanone increases.

If the disorder is diagnosed promptly and proper therapy of protein restriction and correction of acute attacks of acidosis implemented, it is possible for relatively normal development to occur in patients (120,436).

GLUTARIC ACIDEMIA

This autosomal recessive disorder presents as childhood onset mental and motor retardation with glutaric acidemia and aciduria. There may be clinical hypotonia, dystonic posturing, and choreoathetosis. The enzyme defect involves glutaryl-CoA dehydrogenase (349). Minor improvement has been reported with a diet low in lysine and tryptophan, which produces a significant reduction in serum and urinary levels of glutaric acid.

MAPLE SYRUP URINE DISEASE

In 1954 Menkes et al. (394) described a family in which four of six siblings in early neonatal life presented with a syndrome of vomiting, hypertonia, and a urinary odor resembling that of maple syrup. Westall et al. in 1957 (633) described a child with elevated serum and urine levels of leucine, isoleucine, and valine. A late onset form of the disorder was described by Morris et al. in 1961 (410). The incidence of disease is about 1 in 290,000 births. It is an autosomal recessive disorder caused by a defect in the enzyme branched-chain amino acid decarboxylase as measured in leukocytes or fibroblasts. Clinical features include neonatal failure to thrive, vomiting, lethargy, and a maple syrup odor of the urine. Patients may also develop hypotonicity and seizures. Occasionally hypoglycemia will develop that is probably secondary to elevated serum leucine, isoleucine, and valine. There is considerable heterogeneity in clinical severity (113).

Treatment consists of a diet reduced in branched-chain amino acids with careful monitoring of serum leucine, isoleucine, and valine to maintain them within a normal range.

HYPERVALINEMIA

A single patient has been reported to date who presented with failure to thrive and vomiting. The child, who was of Japanese extraction, was mentally retarded, had hypervalinemia (622), and had a disorder of valine transamination (113). The child improved with a low-valine diet. This is an autosomal recessive disorder caused by a defect in the transamination reaction coverting valine to α-keto-isovaleric acid.

ISOVALERIC ACIDEMIA

This is an autosomal recessive disorder in which young children present with mental retardation, a body odor resembling sweaty feet or cheese, and increased levels of isovaleric acid in serum and urine. Such a syndrome was reported originally by Tanaka et al. in 1966 (591) in siblings 2½ and 4 years of age. The initial presentation is similar to that of maple syrup urine disease, with a severe acidosis, failure to thrive neonatally, neurologic deterioration leading to coma, and a high mortality in the first 3 months of life. The abrupt onset of acidosis and neurologic deterioration is often induced by acute infections.

It is presumed that the enzyme defect is isovaleryl-CoA dehydrogenase.

Therapy includes a diet low in leucine enriched with lipid, carbohydrate, and vitamins until the isovaleric acid levels achieve a normal value. With acute therapeutic intervention the outcome is significantly improved.

METHYLCROTONYLGLYCINURIA

This is an autosomal recessive disorder first reported by Eldjarn et al. (155) in a 4-and-a-half-month-old girl whose parents were first cousins. The child presented with a clinical picture of spinal muscular atrophy and excreted excessive levels of β-hydroxyisovaleric acid and β-methylcrotonylglycine. Subsequently Gompertz et al. (227) reported a second case in a 5-month-old infant with acidosis, rash, and vomiting who also had increased urine excretory levels of β-methylcrotonylglycine and diglylglycine. The child improved clinically and biochemically when treated with biotin at 10 mg/day.

Therapy consists of leucine restriction in the diet and biotin administration, and when treatment is begun early in the course the prognosis is favorable.

GLUTAMYL-RIBOSE-5-PHOSPHATE STORAGE

Historical

Williams et al. (638) described a 6-year-old boy with seizures, neurologic deterioration, and proteinuria.

Genetics

This is presumably an X-linked recessive disorder with storage of glutamyl-ribose-5-phosphate caused by a postulated defect of an ADP-ribose protein hydrolase.

Clinical Presentation

A 2-year-old boy developed normally, but then his speech and language deteriorated. He developed seizures at 3 years of age and was microcephalic. He developed proteinuria, and a renal biopsy showed focal segmental and global glomerulosclerosis. There was progressive deterioration in neurologic and renal function, and he died at 8 years of age. A maternal uncle had a similar clinical presentation and died at 7 years of age with seizures, mental retardation, nephrotic syndrome, optic atrophy, hypertension, and hyporeflexia (638).

Pathology

The brain described by Williams et al. (638) was that of an 8-year-old boy which was atrophied, weighing 860 g (normal weight for age = 1,273 g). The cerebral cortex, basal ganglia, cerebellum, dentate nucleus, and pontine and roof nuclei had moderate to marked neuronal loss affecting all layers. There was end-stage renal disease. Electron microscopy of connective tissue cells in a conjunctival biopsy showed lysosomes containing granular and multilamellar material.

Biochemistry

The activities of enzymes in leukocytes and cultured skin fibroblasts known to be responsible for lysosomal storage disease were normal. Chromatography of an acetic acid extract of brain and kidney showed an abnormal carbohydrate-containing peak. The structure of the stored material was shown to be glutamyl-ribose-5-phosphate. The postulated enzyme defect is ADP-ribose protein hydrolase.

Diagnosis

This disorder is identified by the early childhood progressive deterioration of neurologic and renal functions, normal lysosomal enzymes for the common storage disorders, and identification of glutamyl-ribose-5-phosphate on a renal biopsy.

Treatment

No specific therapy is available.

HISTIDINEMIA (HISTIDASE DEFICIENCY)

This is a rare autosomal recessive aminoacidopathy characterized by elevated histidine in serum and urine with a reduced activity of the enzyme histidase. Clinical features include partial deafness, delayed speech development, and moderately severe mental retardation. The metabolic defect is an inability to convert histidine to urocanic acid because of a deficient activity of histidase. A positive urine ferric chloride test is caused by elevated levels of imidazole pyruvic acid. It has an incidence in the United States of about 1 in 18,000 newborns. Some patients have shown some histidase activity in skin, suggesting a heterogeneous syndrome. A dominant pedigree has also been reported. Therapy is limited for practical purposes to a diet low in histidine (78,338).

TRIOSEPHOSPHATE ISOMERASE DEFICIENCY

Triosephosphate isomerase (TPI) (EC 5.3.1.1) deficiency results in a syndrome characterized by chronic hemolytic anemia with progressive neurological dysfunction. It may also be associated with an increased susceptibility to infection. This enzyme (TPI) catalyzes the interconversion of glyceraldehyde phosphate and dehydroxyacetone phosphate in the glycolytic pathway. It was first described as an enzyme deficiency disorder in 1965 by Schneider et al. (534), and its inheritance is autosomal recessive. About 18 cases have now been reported. Clinical features include dystonia, tremor, corticospinal deficits, and muscle atrophy due to anterior horn cell disease. Optic disc pallor may be present. Intelligence is usually maintained. These neurological deficits begin about 2 years of age and continue on a progressive basis through childhood (467). No treatment is available.

HARTNUP DISEASE

This is an autosomal recessive disorder caused by an intestinal transport defect for tryptophan that results in ataxia, mental retardation, and a pellagra-like skin rash. It owes its name to the first patient with this disease, reported by Baron et al. (31). It has as its characteristic amino acid pattern the excretion of increased amounts of neutral amino acids. It occurs in about 1 in 16,000 newborns, thus indicating the mutation is not a rare one. Treatment with nicotinamide, 50 to 300 mg/day, has resulted in improvement in the skin rash and neurologic deficits.

LOWE'S SYNDROME (OCULOCEREBRORENAL SYNDROME)

Lowe et al. (360) described an X-linked recessive syndrome associated with mental retardation, hypotonia, cataract, corneal lesions, glaucoma, and rickets. Renal hypophosphatemic rickets with low normal or decreased serum phosphate and elevated alkaline phosphatase, and normal serum calcium with metabolic acidosis, are typical features. Life span is limited to the late childhood years, and death results from renal insufficiency, metabolic acidosis, or infection.

Urea Cycle Enzyme Defects

OVERVIEW

For each of the five enzymes of the urea cycle, an inherited deficiency has been described, and the overall prevalence of disease is 1 in 30,000 live births (Fig. 24). A child who is born with an absolute deficiency of one urea cycle enzyme appears normal at 24 hr of life, but the symptoms of hyperammonemia begin in about 1 week. These include feeding difficulties, impaired level of consciousness, vomiting, and seizures.

Msall et al. (416) studied the neurologic outcome in 26 children with inborn errors of urea synthesis. There was a 92% survival rate at 1 year with nitrogen restriction therapy and stimulation of alternative pathways of waste nitrogen excretion. Seventy-nine percent of the children had one or several developmental disabilities between 12 and 74 months of age, and their mean IQ was 43 ± 6. Msall et al. further found a direct negative linear correlation between duration of stage 3 or 4 neonatal hyperammonemic coma and IQ at 1 year, and a significant correlation between CT abnormalities and duration of hyperammonemic coma. There was also

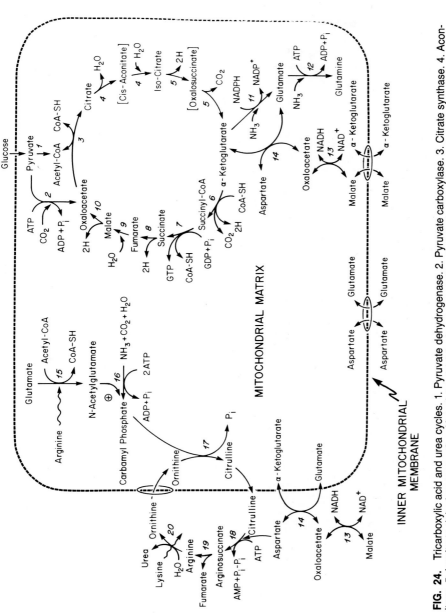

FIG. 24. Tricarboxylic acid and urea cycles. 1. Pyruvate dehydrogenase. 2. Pyruvate carboxylase. 3. Citrate synthase. 4. Aconitase. 5. Isocitrate dehydrogenase. 6. α-Ketoglutarate dehydrogenase. 7. Succinyl-CoA synthetase. 8. Succinate dehydrogenase. 9. Fumarase. 10. Malate dehydrogenase. 11. L-Glutamate dehydrogenase. 12. Glutamine synthetase. 13. Malate dehydrogenase. 14. Aspartate aminotransferase. 15. Glutamate acetyltransferase. 16. Carbamyl phosphate synthetase. 17. Ornithine carbamayl-transferase. 18. Argininosuccinate synthetase. 19. Argininosuccinate lyase. 20. Arginase. (From ref. 505, with permission.)

a good correlation between CT abnormalities and concurrent IQ. They conclude that a poor outcome for children can be prevented by early diagnosis and aggressive therapy.

The urea cycle was described by H. A. Krebs and K. Henseleit in 1932, and a 20-year perspective on it was republished by Krebs in 1951 (331). In summary, the ammonia nitrogen of the body is generated by aspartate, glutamate, glutamine, and asparagine, and the amino derivatives by the purines adenine and guanine. In general, the cycle includes five separate enzyme steps and converts two amino nitrogen moieties and one mole of carbon dioxide to yield one molecule of urea. It is a hepatic cycle for practical purposes, as only the liver has a significant urea production rate. Brain does possess carbamyl phosphate synthetase, ornithine transcarbamylase, and arginase, but in general their activities are too low for practical clinical purposes.

Carbamyl phosphate synthetase and ornithine transcarbamylase are associated with mitochondrial membrane, and the last three cycle enzymes are present in the cell's cytoplasm. Energy-specific transport systems are utilized for ornithine transport into the mitochondria and for citrulline transport from it. Shih and Efron (550) reported that acetylglutamate synthesis may be regulatory for ammonia entry into the urea cycle initially. This subject was recently reviewed by Walser (623a).

CARBAMYL PHOSPHATE SYNTHETASE DEFICIENCY

It was relatively recently that Freeman et al. (202) reported the first case of carbamyl phosphate synthetase (CPT) deficiency in a patient who at 5 weeks of age had an elevated blood ammonia of 480 μg/dl and CSF ammonia of 550 μg/dl and who clinically by the second week of life was hypotonic, obtunded, and dehydrated. This is a rare syndrome, with fewer than 10 patients reported.

It is inherited as an autosomal recessive disorder.

Patients have a real dislike of protein-rich food, and clinical improvement occurs on a diet restricted to 1.0 to 1.5 g of protein/kg body weight/day. The keto derivatives of the essential amino acids can be useful as well by providing a substrate source for ammonia fixation. This approach has had clinical utility and may be useful in the future for chronic therapy and resolution of acute attacks of lethargy, seizures, and dehydration.

ORNITHINE TRANSCARBAMYLASE DEFICIENCY

Ornithine transcarbamylase (OTC) deficiency is more common than CPT deficiency, as 38 patients in 33 families had been described by 1972 (550).

Clinical Features

Patients appear normal at birth but rapidly a syndrome of obtundation, failure to thrive, seizures, and altered muscle tone develops. Coma and neurologic deterioration to death may rapidly ensue in the first week of life. It is inherited as an

X-linked dominant disorder, with a severe clinical expression and total absence of OTC activities in males and a variation in clinical severity and enzyme activity in heterozygous women. Short et al. (551) described two populations of hepatic cells in a heterozygous female, of which one did not have OTC activity and the other had normal OTC activity. Presumably the variation in clinical severity in heterozygous women is related to random inactivation of the X chromosome by the Lyon hypothesis, which in turn determines cell population distributions for normal and OTC-deficient cells.

Neuropathology

Two brains have been reported by Brutton et al. (79) in which there was ventricular enlargement associated with cerebral cortical neuronal loss, white matter loss, and increased numbers of Alzheimer type II astrocytes, which are a reflection of hyperammonemia.

Biochemistry and Genetics

The mammalian hepatic enzyme OTC is a nuclear-coded mitochondrial protein. It is synthesized on cytosolic ribosomes as a precursor molecule (40 kD) and transported into the mitochondria and processed into its final, active form (36 kD). It is a trimer of identical subunits and catalyzes the second step of the urea cycle, the condensation of carbamyl phosphate with ornithine to form citrulline. The structural gene is located on the X chromosome in human and mouse. The transport of precursor OTC is energy dependent, and cleavage of the leader sequence is catalyzed by a Zn^{2+}-dependent matrix protease (284).

Horwich et al. (284) further have deduced the complete primary structure of the precursor from the nucleotide sequence of cloned cDNA. They found the sequence of mature human OTC resembles that of the subunits of both OTC and aspartate transcarbamylase from *Escherichia coli*. They tested the biological activity of the cloned OTC cDNA by joining it with SV40 regulatory elements and transfected cultured HeLa cells, which do not normally express OTC. Both precursor and processed OTC subunit were identified and enzyme activity detected (284).

Lindgren et al. (357) have mapped the OTC gene to the short arm of the X chromosome by *in situ* hybridization experiments with DNA complementary to the human OTC gene as their probe (see Chapter 1; Figs. 8 and 9). A series of cell lines having X chromosome abnormalities were instrumental in localizing the gene to band Xp21.1. They point out that this locus is also near the Duchenne's muscular dystrophy locus, and so the cDNA probe for the OTC gene may be useful in carrier detection and prenatal diagnosis of Duchenne's muscular dystrophy as well as of OTC deficiency.

Old et al. (442), using a cDNA probe for OTC and two other X-chromosome-specific probes, hybridized them to fetal DNA obtained from cultured amniocytes. In one family in which a son was born with OTC, the next pregnancy was monitored using the probes, and the fetus was shown to be a normal male. Rozen et al. (512), using a full-length human cDNA for OTC, found a partial deletion of the OTC gene in one of 15 affected males.

Therapy is similar to that for CPT deficiency, including protein restriction, keto acid derivative administration to provide a substrate for ammonia fixation, and intravenous fluids for dehydration.

ARGININOSUCCINIC ACID SYNTHETASE DEFICIENCY (CITRULLINEMIA)

Clinical Features

This is an autosomal recessive disorder caused by the deficiency of the enzyme argininosuccinic acid synthetase (ASA). The clinical syndrome, which emphasized severe vomiting and mental retardation, was described initially by McMurray et al. in 1962 (389), and the enzyme abnormality was described by Tedesco and Mellman in 1967 (594).

The clinical manifestations include neonatal, late infantile, childhood, and early adult onset forms. The neonatal form presents with the onset in the first few days of life with lethargy, tachypnea, vomiting, irritability, and failure to thrive, proceeding to seizures, coma, and death. Citrulline is significantly elevated in serum, urine, and CSF. Hyperammonemia is also an important feature. Associated laboratory findings include metabolic acidosis, hypocalcemia, hypoglycemia, elevated serum glutamic-oxaloacetic transaminase, and hyperammonemia. Episodes of lethargy, acidosis, and hyperammonemia may be severe and carry a high mortality. Similar presentations have been reported in the late infantile period. A 4-year-old child with normal development was detected by a routine screening program. A 21-year-old patient with ASA deficiency and hyperammonemia was evaluated for episodes of dysarthria, irritability, insomnia, visual defects, and delirium. Mental evaluation indicated a normal intelligence and a minor hand tremor. He developed a spastic paraparesis but no episodic neurologic dysfunction while treated with a protein-restricted diet along with neomycin and L-arginine.

Neuropathology

There is neuronal loss, demyelination, and Alzheimer type II astrocytosis.

Biochemistry and Genetics

ASA was reduced in activity and had an altered K_m or Michaelis constant. The enzyme has been mapped to chromosome 9. A cDNA probe for ASA (40) was developed, and 10 gene copies have been found per haploid genome, spread over 8 chromosomes, including the X and the Y.

ARGININOSUCCINASE DEFICIENCY

Clinical Features

This is an autosomal recessive disorder caused by argininosuccinase deficiency with associated argininosuccinic aciduria (4,602). It has been diagnosed antenatally (228), and normal brain and kidney enzyme activity have been reported, with absent liver enzyme activity (222).

Neonatal, subacute, and late onset forms have been reported. The neonatal type begins in the first few weeks of life, and its features include failure to thrive, lethargy, seizures, coma, hepatomegaly, and dry brittle hair, referred to as trichorrhexis nodosa. The hair disorder may be related more directly to the low-protein diet. Older children develop delayed motor and mental milestones, with IQs usually in the 30 to 60 range. Ataxis of gait and seizures develop in one-third of patients.

Patients have hyperammonemia with elevated amounts of argininosuccinic acid in serum, urine, and CSF. Argininosuccinase is deficient in liver, fibroblasts, and amniotic fluid cells.

Neuropathology

There is neuronal loss, degeneration of myelin, and a proliferation of Alzheimer type II astrocytes.

Therapy

The conventional therapy for acidosis, dehydration, and hyperammonemia is employed. Use of arginine has been successful to aid in the formation of argininosuccinic acid.

Genetics

The several clinical forms are probably caused by allelic modifications of the enzyme. The enzyme locus has been assigned to chromosome 7 by Naylor et al. (427).

ARGINASE DEFICIENCY (ARGININEMIA)

Clinical Features

This is an autosomal recessive disorder, and patients present with seizures, vomiting, and failure to thrive proceeding to mental retardation, spastic paraplegia, ataxia, and hepatomegaly. The syndrome was reported initially by Terheggen et al. (595), who described two sisters with hyperargininemia and arginase deficiency. Arginine values were intermediate in both parents and in two normal siblings. Arginase activity was also intermediate in the parents.

Therapy

The fact that research workers using the Shope virus had low blood arginine levels led to the use of the Shope virus as a means of therapy (491). Although Shope virus can induce arginase activity in patient fibroblast cultures, its practical value apparently is limited, and the mainstay of therapy is to treat hyperammonemia in the conventional manner.

Glycogen Storage Diseases

A series of enzyme defects involving glycogen degradation have been described in a group of autosomal recessive or X-linked recessive disorders. As a result of these enzyme abnormalities, glycogen accumulates in liver to values much in excess of the normal 5 to 7 g/100 g wet weight or in muscle to values greater than 2 g/ 100 g wet weight. The human fetus begins to store some glycogen in liver in the last trimester of pregnancy, and adult glycogen values are achieved by the first month of age (132,285,297) (Fig. 25). Howell and Williams have recently reviewed this subject in detail (286a).

TYPE I GLYCOGEN STORAGE DISEASE (GLUCOSE-6-PHOSPHATASE DEFICIENCY, VON GIERKE'S DISEASE)

This is a rare autosomal recessive disorder described by von Gierke in 1929 (619), with an incidence of 1 in 50,000, caused by a defect in the enzyme glucose-6-phosphatase.

Clinical Features

Patients present in the newborn period with severe hepatomegaly, hypoglycemia, seizures, and failure to thrive. Older children are short in stature and tend to appear slightly obese with muscle hypotonia. Yellow-appearing, paramacular retinal lesions are noted in some patients. Some patients have a bleeding disorder caused by reduced platelet adhesiveness and prolonged bleeding time. Patients have significant hypolglycemia that is nonresponsive to epinephrine and glucagon but that results in elevations in blood lactate, pyruvate, triglycerides, phospholipids, cholesterol, and uric acid. Hyperlipidemia is a significant finding in the disorder. Glycogen deposition in the renal tubules can also result in a Fanconi's syndrome of glucosuria, aminoaciduria, and phosphaturia.

A diabetic type of glucose tolerance test, with reduced basal plasma insulin levels and reduced output of insulin to stimuli of glucose or arginine, is reported. Hyperuricemia with attendant gouty arthritis and gouty nephropathy is described in older children.

Genetics

This is an autosomal recessive disorder caused by a defect in the activity of the enzyme glucose-6-phosphatase obtained on a liver biopsy.

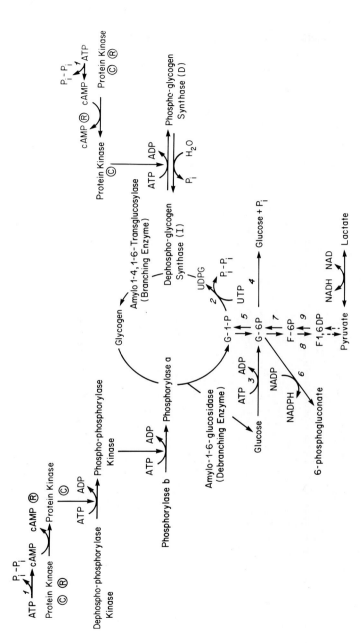

FIG. 25. Glycogen synthesis and breakdown. 1. Adenylate cyclase. 2. Uridine diphosphate glucose pyrophosphocyclase. 3. Glucokinase, hexokinase. 4. Glucose-6-phosphatase. 5. Phosphoglucomutase. 6. Glucose-6-phosphate dehydrogenase. 7. Phosphoglucoisomerase. 8. Phosphofructokinase. 9. Diphosphofructose phosphatase. (From ref. 505, with permission.)

Therapy

Frequent feedings to avoid hypoglycemia are recommended. Diazoxide has been useful to increase glycogenolysis, depress insulin release, and inhibit glucose uptake by the liver. A surgical approach may be necessary in some patients to produce a portacaval shunt to reduce variceal bleeding, reduce liver size, and reduce serum lipids and uric acid. Some patients have had a meaningful improvement in growth postsurgically (575).

TYPE II GLYCOGEN STORAGE DISEASE (α-1,4-GLUCOSIDASE DEFICIENCY, ACID MALTASE DEFICIENCY, POMPE'S DISEASE)

This is an autosomal recessive disorder with an incidence of 1 in 50,000 caused by a defect in the enzyme α-1,4-glucosidase (468).

Clinical Features

The disease has been described in infantile, early childhood, and adult forms. The infantile type begins in the first year of life with muscular atrophy, hypotonia, hyporeflexia, cardiomegaly, and also heart failure (Fig. 26). An early childhood type progresses more slowly, and muscle atrophy and weakness are less severe, but

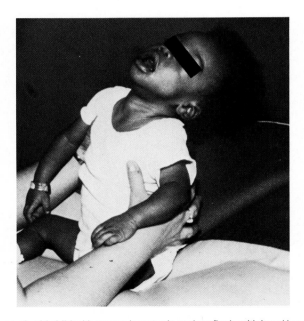

FIG. 26. A 6-month-old child with severe hypotonia and areflexia with head lag and floppy arms due to hypotonia and weakness. The child has a denervation syndrome of striated skeletal muscle caused by glycogen deposition in motor neurons as a result of Pompe's disease (glycogenosis type II). (Courtesy of Dr. Jay Cook, University of Texas Southwestern Medical School at Dallas; from ref. 505, with permission.)

eventually all patients expire by age 20 from severe atrophy and weakness leading to aspiration pneumonia. The adult variety presents with a slowly evolving proximal myopathy with weakness and atrophy. Glycogen storage occurs in skeletal muscle, heart, tongue and also liver. Motor neurons present in cranial nuclei and anterior horn cells of the spinal cord are also involved in storage of glycogen resulting in their dysfunction and demise producing a denervating neurogenic process.

Genetics

This is an autosomal recessive disorder with glycogen storage because of reduced activity of the enzyme α-1,4-glucosidase. Fibroblasts obtained from amniocentesis can be cultured and assayed for enzyme activity and provide a prenatal diagnosis (15,285). Miranda et al. (402) examined immunocytochemically infantile and adult onset muscle cells for acid maltase enzyme activity. Adult muscle cultures showed normal intracellular localization of enzyme activity, and infantile patient cultures showed no activity. Adult-type patients show about 20% enzyme activity compared with controls.

Therapy

There is no specific therapy available.

TYPE III GLYCOGEN STORAGE DISEASE (AMYLO-1,6-GLUCOSIDASE OR DEBRANCHER DEFICIENCY, CORI'S DISEASE)

This is an autosomal recessive disorder with an incidence of 1 in 50,000, caused by a defect in the enzyme amylo-1,6-glucosidase or debrancher enzyme, as originally described by Forbes in 1953. It was Cori in 1954 (103) who showed the form of glycogen stored was an abnormal type with very short outer branches.

Clinical Features

Patients develop hepatomegaly early in life, and eventually in early adulthood muscle atrophy and weakness develop, along with cardiomegaly due to glycogen storage. Occasionally hypoglycemia and seizures develop. Serum lipids may become elevated, but serum urate levels are usually normal (285,621).

Genetics

This is an autosomal recessive disorder in which glycogen is significantly stored in skeletal muscle, heart, and liver. Glycogen is of an abnormal form, with short outer branches, because of a deficiency in the activity of amylo-1,6-glucosidase as measured in liver.

TYPE IV GLYCOGEN STORAGE DISEASE (α-1,4-GLUCAN-6-GLUCOSYL TRANSFERASE OR BRANCHER DEFICIENCY, ANDERSON'S DISEASE)

This is an autosomal recessive disorder with an incidence of 1 in 50,000. The disease process is caused by the storage of an abnormal glycogen with long outer chains as a result of a deficiency in α-1,4-glucan-6-glucosyl transferase (brancher) enzyme in liver. Alternatively, it has been referred to as amylopectinosis (10,74). A defect in the activity of this enzyme has been found and measured in fibroblasts, which makes prenatal detection of disease feasible (286).

Clinical Features

Patients present in infancy with hepatosplenomegaly, failure to thrive, and hypotonia. Cirrhosis, portal hypertension, and liver failure occur, with death resulting in the first few years of life.

Genetics

This is an autosomal recessive disorder caused by the storage of abnormal glycogen with long outer chains because of a deficiency in brancher enzyme, amylo (1,4 to 1,6) transglucosidase.

Therapy

Therapy is directed at improvement of liver failure and ascites.

TYPE V GLYCOGEN STORAGE DISEASE (MUSCLE PHOSPHORYLASE DEFICIENCY, McARDLE'S DISEASE)

This is an autosomal recessive disorder with an incidence of 1 in 50,000 caused by a deficiency in the enzyme muscle phosphorylase (285,381,404,532).

Clinical Features

Patients begin to have symptoms of easy fatigability in childhood followed by muscle cramps and myoglobinuria with exercise in the second to fourth decades. Thereafter progressive muscle weakness and atrophy occur. Ischemic exercises, such as forearm and hand exercises with an inflated cuff on the upper arm, characteristically produce an electrically silent contracture in which no lactate rise occurs in sampled venous blood. Normal exercising muscle releases alanine, but these patients take up alanine, probably so that it can be a substrate for the tricarboxylic acid cycle. An increase in muscle phosphoenol-pyruvate supports such a view (511).

It is interesting that phosphorylase activity is present in muscle cultures from patients with McArdle's disease and also in biopsied samples containing regenerating fibers. It is felt this enzyme activity is due to a fetal isoenzyme under different regulatory control than the adult species (135,390).

Clinical features of this disorder are virtually identical with those of phospho-fructokinase deficiency (334).

Genetics

This is an autosomal recessive disorder caused by a defect in muscle phospho-rylase assigned to chromosome 11 (345). Muscle glycogen levels are significantly increased.

Therapy

In 1985 Slonim and Goans (564) hypothesized that the myopathy in this syndrome was caused in part by an increased demand by muscles for amino acids as fuel that precluded their availability for normal synthesis of muscle protein. Thus a decrease in synthesis of muscle protein with a normal rate of muscle protein degradation produces muscle weakness and atrophy. They postulated that a high-protein diet would provide adequate amounts of amino acids for both energy and protein synthesis. They fed a patient a high-protein diet and compared the result with that of diets high in carbohydrate or fat. On the high-protein diet the patient had a marked increase in muscle endurance. If this observation by Slonim and Goans on a single McArdle's patient can be extended to others, it will be a significant advance in providing the first effective treatment for this rare metabolic myopathy, and it may open the way to provide therapy for other disorders of muscle carbohydrate metabolism.

TYPE VI GLYCOGEN STORAGE DISEASE (HEPATIC PHOSPHORYLASE DEFICIENCY, HERS'S DISEASE

This is an autosomal recessive disorder with glycogen storage in liver caused by a deficiency of liver phosphorylase (272,285). It has an incidence of about 1 in 50,000.

Clinical Features

It presents in a manner similar to type I glycogenosis but in a milder form.

Genetics

It is inherited as an autosomal recessive disorder caused by a defect in hepatic phosphorylase with an increase in liver glycogen.

TYPE VII GLYCOGEN STORAGE DISEASE (MUSCLE PHOSPHOFRUCTOKINASE DEFICIENCY, TARUI'S DISEASE, LAYZER'S DISEASE)

This is an autosomal recessive disorder with an estimated incidence of 1 in 50,000 caused by a defect in the muscle enzyme phosphofructokinase (344,592).

Clinical Features

Presenting symptoms are identical to those of McArdle's disease, with childhood onset of easy fatigability followed by muscle cramps and myoglobinuria. In the early adult years muscle weakness and atrophy develop.

Genetics

This is an autosomal recessive disorder caused by a defect in muscle phosphofructokinase. Muscle glucose-6-phosphate and fructose-6-phosphate are increased and fructose-1,6-diphosphate is markedly reduced from the enzyme defect. Muscle glycogen is increased. Phosphofructokinase is absent in activity in muscle, 50% of normal activity in red blood cells, and normal in activity in leukocytes. It is thought that the muscle enzyme is composed of identical muscle type (M) subunits, whereas the red blood cell isoenzyme is composed of both muscle and red blood cell type (R) subunits. Thus the absence of enzyme activity in muscle is caused by a defect in the M subunit and a partial loss of activity in erythrocytes (91). A late onset adult form of the disease has also been recently described (117).

TYPE VIII GLYCOGEN STORAGE DISEASE (HEPATIC PHOSPHORYLASE KINASE DEFICIENCY)

This is an X-linked recessive disorder with an incidence of 1 in 50,000 in which glycogen is stored in liver because of a 90% deficiency in phosphorylase *b* kinase activity (285,289).

Clinical Features

Patients present with an asymptomatic hepatomegaly. The diagnosis depends on finding low activity of phosphorylase *b* kinase in liver.

Genetics

This is an X-linked recessive disorder caused by a deficiency in the activity of phosphorylase *b* kinase in liver, with resultant glycogen storage of normal structure in liver.

GALACTOSEMIA (GALACTOSE-1-PHOSPHATE URIDYLTRANSFERASE DEFICIENCY)

This is an autosomal recessive disorder caused by a deficiency of the enzyme galactose-1-phosphate uridyltransferase. Its incidence varies between 1 in 35,000 and 1 in 190,000. It was described clinically in 1935 (376), and the increase in erythrocyte galactose-1-phosphate was reported in 1956 (326). The enzyme defect was first reported by Isselbacher et al. in 1956 (298), and an erythrocyte uridine diphosphate glucose consumption test was described in 1957 by Anderson et al. (11). This test made it possible to identify heterozygotes for carrier detection purposes in addition to homozygotes. Variation in clinical and biochemical features of the disorder has been noted (288,546).

Clinical Features

The disease presents early in infancy with jaundice, hepatomegaly, ascites, vomiting, diarrhea, and failure to thrive. These clinical features have their onset shortly after milk ingestion occurs. Nascent cataracts can be detected in the neonatal period, and progressive mental retardation is noted in the first few months of life. Associated clinical chemical abnormalities include galactosemia, galactosuria, hyperchloremic acidosis, albuminuria, and occasionally aminoaciduria; other routine liver chemical studies may be abnormal.

Genetics

This is an autosomal recessive disorder caused by a deficiency in the activity of the enzyme galactose-1-phosphate uridyltransferase. It has been mapped to chromosome 9p12-p13. Cataract formation occurs because of accumulation in the lens of dulcitol, which is the product of aldose reductase in the lens from the substrate galactose. Dulcitol and galactose-1-phosphate are stored in liver, kidney, and brain as well. The neural toxicity of galactose feeding has been described by Wells and Wells (632), and effects include decreased brain ATP, glucose, and glycolytic metabolic intermediates and a decrease in fast axoplasmic transport.

Therapy

This is one neurogenetic disorder that responds to specific therapy, in this instance, the elimination of dietary galactose. The casein hydrolysate nutramigen and soybean milks are used early in life to avoid the development of mental retardation and cataracts. Dietary galactose should also be eliminated by women who already have one galactosemic child so that fetal toxicity can be eliminated. The earlier the onset of the galactose dietary restriction, the better the clinical outcome.

GALACTOKINASE DEFICIENCY

This is an autosomal recessive disorder with an incidence of 1 in 40,000 caused by a deficiency in the enzyme galactokinase.

Clinical Features

The brain feature is juvenile cataract formation without mental retardation and liver disease. The absence of liver and gastrointestinal disease separates it from the transferase deficiency. Elevated galactose levels in serum and urine, normal activity of galactose-1-phosphate uridyltransferase, and absence of galactokinase activity in erythrocytes or fibroblasts establish the diagnosis. The formation of cataracts is caused by dulcitol and the absence of mental retardation is probably caused by the lack of galactose-1-phosphate production.

Genetics

This is an autosomal recessive disorder caused by galactokinase deficiency and the resultant presence of elevated amounts of galactose in body tissue. The enzyme has been mapped to chromosome 17 near the thymidine kinase locus.

Therapy

As with the transferase deficiency, dietary elimination of galactose is effective to reduce tissue levels of galactose and prevent cataract formation.

UNVERRICHT-LUNDBORG SYNDROME (MYOCLONUS EPILEPSY)

This is a rare glycoprotein-mucopolysaccharide storage disease described as an autosomal recessive disorder. Clinical features include myoclonus epilepsy, mental retardation, spasticity, extrapyramidal rigidity, and ataxia. Life span is usually limited to the second decade of life. The neuronal inclusions are referred to as Lafora bodies. A Hartung variety has been inherited as an autosomal dominant trait. It has also been referred to as Lafora's disease when the inclusions are present. There is no known biochemical defect described and no specific metabolic therapy is available (83,543).

Disorders of Lipid Metabolism

Lipid metabolism is summarized in Fig. 27 (505).

LIPID STORAGE DISORDERS

GM₁ Gangliosidosis

This is an autosomal recessive disorder caused by a deficiency of the enzyme β-galactosidase, resulting in the storage of the lipid GM_1 ganglioside. Norman et al.

---------------------------------->

FIG. 27. Sphingolipid metabolism. 1. 3-Dehydrosphingosine synthase. 2. Reductase. 3. Flavin dehydrogenase. 4. Sphingosine *N*-acyl transferase. 5. Sphingosine galactosyl transferase (anabolic). 6. Galactosylsphingosine sulfokinase (anabolic), galactosylsphingosine sulfatase (catabolic). 7. Galactosylceramide (cerebroside) sulfokinase (anabolic), cerebroside sulfatase (catabolic). 8. Galactosylsphingosine *N*-acyl transferase. 9. Ceramide galactosyl transferase (anabolic) galactosylceramide (cerebroside) galactosidase (catabolic). 10. Ceramide cholinephosphotransferase (anabolic), sphingomyelinase (catabolic). 11. Ceramide glucosyl transferase (anabolic), glucosylceramide (cerebroside) glucosidase (catabolic). 12. Glycolipid galactosyl transferase (anabolic), lactosylceramide galactosidase (catabolic). 13. Glycolipid sialyl transferase (anabolic), glycolipid sialidase (catabolic). 14. Glycolipid *N*-acetyl galactosamine transferase (anabolic), glycolipid β-*N*-acetyl galactosaminidase (hexosaminidase) (catabolic). 15. Glycolipid galactosyl transferase (anabolic), glycolipid β-galactosidase (catabolic). 16. Glycolipid sialyl transferase (anabolic), glycolipid sialidase (catabolic). Defects in the following catabolic enzymes give rise to the following clinical disorders: 7, metachromatic leukodystrophy; 9, Krabbe's; 10, Niemann-Pick; 11, Gaucher's; 12, lactosylceramidosis; 14, GM₂ type I (Tay-Sachs); 15, GM₁ (generalized gangliosidosis). (From ref. 505, with permission.)

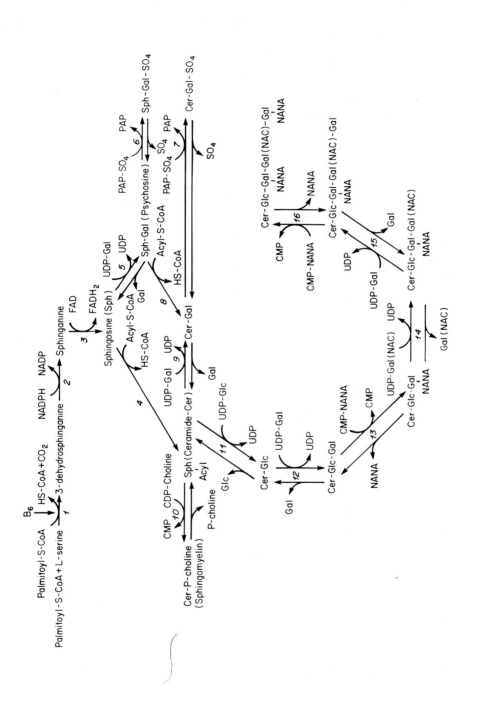

(434) first described it clinically as a variant of Tay-Sachs disease with visceral involvement. Infantile, juvenile, and adult forms have been described (58,59,128).

Infantile Form or Type I

Clinical features

The disorder has as its main features severe mental retardation, seizures, early hypotonia, and hepatosplenomegaly. Hurler-like features clinically and roentgenographically also occur. The newborn is hypoactive, hypotonic, and has coarse facial features. These facial abnormalities include hirsutism, macroglossia, prominent maxilla, frontal bossing, depressed nasal bridge, long philtrum, and hypertrophied alveolar ridges.

The infant gradually develops motor and mental retardation. Gradually increased tone, increased deep tendon reflexes, and Babinski signs develop, indicating impairment of the corticospinal tract. Seizures occur early in development as well. By 12 months of age the child is severely retarded, has optic atrophy and blindness, may be deaf, and shows spasticity, quadriparesis, and often decortication or decerebration. Hepatosplenomegaly and skeletal defects are also present. Malformations of the wrist and ankles occur and a progressive dorsolumbar kyphosis also develops.

Roentgenographic findings are those of a dysostosis multiplex. The long tubular bones are shortened and widened in the midshaft area and tapered at the proximal and distal ends. The lumbar vertebrae are hypoplastic and beaked anteriorly. The ribs are spatula-like and thickened. The ilea are flared and the sella turcica is elongated and shallow, giving it a shoe-shaped appearance.

Laboratory findings include vacuolated lymphocytes in the peripheral blood, foam cells in the bone marrow, and a normal or slightly elevated quantity of mucopolysaccharides in the urine.

The deteriorating clinical course continues until death, which occurs about age 2 years.

Genetics and biochemistry

GM_1 gangliosidosis is an autosomal recessive disorder in which a deficiency of the enzyme β-galactosidase occurs, resulting in the storage of GM_1 ganglioside in neurons and glia of the brain, brainstem, and spinal cord. In addition, all organs contain foam cells. Their cytoplasm is filled with periodic acid-Schiff- and Alcian blue-positive metachromatic granules, which are probably keratin sulfate. Gangliosides are glycolipids that contain sialic acid moieties attached to their oligosaccharide chains. Gangliosides are localized primarily in neuronal synaptic membranes (587), although they are found in most cell types.

The biosynthesis of GM_1 gangliosides is by a multiglycosyltransferase system, which has highest activity in synaptosomal membranes. On the catabolic side all the glycosidases appear to be localized in lysosomes, except for some sialidases, which are extralysosomal (19,46).

The stored material in brain is identical to normal GM_1 ganglioside and is elevated to 10 times normal in the gray matter in types I and II and to 20 to 50 times normal in the liver of type I patients. The asialo-derivative of GM_1 accumulates to 10 times normal in the brain, and galactose-containing glycoproteins accumulate in viscera of both types I and II.

There are two acid β-galactosidase isoenzymes: A and B. Both are sialoglycoproteins with an acid pH optimum (4.2–4.4), and both are heat-labile and stimulated by chloride. The enzyme is mapped to chromosome 22q13-22qter.

In 1981 Farrell and Ochs (181) suggested more precisely that the phenotypic variation found in GM_1 gangliosidosis resulted from different allelic mutations affecting the GM_1 ganglioside β-galactosidase locus, and that different combinations of these mutations determined the clinical heterogeneity of this illness. They reported a family that supported their hypothesis in which both the infantile and juvenile forms of GM_1 gangliosidosis were found. They reported that acid β-galactosidase activity could be separated into multiple molecular forms by isoelectric focusing on cellulose acetate membranes. The residual acid β-galactosidase in the juvenile form of GM_1 gangliosidosis had three bands of enzyme activity with an apparent isoelectric pH (pI) range from 4.9 to 5.2. The infantile form of the enzyme had a single band with an apparent pI of 5.2. Thus they were able to show that separation of residual acid β-galactosidase into multiple molecular forms by isoelectric focusing demonstrated that enzymatic differences can be correlated with the allelic mutations that affect the GM_1 ganglioside β-galactosidase locus (179).

Therapy

There is no specific therapy that has been useful.

Juvenile Form or Type II

This is similar to type I disease but it is less aggressive and less severe, beginning at about 1 year of age and progressing to death at about age 5 years. Motor and mental retardation occur associated with mild Hurler-like features of facial coarsening. Seizures, spasticity, and mental retardation complete the clinical picture. The biochemical, enzymatic, and pathologic features are similar to those of type I disease.

Tay-Sachs Disease (GM₂ Gangliosidosis Type I)

This is an autosomal recessive disorder first described as a clinical entity by Tay (593), who reported the retinal degeneration, and by Sachs (515), who described the neurologic and neuropathologic findings in an affected infant having blindness and dementia. It was Klenk (323,324) who first showed increased concentrations of gangliosides in brain tissue from patients, and in 1961 Svennerholm and Raal (587) found the stored ganglioside was a monosialoganglioside. Hexosaminidase A was first reported as being the specific molecular defect in this disorder almost simultaneously by Sandhoff et al. in 1968 (520), Sandhoff in 1969 (519), Hultberg in 1969 (290), and Kolodny et al. in 1969 (325). There have been other similar reports. Further characterization of the enzyme defect was provided by Sandhoff and Jatzkewitz in 1972 (521). The mutant gene has a frequency in the New York City Jewish population of 0.016, with a carrier rate of 1:30 in the Jewish population and 1:300 in the non-Jewish population.

Clinical Features

Seizures, blindness, and motor and mental retardation are cardinal features. These features begin within the first 6 months of life, and the child gradually loses interest in visual stimuli, moves less, and startles easily to sound. Milestones for sitting and standing are delayed, and the child usually never learns to walk. Optic atrophy and macular degeneration, with the generation of a cherry-red spot when increased vascularity becomes visible as the ganglion retinal cells are lost, appear early. Seizures, which are absence, fragmentary motor, myoclonic, or generalized major-motor, occur in the first year of life. By 1 year, spasticity with decortication or decerebration may develop. Because of progressive lipid storage, megalencephaly develops but hepatosplenomegaly does not occur.

Neuropathology

Neurons are characterized by the lysosomal storage of ganglioside. The presence of a lipidosis is evident in all neurons of the central and peripheral nervous system, but the degree of storage is most evident in Ammon's horn of the temporal lobe.

Neuronal loss, gliosis, demyelination, and brain atrophy are features of the disorder. Elevated levels of gangliosides are present in liver.

Genetics and Biochemistry

GM_2 monosialoganglioside is increased in brain between 100 and 300 times normal. Asialo-GM_2 is elevated about 20 times normal. Hexosaminidases A and B are isoenzymes possessing both β-D-N-acetylglucosaminidase and β-D-N-acetylgalactosaminidase activity. Both isoenzymes are found in all normal human tissues except erythrocytes. Hexosaminidase A is more heat-labile and more negatively charged than hexosaminidase B. These hexosaminidase isoenzymes act on the widely used artificial fluorogenic and chromogenic substrates and on all of the natural substrates except GM_2 ganglioside. GM_2 ganglioside is cleaved rapidly only by hexosaminidase A in the presence of a heat-stable cofactor protein or activator protein. The activator protein binds to GM_2 ganglioside in such a way that it can be rapidly cleaved by hexosaminidase A (307). In GM_2 gangliosidosis type I, hexosaminidase A activity is nearly absent, but activity of hexosaminidase B in brain is increased 10 times normal, possibly because of lysosomal stimulation secondary to ganglioside storage. A heat-denatured serum assay for hexosaminidase A is 96% accurate in detecting homozygotes as well as heterozygotes. False positives in the heterozygote range may occur in patients with diabetes mellitus, myocardial infarction, hepatitis, and pancreatitis. False positives also occur in normal pregnant women and women taking birth control pills. Leukocyte hexosaminidase A activity, however, remains unaltered in these disorders and is accurate in more than 99% of patients tested. For the most reliable results, and especially for some of the variants, the natural GM_2 ganglioside should be used as substrate. Hexosaminidases A and B both cleave asialo-GM_2 and globoside (Cer-Glc-Gal-Gal-Gal) (NAc), but kinetic studies indicate that only hexosaminidase A cleaves GM_2 ganglioside. Hexosaminidase A has a molecular weight of 100,000 daltons and hexosaminidase B a molecular weight of 108,000 daltons. Both isoenzymes may be dissociated into four subunits with hexosaminidase A (composed of two α and two β: $\alpha_2\beta_2$ polypeptide chains) and hexosaminidase B (four β: $\beta_2\beta_2$ chains). At this time it appears that the α chain is coded by chromosome 15 and the β chain by chromosome 5. This would indicate the genetic defect is on chromosome 15 for GM_2 gangliosidosis type I and on chromosome 5 for GM_2 gangliosidosis type II.

Treatment

At the present time no definitive treatment is available. Enzyme infusion intravenously, intracisternally, and intrathecally has produced no clinical improvement (59). Screening for heterozygotes and genetic counseling is the most logical approach. Since the enzyme deficiency is manifest in amniotic fluid cells, therapeutic abortion is possible. Supportive care is all that is presently available for the affected homozygote.

GM_2 Gangliosidosis Type II (Sandhoff's Disease)

Sandhoff et al. described a form of GM_2 gangliosidosis in 1968 (520) in a non-Jewish infant in which the clinical features and natural history of disease are almost identical to GM_2 gangliosidosis type I or Tay-Sachs disease. The one clinical difference between the two syndromes is that some GM_2 type II patients may have hepatosplenomegaly. The enzyme defect is characterized by decreased activity of both hexosaminidase A and B in serum, fiborblasts in culture, white blood cells, and amniotic fluid cells.

GM_2 Gangliosidosis Type III

This is a rare clinical entity first reported by Bernheimer and Seitelberger in 1968 (45). Children, all of whom are reported to be non-Jewish, begin with cerebellar ataxia between 3 and 7 years of age with slowly progressive psychomotor retardation, spasticity, and seizures. These children develop optic atrophy, retinitis pigmentosa, and clinical blindness. The course is progressive with decortication, decerebration, and death within the first decade of life. Hexosaminidase A activity is about 25% of normal, and serum levels are severely reduced.

Hexosaminidase Variants and Neuromuscular Syndromes

Johnson and associates in recent years have described disorders of the neuromuscular system in association with deficiencies of β-D-N-acetylhexosaminidase and β-methylcrotonylglycinuria I (307). Hexosaminidase deficiencies have been associated with recognized clinical phenotypes, including infantile encephalopathy, late infantile or juvenile encephalopathy, cerebellar or spinocerebellar ataxia, Kugelberg-Welander syndrome, a disorder similar to ALS, and even an adult onset type of dementia. Johnson points out that motor neuron syndromes are encountered mainly in α-locus defects of hexosaminidase rather than in β-locus or protein activator disorders. However he points out also that α locus disorders are more common than β- or activator locus defects.

A patient reported by Johnson (307) with the Kugelberg-Welander disease phenotype was in actuality a true genetic compound, as the patient had a severe deficiency in hexosaminidase A and a partial deficiency in both parents. The father of this patient carried the HEX α_2 allele, as a paternal relative had classic infantile Tay-Sachs disease and the mother carried a milder hexosaminidase α-locus allele (307). Rectal ganglion cells from the patient contained classic membranous cytoplasmic bodies seen in the other GM_2 gangliosidoses, and most likely spinal cord anterior horn neurons were similarly affected to explain the denervating clinical syndrome.

Another patient reported by Johnson (307) had an ALS-like syndrome with hexosaminidase A deficiency. He was a 22-year-old man with a 2-year history of progressive weakness and proximal muscle wasting with increased reflexes and bilateral Babinski signs. Electromyographic studies and a muscle biopsy were consistent with the diagnosis. He had a severe deficiency of hexosaminidase A, and partial deficiencies were present in his parents. Thus he had upper and lower neuron involvement clinically and a rectal ganglion cell disorder caused by inclusions of membranous cytoplasmic bodies typical of GM_2 gangliosidoses, and presumably his motor neurons were similarly affected. It is important to point out that most patients with motor neuron disease do not have a hexosaminidase A deficiency, especially those with rapidly advancing disease over 40 years of age. It should be considered in younger patients with a slowly progressive form of disease and a recessive pattern of inheritance.

A cerebellar ataxia syndrome has been associated with an α-locus defect of hexosaminidase A, and a juvenile cerebellar ataxia form (a Ramsay-Hunt phenocopy) and an adult onset spinocerebellar ataxia syndrome have been associated with a β-locus defect. A protein activator locus defect has been described with adult GM_2 gangliosidosis with dementia, seizures, and normal pressure hydrocephalus.

Mitsumoto et al. (403) have recently described two families with an adult hexosaminidase A deficiency syndrome with a multisystem degeneration. The clinical picture included a mild dementia, ataxia, and an axonal motor-sensory peripheral neuropathy associated with a juvenile ALS syndrome. Marked cerebellar atrophy was detected by head scans in all patients.

Thus the clinical spectrum seen in various hexosaminidase deficiencies has widened considerably in recent years and the story has become more complex. About two dozen hexosaminidase deficiency types now exist and the number is bound to increase. Similar allelic mutations, activator defects, and genetic compounds exist for other lysosomal enzymes as well; thus Johnson, by making us aware of the multiple genotypes and associated phenotypes for this enzyme in particular as a model approach to other lysosomal enzymes, has made an extremely important contribution that has moved molecular neurogenetics forward in a most elegant fashion (306,307).

One interesting clinical note along these lines is the report by Johnson and associates on a child who developed classic late infantile GM_2 gangliosidosis; the biological father was a donor for artificial insemination and both he and the mother were carriers of an α-locus hexosaminidase deficiency. Thus here is another gene product for which insemination screening is needed to avoid a lethal genetic disease (310).

Gaucher's Disease (Glucosyl Ceramidase Deficiency)

Gaucher (216) published a description of a chronic, progressive disorder characterized by hepatosplenomegaly that he believed was caused by an epithelioma of the spleen. Tuchman et al. (605) reported elevation of serum acid phosphatase in patients with Gaucher's disease. Brady et al. (62) demonstrated glucocerebrosidase deficiency (Fig. 27) in Gaucher's disease, and later they demonstrated that both the heterozygote carrier and the intrauterine presence of Gaucher's disease could be diagnosed. The adult form of the disease is approximately 30 times more frequent in Ashkenazic Jews, and the incidence in this population has been reported to be as high as 1 in 2,500, with a reported carrier frequency in Ashkenazic Jews from 1 in 100 to 1 in 20. It is an autosomal recessive disorder.

Clinical Features

Gaucher's disease has been divided into three clinical forms: type I (chronic, nonneuronopathic), type II (acute neuronopathic), and type III (subacute neuronopathic).

Type I

The type I disorder usually presents late in the first or early in the second decade, frequently with the onset of episodic pains in the legs, arms, or back, which may be accentuated by fever or by a minor illness. There is also abdominal distention with hepatosplenomegaly, hypotonic colon, respiratory difficulties, and the beginning of yellow pallor and a diffuse yellow-brown discoloration of the face and legs. A mild microcytic anemia with thrombocytopenia may occur. The hematologic abnormalities may be severe at times. Bone marrow examination reveals many Gaucher's cells. The course is one of frequent painful and hemorrhagic episodes that progress in severity over the years. The hepatosplenomegaly increases but is usually associated with normal liver function tests. There is worsening of pulmonary function and appearance of bony changes including rarefaction of the bony cortex, pathologic fractures of the femur, and compression fractures of the vertebral bodies.

Type II

Type II infants are usually normal up to 6 or 7 months of age, when they develop hepatosplenomegaly, pulmonary deterioration, and marked brain degenerative findings. It involves the brainstem neurons and clinically is manifested by strabismus, retroflexion of the head, dysphagia, and laryngeal stridor. Hypertonicity, hyperreflexia, Babinski signs, and seizures occur. The course is progressively downhill, with death usually occurring at 9 to 12 months of age.

Type III

The type III disorder includes a small number of patients who have been described with hepatosplenomegaly and Gaucher's cells in their bone marrow in whom the onset of brain deterioration occurs in the childhood years.

The diagnosis is suspected in the presence of the constellation of hepatosplenomegaly, brain degenerative findings, hemorrhagic tendencies, a marked increase in the serum non-tartrate-inhibitable acid phosphatase, and the presence of Gaucher's cells in the bone marrow.

The diagnosis is supported by the findings of increased glucocerebroside levels in tissues and markedly decreased glucocerebrosidase activity in leukocytes, skin fibroblasts, and amniotic fluid cells. Heterozygotes may be identified by enzymatic assay of either skin fibroblasts or leukocytes, and intrauterine diagnosis is possible.

Gaucher's Cells

A Gaucher's cell is an enlarged, lipid-laden histiocyte that stains positively with periodic acid-Schiff, indicating the presence of glycolipid. The cells range from 20 to 100 μm in diameter, with an eccentrically placed nucleus. The cytoplasm has the appearance of crinkled tissue paper. The cells react readily with phenylphosphate, demonstrating the presence of acid phosphatase. Gaucher's cells contain spindles or rod-shaped membrane-bound inclusions, which in cross section appear to be tubules with a diameter between 130 and 150 Å.

Therapy

Patients with Gaucher's disease need careful follow-up and supportive care of any hematologic difficulties that may arise. Splenectomy may become necessary for hypersplenism, but it is usually postponed as long as possible because of the danger of accelerating bone and liver involvement after splenectomy. Corrective orthopedic surgery may be indicated in certain cases.

At this time enzyme replacement therapy has been shown to be inconsistently effective in ameliorating the nonneurologic signs and symptoms in patients with type I disease. There was a 26% reduction in the first two patients in the quantity of glucocerebroside in liver, and serum concentrations returned to normal in 3 days in both patients. By modifying glucocerebrosidase through deglycosylation, it has been possible to increase the amount of enzyme delivery to Kupffer cells fivefold and thus more effectively mobilize substrate (59). Preliminary evidence in one patient using modified enzyme again shows significant clinical improvement in patients in terms of reduction of the glucocerebroside burden of hepatic Kupffer cells, normalization of serum concentrations of glucocerebroside, and improvement in the patients' hematologic status (Dr. Robin Ely Berman, *personal communication*).

As reviewed by Brady (59), most Gaucher's patients have type I disease, in which the nervous system is minimally, if at all, involved. There is extensive brain damage in types II and III Gaucher's patients, and so special considerations must be employed to possibly mobilize substrate on the brain side of the blood-brain barrier. As has been mentioned previously for Tay-Sachs disease, intravenous, intrathecal, and intracisternal administration of enzyme is not effective for this purpose. Brady, Neuwelt, and associates (59) approached this problem by attempting to open the blood-brain barrier with hyperosmolar solutions of mannitol or arabinose just prior to enzyme infusion. This approach is being attempted for both Tay-Sachs and Gaucher's patients (types II and III), and the results, although preliminary, are probably not going to indicate meaningful clinical improvement. Additional new approaches, such as plasmapheresis and bone marrow transplantation with recombinant DNA techniques that transfect the normal gene into patient cells, will be necessary for therapy to be effective. There is no evidence that replacement enzyme crosses the blood-brain barrier, and therefore replacement therapy is not effective against the neurologic manifestations (32).

Two cases of transplantation, one of a spleen and the other of a kidney, were not shown to be effective. However, bone marrow transplants may be clinically helpful in selected patients.

Niemann-Pick Disease (Sphingomyelinase Deficiency)

Niemann, a German pediatrician, described an 18-month-old infant of Jewish extraction with hepatosplenomegaly, lymphadenopathy, edema, pigmentation of the face, and brain impairment (431). The infant died before 2 years of age. Pathologic examination revealed yellow deposits in the liver, spleen, lymph nodes, kidneys, and adrenals, and large sudanophilic cells were seen throughout these organs. Between 1922 and 1927, Pick (461) provided histologic evidence that differences existed between this disease and Gaucher's disease. Brady et al. presented evidence that the deficient enzyme was sphingomyelinase (61). The incidence of this disorder is high for Ashkenazic Jews, but the disorder has been described in other ethnic groups. It is an autosomal recessive disorder.

Clinical Features

Five clinical types of Niemann-Pick disease are now recognized: type A (acute neuronopathic), type B (chronic nonneuronopathic), type C (chronic neuropathic), type D (Nova Scotia variant), and type E (adult nonneuronopathic) (111).

Type A

The type A patient presents with visceral and brain involvement in early infancy, with rapid deterioration. Hepatosplenomegaly is usually recognized by 6 months of age with concomitant feeding difficulties and failure to thrive. A brownish-yellow discoloration of the skin may be observed, and approximately 50% of the patients have a cherry-red spot in the macula. Neurologically there is a rapidly progressive deterioration with loss of motor and intellectual functions.

Type B

In the type B variant visceromegaly may appear as early as in type A, but there is no brain involvement. Splenomegaly is usually apparent first, followed by hepatomegaly, with little or no impairment in liver function tests. There is often a diffuse infiltration of the lung fields with secondarily increased susceptibility to pneumonia.

Type C

The patient with type C variant is usually normal for the first 1 to 2 years of life. There is then a gradual onset of neurologic degeneration originally manifested by moderate ataxia, grand mal seizures, and loss of language. The hepatosplenomegaly is less striking than in the type A or B variants. There is progressive gray matter deterioration followed by the onset and progression of white matter deterioration.

Type D

The patients with the type C variant share a common ancestry and live in a coastal area in western Nova Scotia. Clinically they have the onset of a neurologic gray matter deterioration between 2 and 4 years of age that resembles type C. There then occurs progressive hepatosplenomegaly and the onset and progression of a neurologic degeneration.

Type E

The type E variant is represented by adults with moderate hepatosplenomegaly without brain abnormalities. These patients also have foamy lipid-laden cells in their bone marrow.

Type C-E hybrid

This variant is represented by adults with minimal hepatosplenomegaly but with foam cells in their bone marrow, cerebellar ataxia, and cherry-red spots in the macula. The presumptive diagnosis can be made on the basis of clinical presentation and presence of lipid-laden cells with foamy cytoplasm in the bone marrow. The diagnosis is supported by finding increased levels of sphingomyelin in tissues.

Niemann-Pick Cell

The Niemann-Pick cell is a large, foamy, lipid-laden cell found throughout the reticuloendothelial system. Brain neurons undergo similar changes. Niemann-Pick cells range from 20 to 90 μm in diameter, with an eccentric nucleus and cytoplasm filled with many droplets, giving them a "mulberry" appearance.

Neuropathology

The brain is usually reduced to 50 to 90% of its normal weight, and there is a marked firmness in its consistency. Neurons in the brain are swollen with foamy cytoplasm, within which are found membrane-bound inclusions. These may appear loosely arranged or in concentric lamellar structures. With neuronal cell loss there is disorganization of the cerebral and cerebellar architecture. The neuronal cell loss is followed by gliosis and secondary demyelination.

Genetics and Biochemistry

This is an autosomal recessive disorder. The predominant lipid accumulating throughout the reticuloendothelial system and the CNS is sphingomyelin. There is also a substantial increase in unesterified cholesterol and lyso-bis-phosphatidic acid. The latter two lipids may be derived from uncatabolized membrane fragments.

The underlying biochemical abnormality is a result of sphingomyelinase deficiency. At the present time, on the basis of isoelectric focusing studies, there appear to be two sphingomyelinase isoenzymes. Further studies have revealed a virtual absence of both isoenzymes (I, II) in type A, marked decrease in both I and II in type B, and absence of isoenzyme II in type C. Further studies are needed to confirm and further clarify this point. However, if different isoenzyme preponderances are found in different organ systems, one can begin to understand the variety of clinical presentations in Niemann-Pick disease.

Therapy

At the present time there is no specific treatment available for Niemann-Pick disease. Splenectomy is occasionally performed for the rare Niemann-Pick patient with symptomatic hypersplenism.

Cerebrotendinous Xanthomatosis

Cerebrotendinous xanthomatosis is a rare familial autosomal recessive disease characterized by elevated plasma cholestanol and accumulation of cholestanol in xanthomas of the tendons, lungs, and brain in spite of a normal or low plasma cholesterol level. The neurologic manifestations include subnormal intelligence, progressive cerebellar ataxia, dementia, paresis, and cataracts. Schneider (535) described xanthomatous lesions in the nervous system of a mentally retarded and epileptic patient. Menkes et al. (395) reported greatly increased cholestanol levels in the cerebellum and cerebrum of two patients with cerebrotendinous xanthomatosis. Since then cholestanol has been found in the blood and tissues in greatly increased amounts in several patients.

Clinical Features

Cerebrotendinous xanthomatosis has an insidious onset and unpredictable course and was arbitrarily divided into three stages by van Bogaert et al. (611):

1. The initial stage usually begins in childhood and is characterized by borderline intelligence and mental deterioration. In some patients, however, mentation remains normal well into the third and fourth decades.
2. During adolescence and young adulthood, white matter degeneration develops and is manifested as progressive spasticity and ataxia. At this time juvenile cataracts and tendon xanthomas are observed, which become progressively worse.
3. The final stage of this disease is characterized by enlargement of the xanthomas and severe neurologic deterioration. The neurologic deterioration is manifested as a mixed gray and white matter degeneration involving the cerebrum, cerebellum, and spinal cord.

The diagnosis of cerebrotendinous xanthomatosis is difficult to establish in the first stage of the illness. However, the disease should be considered in any young adult with tendon xanthomas, cataracts, low or borderline intelligence, and cerebellar findings. The diagnosis is confirmed by measuring the concentration of cholestanol in plasma and particularly in xanthomas, skin, or adipose tissue (459).

Plasma lipid studies reveal that in most patients the plasma cholesterol level is within the normal range, as are plasma triglyceride and plasma phospholipid concentrations; however, the plasma cholestanol is greatly increased. In 13 patients studied the range of plasma cholestanol was between 1.3 and 4.0 mg/dl, compared with a normal plasma cholestanol level of 0.1 to 0.6 mg/dl. In the brain free esterified cholestanol is greatly increased from its normal trace amounts to 20 to 25% of the total free sterols. Cerebral and cerebellar cholesterol content is also increased, mostly because of increased cholesterol esters. Peripheral nerves reveal 20% of the total sterols is cholestanol, and of this 59% is esterified cholestanol. Tendon xanthoma studies have revealed that 90% of the total sterols is in the form of cholesterol and the other 10% in the form of cholestanol. Some studies have revealed that from 47 to 86% of the total cholestanol content is in the esterified form.

Normal bile contains a very small amount of cholestanol (less than 1%) and a trace (0.2%) of lanosterol, an intermediate in the pathway of cholesterol biosynthesis. In cerebrotendinous xanthomatosis the amount of cholestanol excreted in the bile is greatly increased to 4 to 11% of total biliary neutral sterols. Whereas in normal individuals approximately 90% of the bile acids are equally divided between cholic and chenodeoxycholic acids, in cerebrotendinous xanthomatosis cholic acid predominates and represents approximately 80% of the total bile acids.

Neuropathology

Xanthomas are found in the white matter of the cerebral hemispheres, globus pallidus, and cerebral peduncles. The most striking and consistent findings are in the cerebellum, where yellowish granulomatous lesions may attain 1.5 cm in diameter and may replace most of the white matter. Microscopic examination reveals extensive demyelination of the cerebellar white matter lateral to the dentate nucleus and in the superior cerebellar peduncles, while the white matter adjacent and medial to the dentate nucleus is spared.

Therapy

Specific treatment for cerebrotendinous xanthomatosis was recently described by Berginer et al. (43), who reported that after 1 year of treatment with oral chenodeoxycholic acid (750 mg/day), dementia cleared in 10 of 13 patients and pyramidal and cerebellar signs resolved in five and improved in another eight of a total of 17 patients studied. Cerebral CT scans improved in seven patients. Thus, as commented on by Grundy in an accompanying editorial, Beringer et al. have provided evidence that therapeutic intervention can reverse the entire process by changing the course of sterol deposition in the nervous system (241). Cataract extraction may partially relieve the visual symptoms, and surgical removal of tendon xanthomas may help relieve pain and discomfort.

This disease has a deteriorating course that eventually leads to death, usually between the fourth and sixth decades, unless long-term therapy with chenodeoxycholic acid is instituted. This therapy may correct and even possibly reverse the progression of disease.

Acid Cholesterol Ester Hydrolase Deficiency (Wolman's Disease) and Cholesterol Ester Storage Disease

Wolman's disease and cholesterol ester storage disease are two disorders in which there is tremendous storage of cholesterol esters and often triglycerides in lysosomes secondary to a deficiency of an acid lipase or acid esterase enzyme. Wolman's disease is the more severe of these disorders; cholesterol ester storage disease follows a more benign protracted course.

Wolman's Disease

Wolman's disease is an abnormality of lipid metabolism that usually becomes clinically evident in the first weeks of life and is characterized by GI symptoms, failure to thrive, hepatosplenomegaly, steatorrhea, and adrenal enlargement and calcification. It is inherited as an autosomal recessive disorder. This disease is invariably fatal, usually by 6 months of age. Nearly every organ contains cells loaded with neutral lipids, particularly cholesterol esters and glycerides. The presence of calcified adrenals associated with tissue lipid storage in a seriously ill infant is nearly pathognomonic of Wolman's disease.

Abramov et al. (1) described an infant with abdominal distention, hepatosplenomegaly, and massive calcification of the adrenal glands. This child expired at the age of 2 months following a short illness. The child was noted to have accumulation of both cholesterol and triglycerides in the liver, adrenal glands, spleen, and lymph nodes. Patrick and Lake (450) demonstrated that an acid lipase that catalyzes the hydrolysis of both cholesterol esters and triglycerides was severely deficient in the liver and spleen of patients with Wolman's disease. This has been confirmed in other tissues, including cultured fibroblasts, in other patients.

Clinical features

Wolman's disease has its onset in the first weeks of life with persistent and forceful vomiting associated with marked abdominal distention, steatorrhea, failure to thrive, and adrenal calcification. Anemia usually appears by 6 weeks of age and becomes more severe as the disease progresses. Lymphocytes have been repeatedly noted to be vacuolized, with the vacuoles being both intracytoplasmic and intranuclear. Lipid-laden histiocytes have been observed in bone marrow aspirates. The plasma lipids are usually in low concentration. Neurologically the infants are frequently bright and alert at age 5 to 6 weeks. By age 9 weeks there is usually a marked reduction in their activity. The hepatosplenomegaly, abdominal distention, anemia, vomiting, diarrhea, and inanition continue in a progressive fashion, and the child usually expires by age 3 to 6 months.

Neuropathology

Abramov et al. observed sudanophilic droplets in the capillary endothelium of the gray matter and swollen neurons in the medulla and retina. Lipid storage in neurons, including Purkinje cells, and sudanophilic granules within swollen microglia, periadventitial histiocytes, and possibly astrocytes have been observed. Ganglion cells of both Auerbach's and Meissner's plexuses were filled with sudanophilic granules.

Genetic and biochemical abnormalities

This is an autosomal recessive disorder. In Wolman's disease the enzyme deficiency is caused by a selective loss of lysosomal acid lipase.

Burton et al. (81) recently demonstrated abnormal cholesterol ester and triglyceride metabolism in intact fibroblasts from both patients with Wolman's disease and those with cholesterol ester storage disease. The differences in these two disorders could be related to the specific abnormalities they described (81).

Treatment

At the present time there is no specific treatment for this disorder. The prognosis for Wolman's disease is extremely poor, and the majority of infants die within the first 3 to 6 months of life.

Cholesterol Ester Storage Disease

Cholesterol ester storage disease is a rare familial autosomal recessive disease characterized by hepatomegaly and accumulation of cholesterol esters and triglycerides mainly in lysosomes in liver, spleen, intestinal mucosa, lymph nodes, and other tissues. Cholesterol ester storage disease is believed to be an allelic disorder to Wolman's disease. The distinction between Wolman's disease and cholesterol ester storage disease is that the latter has a much more benign course because of a defect in lysosomal acid lipase. In 1972 it was reported that patients with cholesterol ester storage disease were severely deficient in acid lipase or cholesterol ester hydrolase activity (563).

Clinical features

Of the cases reported to date, hepatomegaly appears to be a common early clinical finding that may not manifest until the adult years, although it may be discovered within the first decade of life. Hypercholesterolemia is common, and premature arteriosclerosis may be severe. A child with marked hepatomegaly and hyperlipidemia without splenic enlargement, with otherwise normal mental and physical development, should be considered a possible candidate for cholesterol ester storage disease.

Neuronal Ceroid Lipofuscinoses

These disorders present with progressive mental retardation, blindness, and seizures. This class of disease was first recognized by Batten in 1903 (37) and was reclassified and established as separate and distinct from the gangliosidoses by Zeman in 1976 (656). This is a group of heterogeneous genetic diseases inherited as autosomal recessive diseases, although autosomal dominant inheritance has been reported in the late onset form (366).

Clinical Features

Santavuori or Finnish form

This form begins as an autosomal recessive disease between 6 months and 2 years of age with insidious mental retardation, hypotonia, and ataxia. Seizures eventually occur with early onset amaurosis. Optic atrophy and vascular discoloration occur. The course is one of rapid deterioration with severe brain atrophy.

Jansky-Bielschowsky form

This form is also inherited as an autosomal recessive disease with onset between 2 and 4 years. Seizures, blindness, and mental retardation with associated optic atrophy, retinitis pigmentosa, and a rapid deterioration in neurologic function characterize the disorder (Fig. 28).

Spielmeyer-Vogt Sjögren form

This form has a later onset with a range between 2 and 10 years. Seizures and blindness with subsequent mental retardation occur, with associated vascular degeneration and pigmentary retinal degeneration. This form of disease is more slowly progressive and patients survive to puberty.

Kufs form

This form presents in young adulthood as an autosomal recessive or dominant with mental retardation and seizures. The optic fundus usually is normal and blindness does not occur. The course is slowly progressive and compatible with life until about age 40 years. The main clinical deficits are those of a progressive dementing disorder with seizures.

Biochemical Findings

All of these forms have in common the presence of autofluorescent lipopigments in neurons, glia, and endothelial cells of cerebral cortex, cerebellum, and hypothalamus. Liver and kidney also contain lipopigments. These two pigments, ceroid and lipofuscin, have different chemical properties and probably represent peroxides of cross-linked polymers of polyunsaturated fatty acids. The basic biochemical defect in these disorders that results in the deposition of the lipid peroxides remains unknown. Recently Ivy et al. (299) reported that injections of leupeptin (a thiol proteinase inhibitor) or chloroquine (a general lysosomal enzyme inhibitor) into the brains of young rats induced the formation of lysosome-associated granular aggregates or dense bodies that closely resembled the ceroid-lipofuscin that accumulates in the ceroid lipofuscinoses. These observations provide insights into the origin of these syndromes and a means to study them experimentally. Perhaps endogenous inhibitors of lysosomal enzymes or processing defects that prevent their lysosomal addressing might be areas for future research based on these findings.

Neuropathology

The neuropathology is characterized by neuronal loss, spongiform change of the brain, and the cytoplasmic inclusion of lipopigments. By electron microscopy the lipopigments appear as lamellar aggregates referred to as curvilinear bodies, and others appear as fingerprint bodies. Often a limiting membrane can be identified around these bodies suggestive of tertiary lysosomes. Several reports have described that the lipopigment bodies have acid phosphatase activity.

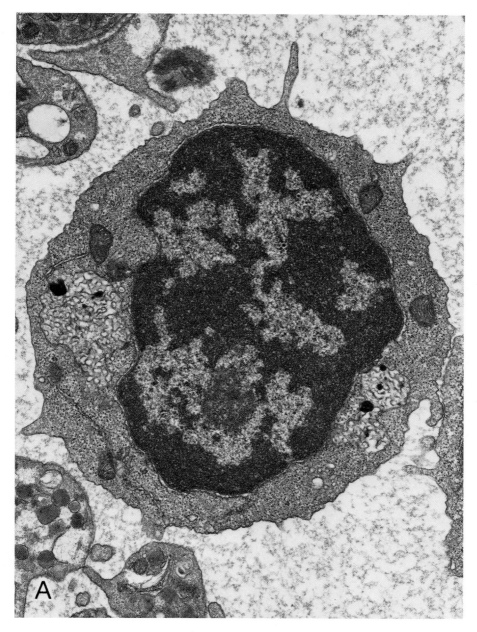

FIG. 28. Electron micrograph of a lymphocytic inclusion from a 6-year-old girl with the Jansky-Bielschowsky (late infantile) form of ceroid lipofuscinosis. The cell has several curvilinear profiles contained in membrane-bound cytosomes. These inclusions are easily seen using this technique and assist greatly in making this diagnosis. (Courtesy of Dr. Sidney Schochet, University of Oklahoma School of Medicine; from ref. 505, with permission.)   **A:** ×6000. *(Continued.)*

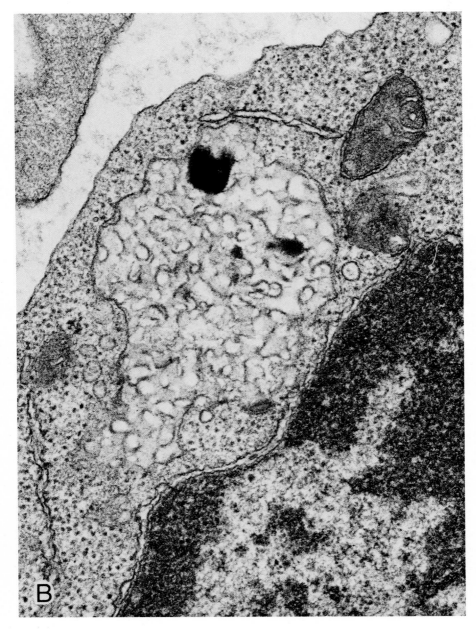

FIG. 28. *(Continued.)*   **B:** Higher resolution of Fig. 28A. ×60,000.

Lymphocytes can be of diagostic value, as they may contain cytoplasmic lipo-pigment inclusions, as seen in Fig. 28. Similarly, as shown by Farrell and Sumi (182), epithelial cells in the urinary sediment, peripheral nerve, skin, and muscle biopsies may contain cells with lipopigment inclusions.

Phytanic Acid Storage Disease (Refsum's Syndrome)

In 1946 Sigvald Refsum published a monograph identifying a new familial neurologic syndrome that he designated heredopathia atactica polyneuritiformis, and in 1963 the postmortem tissues from a 7-year-old girl diagnosed with Refsum's syndrome were biochemically analyzed. The liver and kidneys were grossly infiltrated with lipid, mostly neutral lipid. Gas chromatographic analysis revealed a 20-carbon branched-chain fatty acid that was fully characterized as phytanic acid. Whereas normal human plasma contains only traces of phytanic acid (less than 0.3 mg/dl), patients with Refsum's syndrome have 5 to 30% of their total plasma fatty acids present as phytanic acid. A series of studies has pointed to an exogenous origin for the accumulated phytanic acid and a defect in its catabolism as a basis for its accumulation. Steinberg and co-workers, in a series of studies, established that the major pathway for phytanic acid oxidation in human subjects and experimental animals involved the unusual initial α-oxidation to yield α-hydroxy-phytanic acid and then the (*n*-l) fatty acid pristanic acid. Through a series of successive β-oxidation steps, pristanic acid is further degraded. Evidence from clinical observation and cell culture studies now indicates the primary enzyme defect lies at the first step in this metabolic pathway, the α-oxidase. It is inherited as an autosomal recessive disorder (476).

Clinical Features

Refsum's disease presents with the tetrad of retinitis pigmentosa, peripheral polyneuropathy, cerebellar ataxia, and high CSF protein concentration in the absence of pleocytosis.

The onset of the disease has been detected in early childhood in some, but not until the fifth decade in others. The most frequent initial manifestation is night blindness. This is followed by decreased vision, signs of peripheral polyneuropathy, and cerebellar ataxia.

The course of the disease is one of gradually progressive deterioration, interrupted in approximately half of the patients by unexplained and sometimes lengthy periods of remission. Dramatic exacerbation associated with an ill-defined febrile illness, a surgical procedure, or pregnancy has been noted. Gradual recovery of function following such episodes is the rule, but residual neurologic deficits may remain.

At the present time the diagnosis is based on the constellation of clinical findings, demonstrated accumulation of phytanic acid in serum and tissue, or demonstrated reduction in capacity to oxidize phytanic acid. The carrier state can be diagnosed using the fibroblast cell culture methods. Normal amniotic cells have the capacity to oxidize phytanic acid, so intrauterine diagnosis is possible.

Neuropathology

The changes in peripheral nerves are those of a hypertrophic neuropathy. Electron microscopy reveals Schwann cell hyperplasia with osmophilic droplets in their cytoplasm and crystalline-like inclusions in their mitochondria.

In the brain axonal reaction in anterior horn cells and degeneration of the posterior columns appear to be secondary to the peripheral lesions. There also is tract degeneration in the medial lemniscus and cerebellar connections, particularly the olivocerebellar fibers. Droplets of sudanophilic lipid have been found in the leptomeninges, choroid plexus, ependyma, glial cells of the globus pallidus, and reticulata of the substantia nigra. Only in one instance has sudanophilic lipid been found in neurons. Degenerative changes in the cerebellar Purkinje cells are rarely seen.

Skeletal muscles show denervation atrophy. The heart may show a cardiomyopathy with focal scarring, reminiscent of the lesions found in Friedreich's ataxia. The liver and kidney show fatty infiltration.

Genetics and Biochemistry

This is an autosomal recessive disorder. Biochemical studies to date have revealed that there is little or no endogenous biosynthesis of phytanic acid and that phytol and phytanic acid are potential dietary precursors, since the metabolic error in Refsum's disease lies in a degradative pathway of phytanic acid. It has also been shown that the defect in phytanic acid storage disease persists in cultured fibroblasts. Normal human fibroblasts derived from skin biopsies oxidize added phytanate at rates comparable to those for added palmitate. Cells derived from patients with phytanic acid storage disease, however, oxidize palmitate at a normal rate but oxidize phytanate at only approximately 1% of the normal rate. Further biochemical studies have shown that the metabolic defect is localized to the initial α-oxidation of phytanate and probably to the α-hydroxylation step itself. The α-hydroxylation step has been shown to occur in mitochondria. The reaction is stimulated by NADPH and requires molecular oxygen. The reaction shows a marked stimulation by added ferric iron, whereas ferrous iron inhibits. This further distinguishes the phytanate oxidizing system in the liver from the straight-chain α-oxidation system in the brain, as the latter is primarily a microsomal enzyme and is stimulated by ferrous iron.

At the present time it is not known how the accumulation of phytanic acid leads to clinical manifestations of the disease. Indeed, it is not firmly established whether or not phytanic acid accumulation *per se* is necessary and sufficient for the clinical manifestations.

Therapy

If it is true that stored phytanate is exclusively of exogenous origin, elimination of phytanate and its potential precursors from the diet should prevent further accumulation. Patients adhering well to a rigorous diet have brought plasma phytanate levels down to 10% of pretreatment values and even normalized them in some instances. In those patients responding with a good fall in plasma phytanate, there has been an arrest in the progress of the peripheral neuropathy. Improvement in nerve conduction velocity has been documented in five patients followed in three different clinics. Cranial nerve functions have not shown improvement. Two patients have been studied whose symptoms and ulnar nerve conduction velocities improved on the diet, worsened when they went off the diet, and again improved when they went back on the diet.

Lundberg et al. (362) called attention to a potential hazard in dietary management. They followed two patients whose plasma phytanate levels paradoxically increased and whose neurologic status deteriorated markedly over a period of 1 to 2 months on a reduced caloric and reduced phytanate diet. This was attributed to the marked rise in plasma phytanate secondary to mobilization of tissue storage during rapid weight loss. At this time the evidence available indicates that any patient with a diagnosis of phytanic acid storage disease deserves an intensive trial of dietary treatment.

The untreated disease has a progressive course, with periods of exacerbation followed by improvement. How much dietary management will alter the progression of this disease is not clear at the present time, but hopefully it will slow the long-term deterioration.

LEUKODYSTROPHIES

Krabbe's Disease (Galactosyl Ceramidase Deficiency, Globoid Cell Leukodystrophy)

Krabbe described clinical and histologic findings in two siblings who presented with early onset of spasticity culminating in a rapidly fatal course (330). Krabbe described the globoid cells that are a hallmark of the disease. In 1970 Suzuki and Suzuki (585) demonstrated that galactocerebroside β-galactosidase is deficient in this disorder and that it is autosomal recessive. In 1971 Suzuki et al. (586) made the first intrauterine diagnosis and subsequently were able to detect the heterozygous condition by enzymatic assay. Hagberg (251) reported 32 Swedish cases during the period from 1953 to 1967 and calculated the incidence for that series as 1.9 per 100,000 births. Although the geographic distribution of the cases is widespread, the incidence in Scandinavian countries appears to be higher than in the rest of the world.

Clinical Features

In the majority of patients this disorder manifests between 3 and 6 months of age and presents as a degenerative disease involving predominantly the CNS. Hagberg (251) has divided the disease into three arbitrary stages:

Stage 1

A child who has been normal for the first few months of life develops hyperir-ritability, hypertonia, and hypersensitivity to tactile, visual, and auditory stimuli. There are episodes of fever of unknown origin. Psychomotor delay becomes apparent, with feeding difficulties appearing and seizures occasionally being manifested. The CSF protein level is elevated without pleocytosis, even at this early stage.

Stage 2

There is an acceleration of the brain degeneration with marked hypertonia, hyperreflexia, and optic atrophy. Minor motor seizures may occur.

Stage 3

This stage is characterized by decerebration, blindness, and sometimes complete deafness. Patients rarely survive for more than 2 years. The head is usually micro-cephalic, reflecting the destruction of brain myelin, although occasionally macro-cephaly may be seen (Fig. 29A).

Peripheral nerve involvement may be demonstrated electrophysiologically by diminished nerve conduction velocities and findings of denervation on electro-myography. The peripheral neuropathy is almost always completely overshadowed clinically by the prominent brain white matter degeneration. There is no visceral involvement in this disorder.

A later onset form of the disease has been described in more than 10 patients, who also have a slow progression of this disorder. Again, the clinical manifestations are those of a white matter degeneration, with the brain manifestations being visual impairment secondary to optic atrophy and/or cortical blindness, hypertonia, hy-perreflexia, and pathologic plantar responses. A peripheral neuropathy may be demonstrated by nerve conduction velocity studies but is clinically almost always overshadowed by the brain white matter degenerative findings. The CSF protein level is usually normal. The diagnosis is confirmed by finding decreased galactosyl ceramide-β-galactosidase activity in serum, leukocytes, cultured fibroblasts, or cultured amniotic fluid cells.

Neuropathology

All the important pathologic findings are limited to the nervous system, both central and peripheral. Peripheral nerve lesions consist of minimal to severe axonal degeneration, myelin breakdown associated with endoneural fibrosis, and accu-

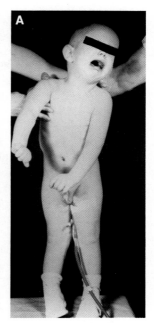

FIG. 29. A: A child with Krabbe's globoid cell leukodystrophy has evidence of quadriparesis and decerebrate posturing.   B: A brain biopsy of a patient with Krabbe's globoid cell leukodystrophy showing the large globoid cell characteristic of the disease. (Courtesy of Dr. M. E. Blaw, University of Texas Health Science Center at Dallas.)

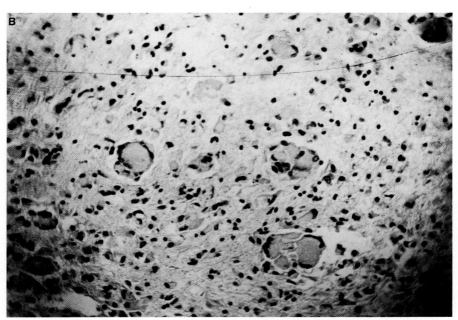

mulation of foamy histiocytes around endoneural blood vessels and endoneural trabeculae. Although typical globoid cells are not seen, straight or curved tubular inclusions are ultrastructurally seen within histiocytes.

Two types of globoid cells occur in the brain: mononuclear and multinuclear. At the present time available evidence strongly suggests the globoid cells originate from nonneural mesodermal cells, which is in keeping with their predominantly perivascular location and numerous fine tortuous cytoplasmic processes (Fig. 29B).

By light microscopy the globoid cells are seen to contain pale nuclei with prominent nucleoli. The abundant cytoplasm stains moderately positive with periodic acid-Schiff and faintly positive with Sudan black B and Sudan IV, which taken together indicate the presence of glycolipid. The cytoplasm is not metachromatic, with toluidine blue stain at acid pH. The globoid cell has many morphologic and histochemical characteristics in common with Gaucher's cells.

Ultrastructurally, mononuclear and multinuclear globoid cells appear identical except for the number of nuclei, and both have pseudopods, prominent rough endoplasmic reticulum, many free ribosomes, abundant fine cytoplasmic filaments, and scattered or clustered abnormal cytoplasmic inclusions. Globoid cells produced experimentally secondarily to intracerebral galactoceramide injection contain both types of tubules.

Grossly, the brain is usually markedly and uniformly reduced in size, with shrunken gyri and widened sulci. On cut section the white matter is grayish-white with a firm rubber-like consistency. The phylogenetically newer myelinated tracts are usually more severely affected and the subcortical U fibers are usually spared.

The prominent light microscopy findings are myelin deficiency (with sparing of the subcortical U fibers), loss of the oligodendroglial cells, and an astrocytic gliosis. The gray matter is typically only minimally affected, with mild focal or laminar degenerative changes in the cerebral cortex and mild degenerative changes in neurons elsewhere. No neuronal storage cells are seen.

Genetics and Biochemistry

The disease is inherited as an autosomal recessive. The most consistent finding in the white matter is an increased ratio of galactocerebroside to sulfatide, although both are much lower than normal. This is because there is more of an increase in galactocerebroside than a decrease in sulfatide. Another important observation has been the presence of 10 to 100 times more than the normal amount of galactosyl sphingosine (psychosine), which is galactosyl ceramide minus the fatty acid. Galactosyl sphingosine has been shown to be highly cytotoxic. Further studies have shown that the myelin formed in globoid cell leukodystrophy is normal ultrastructurally and biochemically.

Galactocerebroside is characteristically a lipid of the nervous system. The kidney is the only extraneural organ with significant amounts of this glycolipid. In brain galactocerebroside is almost exclusively localized in oligodendroglial cell membranes and therefore in myelin. It is now postulated that during the period of active myelination, both galactosyl ceramide and galactosyl sphingosine accumulate owing to the deficiency of galactocerebroside β-galactosidase. Galactosyl sphingosine is highly cytotoxic and leads to oligodendroglial cell death, since the oligodendroglia are predominantly exposed to this toxic glycolipid.

Therapy

At this time there is no effective treatment for this disorder.

Metachromatic Leukodystrophy (Sulfatide Lipidosis)

In 1910 Alzheimer (7) reported a patient with diffuse sclerosis and metachromatic staining of the tissues, and James Austin (23) and Austin et al. (25) demonstrated a large excess of sulfatides in the tissues of patients with metachromatic leukodystrophy. Austin et al. (25) demonstrated markedly low activity of arylsulfatase A and cerebroside sulfatase in the tissue of patients with metachromatic leukodystrophy. It is inherited as an autosomal recessive disorder.

Gustavson and Hagberg (245) reported an incidence of approximately 1 in 40,000, and in the juvenile form an incidence between 1 in 160,000 and 1 in 200,000.

Clinical Features

Late infantile form

This form of metachromatic leukodystrophy presents as a peripheral and central white matter degenerative disorder with onset usually between 12 and 18 months of age. The clinical course has been divided into four stages by Hagberg (249):

Stage 1.   This stage is represented by weakness, hypotonia, and hyporeflexia, which may involve all four extremities. Corticospinal tract and cerebellar findings may occasionally be present at this time. The mean duration of this stage is about 1 year.

Stage 2.   This stage is characterized by further progression of white matter degeneration, resulting in dysarthria, ataxia, and onset of hypertonia. The deep tendon reflexes remain diminished to absent. Mental deterioration becomes apparent. Intermittent pain in the arms and legs is a frequent feature that may be a manifestation of peripheral nerve root involvement. This stage usually lasts from 3 to 6 months.

Stage 3.   At this stage the child is usually bedridden and quadriplegic, with decorticate, decerebrate, or dystonic posturing (Fig. 30). Bulbar and/or pseudobulbar palsies are present, and the mental deficiency is severe. The deep tendon reflexes are almost always absent, and optic atrophy may occur. The optic atrophy appears as a gray macula with a red center. This stage lasts from 3 months to 3½ years in Hagberg's series.

Stage 4.   The patients in this final stage are characterized by loss of contact with their surroundings. They must be fed through a nasogastric or gastrostomy tube.

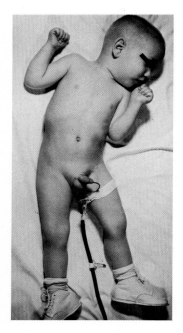

FIG. 30. A 1-year-old boy with advanced metachromatic leukodystrophy, illustrating a decorticate posture associated with a spastic quadriparesis and severe mental retardation. (Courtesy of Dr. M. E. Blaw, University of Texas Health Science Center at Dallas.)

Juvenile form

This form of metachromatic leukodystrophy has onset between 3 and 21 years of age, usually between 5 and 10 years. The initial symptom is usually in mental functioning, such as school problems or emotional lability, or the disorder may appear initially as a gait disorder. Extrapyramidal dysfunction and cerebellar findings are fairly common.

Adult form

The clinical manifestations of this form have their onset between 19 and 46 years of age in the cases described to date. The earliest symptoms are usually in the intellectual or emotional areas. Corticospinal and extrapyramidal symptoms develop and outweigh the peripheral nerve findings. Cerebellar findings of truncal ataxia, intention tremor, and nystagmus are also common. Seizures may occur duing the later stages. An excellent review of the subject is available (90).

The diagnosis of metachromatic leukodystrophy is suspected on the basis of the clinical presentation of the three forms as outlined above. The diagnosis is greatly strengthened by finding decreased activity (almost undetectable in homozygotes and 50% reduced in heterozygotes) of arylsulfatase A in serum, urine, leukocytes, cultured skin fibroblasts, or cultured amniotic fluid cells. Since arylsulfatase activity has been found to be normal to only slightly diminished in two patients with definite clinical symptoms, and has been found to be in the homozygous range in two other clinically normal individuals, one cannot rely entirely on arylsulfatase A activity to make the diagnosis. Therefore, it has been suggested that before the diagnosis is firmly established, one or more of the following confirmatory assays be positive: (a) nonspecific abnormalities such as decreased peripheral nerve conduction velocity, impaired gallbladder function, or elevated CSF protein; (b) above normal sulfatide excretion in the urine; or (c) the accumulation of glycolipid with metachromatic properties in tissues, preferably in peripheral nerve obtained by sural nerve biopsy.

Pathology of Nonneurologic Tissues

Metachromatic material is stored in the renal convoluted tubular epithelia, loops of Henle, and collecting tubules. Metachromatic material is also found in the liver, pancreatic islands, lymph nodes, adrenal glands, ovaries, and gallbladder. In the gallbladder the stored material appears to lead to cellular dysfunction, with a thickened, fibrotic gallbladder wall. No dysfunction is apparent in the other tissues mentioned.

Neuropathology

Grossly, the brain in late infantile metachromatic leukodystrophy usually appears quite normal, although it may be firmer and heavier than normal. Atrophy with reduced weight has also been observed. On cut section, there may be no apparent abnormality of the white matter.

Microscopically, there is a paucity or absence of myelinated fibers, with the deficit most intense in periventricular white matter, diminishing gradually toward the surface, and usually sparing the subcortical U fibers. The maximum changes are in the centrum semiovale, cerebellar white matter, and various brainstem and spinal cord tracts. As a general rule the process is most severe in tracts that are extensively myelinated after birth. Oligodendroglia are absent from areas of severe demyelination and reduced in adjacent apparently well-myelinated areas. Granular masses in the white matter are strikingly metachromatic when stained in frozen section with 1% cresyl violet at pH 3.6 adjusted with acetic acid (42).

In metachromatic leukodystrophy certain neurons also accumulate metachromatic lipids. The dentate nucleus of the cerebellum of all patients examined has been involved.

The peripheral nerve lesion is one of segmental demyelination with accumulation of metachromatic material in the perinuclear cytoplasm of Schwann cells and within macrophages. One study revealed that 80% of all nerve fibers had some damage.

Genetics and Biochemistry

This is an autosomal recessive disorder caused by a deficiency of arylsulfatase A. This enzyme has been mapped to chromosome 22q13. The chemical pathology of metachromatic leukodystrophy caused by this enzymatic defect is the accumulation of sulfatide up to 3 to 10 times normal in the late infantile form, with other myelin lipids, such as cholesterol and sphingomyelin, decreased by 30 to 50%. Cerebroside levels in white matter are decreased by 10 to 50 percent of normal, and this gives rise to an abnormal cerebroside to sulfatide ratio. In normal white matter the ratio is approximately 4. In the late infantile form of metachromatic leukodystrophy, the cerebroside to sulfatide ratio may be decreased to 0.5. All evidence indicates that the chemical structure of sulfatide is normal in metachromatic leukodystrophy (194).

The adult form of metachromatic leukodystrophy shows chemical abnormalities similar to but less severe than those of the late infantile form. The one exception is that in the adult form of the disease, the gray matter sulfatide levels are increased to a greater extent than in the late infantile form. This is interesting in the light of the more prominent intellectual and emotional findings noted earlier in the adult form of the disease.

Immunoassay techniques have revealed slight but significant antigenic differences between normal arylsulfatase A and the mutant enzyme found in metachromatic leukodystrophy.

Porter et al. (470) and Farrell et al. (180), using intact fibroblasts in culture, showed that the amount of arylsulfatase activity in cells from patients with metachromatic leukodystrophy was directly correlated with the age of onset of clinical symptoms and severity of disease. Fibroblasts from patients with the late infantile form of metachromatic leukodystrophy had no detectable cerebroside sulfatase activity, whereas fibroblasts from patients manifesting the disease later in life had appreciable amounts of enzyme activity. One explanation of this finding is that the residual arylsulfatase A may be structurally different in the various clinical forms of the disease, so that in the adult form of the disease the arylsulfatase A may either be physically more stable or possess greater substrate affinity.

In 1983 Hizeidarsson et al. (277) reported low arylsulfatase A levels in two siblings. One sibling had a neurologic disability not typical for metachromatic leukodystrophy, and the other was a healthy 18-year-old woman with a normal developmental history. In both siblings arylsulfatase A levels in white blood cells were 7 to 8% of control values. Other family members had enzyme levels consistent with heterozygote or normal status. Hizeidarsson et al. concluded that the neurologic abnormalities in the one sibling were not the result of the low enzyme activity and that both persons represent examples of "pseudo-arylsulfatase A" deficiency (arylsulfatase A deficiency without metachromatic leukodystrophy). This is an unusual disorder caused by a mutation allelic to the mutation responsible for true metachromatic leukodystrophy.

Therapy

At the present time there is no specific therapy for this disorder. Bone marrow transplantation to provide donor cells capable of enzyme production has not been of clinical value.

Adrenoleukodystrophy

Historical

Adrenoleukodystrophy (ALD) was first described in 1923 by Siemerling and Creutzfeldt (555), who pointed out that skin pigmentation and a progressive leukodystrophy were central features of the disorder. Blaw (51), Schaumberg and associates (526–528), and Moser and associates (415) have provided the important clinical and pathological features.

Genetics

This is an X-linked disease (Xq28) with variable expression beginning in early childhood, teenage years, or early adulthood. Males are principally affected, but carrier females may also show clinical evidence of disease.

Clinical Features

Several phenotypes of ALD are reported. Progressive cerebral degeneration with cortical blindness, spinal cord involvement with spastic quadriparesis, and cutaneous hyperpigmentation in young males are typical features. Variants of the ALD syndrome include X-linked Addison's disease without any neurologic involvement, and spasticity and weakness caused by spinal involvement in female carriers. In the adrenomyeloneuropathy variant, symptoms begin later in the second and third decades and the disease process develops slowly over more than two decades. A peripheral neuropathy, azoospermia, and hypotestosteronemia complete the picture. A neonatal ALD variant has also recently been described that shows the same biochemical defect as in typical ALD but that involves girls as frequently and as severely as boys; it is suggested that it is inherited as an autosomal recessive trait (247,301). Cellular peroxisomes in X-linked ALD are normal in number and size, and the peroxisomes have a characteristic coarsely fibrillar, moderately electron-opaque matrix and are often in clusters. In neonatal autosomal recessively inherited ALD, the peroxisomes are sparse, scattered, and small in size compared with normals. There was a 10-fold decrease in the number and mean volume of hepatocellular peroxisomes in a patient with neonatal ALD. Thus the basis for impaired long-chain fatty acid oxidation in ALD, whether it is X-linked or autosomally recessively inherited, is a defect in peroxisomal availability or function (224). Predilection for parietal lobe and occipital lobe white matter is the basis for early onset cortical blindness. The CT brain scan shows decreased density of cerebral white matter. Clinical and laboratory evidence of hypoadrenalism can be demonstrated at some time during the illness (51), and can precede by many years the onset of neurologic symptoms (525).

O'Neill et al. (444) reported one family having X-linked recessively inherited Addison's disease in men with no other neurologic disease. Carrier heterozygous females may have mild to severe myelopathic findings of a spastic paraparesis

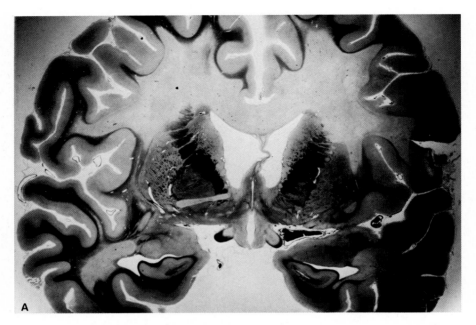

FIG. 31. Adrenoleukodystrophy. **A:** Characteristic demyelination of the central white matter with sparing of the subcortical U-fibers. *(Continued.)*

without cerebral manifestations (444). Presumably the presence of clinical disease in female carriers is explained by the Lyon hypothesis of random inactivation of the X chromosome (363). The disease is inexorably progressive and uniformly fatal. Excellent reviews are offered by Blaw (51) and O'Neill and Moser (444).

Moser et al. (415) recently reported on 303 patients with ALD in 217 kindreds. Their patients showed a broad spectrum of phenotypic variation. Sixty percent of patients had childhood ALD and 17% adrenomyeloneuropathy, a form showing progressive leg spasticity, paralysis, and polyneuropathy without mental status changes. Both ALD and adrenomyeloneuropathy are X-linked recessive and map to Xp28. They found that neonatal ALD, a distinct entity with autosomal recessive inheritance and a resemblance to Zellweger syndrome, was present in 7% of the cases. They concluded that ALD and Zellweger cerebrohepatorenal syndrome belong to a newly formed category of peroxisomal disorders, as in both syndromes the peroxisome to degrade C26:0 very long-chain lipids is defective (ALD) or absent (Zellweger).

Pathology

The cerebral hemispheres undergo a diffuse, symmetrical loss of myelin in the white matter pathways and especially in the posterior quadrants of the hemispheres. There is a sparing of the subcortical U fibers (Fig. 31A). Similar demyelination

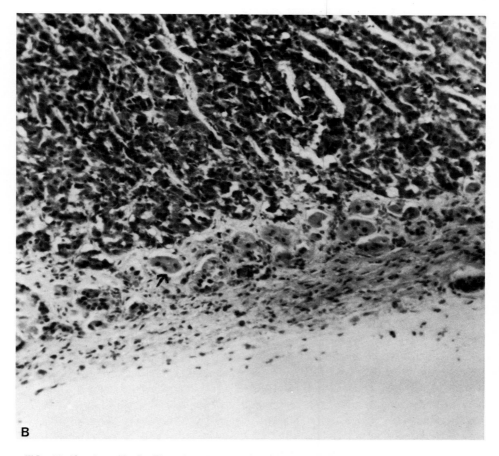

B

FIG. 31. *(Continued.)* **B**: The adrenal cortex also undergoes atrophy with relative preservation of the zona glomerulosa, as shown by the cell with an *arrow*. (Courtesy of Dr. M. E. Blaw, University of Texas Health Science Center at Dallas.)

affects the thoracic spinal cord. There is an associated perivascular mononuclear cell infiltration (526–528). Lamellar lipid profiles are found in adrenal cortical cells and macrophages in brain white matter, indicating a lipid storage disorder. The adrenal cortices are atrophic with relative preservation of the zona glomerulosa (Fig. 31B).

Biochemistry

Brain white matter and adrenal cortex from patients have cytoplasmic inclusions that contain cholesterol esters of saturated very long-chain fatty acids with a carbon chain length of C23 and longer (295,393). Hexacosanoic acid (C26:0) is the most significantly elevated. Cultured fibroblasts accumulate very long-chain fatty acids as well (414,486,603). O'Neill et al. (445) studied 21 women from four ALD kinships, nine of whom had a spastic paraparesis, including two with peripheral neuropathy. Fifteen women were assigned heterozygote status based on abnormal very long-chain fatty acid elevations in plasma, fibroblasts, or both. Singh et al. (559), working with the Mosers, concluded that ALD patients have a defect in the oxidation of very long-chain fatty acids (C24:0 and longer) but not in the degradation of fatty acids with a chain length of 18 carbons or less. The enzymatic basis of the accumulation of very long-chain fatty acids in ALD is unknown.

Therapy

Patients have been treated unsuccessfully by dietary restriction of very long-chain fatty acids, use of carnitine and clofibrate, immunosuppression, and plasma exchange. Adrenal steroid therapy has no effect on neurologic progression. One 13-year-old boy was treated with an allogeneic bone marrow transplant from a normal HLA-identical sibling donor. Complete hematologic recovery occurred but neurologic deterioration continued (415). At present no specific form of therapy exists to treat the progressive neurologic deterioration. Although the excess C26:0 in the brain of patients with ALD is partially of dietary origin, dietary C26:0 restriction did not produce clear benefit (414,415).

Cerebrohepatorenal (Zellweger) Syndrome

Cerebrohepatorenal syndrome (CHRS) has clinical features similar to ALD. The two disorders affect the same general age group, both involve cerebral cortex and white matter, both have similar eye lesions, and peroxisomes are absent in CHRS and defective in ALD (224). CHRS includes craniofacial abnormalities, severe hypotonia, mental retardation, cerebral dysgenesis, cortical renal cysts, and hepatomegaly. It is inherited in an autosomal recessive manner. In 1984 Moser et al. (413) reported that CHRS patients also have abnormalities of very long-chain fatty acids similar to ADL. They found a fivefold increase of C26:0 in plasma, cultured skin fibroblasts, or postmortem brain tissues of 20 CHRS patients. In 1984 Datta et al. (119) reported a marked reduction in the activity of dihydroxyacetone phosphate acyltransferase, a peroxisomal enzyme, in fibroblasts and leukocytes from CHRS patients. Thus the role of peroxisomes in the metabolism of very long-chain fatty acids is an important one and depends on the integrity of the acyltransferase pathway. Both ALD and CHRS are the result of defects in peroxisomal oxidation of very long-chain fatty acids (224).

Fabry's Disease (α-Galactosidase A Deficiency)

Anderson in England (12) and Fabry in Germany (176) independently described patients with angiokeratoma corpus diffusum. In 1947 Pompen et al. (469) described the pathologic findings in two patients known to have angiokeratoma corpus diffusum. The most consistent finding was the presence of vacuoles in the media of abnormal blood vessels throughout the body and similar vacuoles about the nuclei of hypertrophied myocardial fibers.

After a number of reports of a more limited form of the disease in heterozygous females, Opitz et al. (446) in 1965 studied the kindred of 21 carrier females and affected males and confirmed the X-linked transmission of the disease.

On renal autopsy of hemizygote patients, two neutral glycosphingolipids, galactosyl-galactosyl-glucosylceramide (Gal-Gal-Gluc-Cer) and digalactosyl ceramide (Gal-Gal-Cer), have been isolated and characterized. Other studies have shown increased levels of Gal-Gal-Gluc-Cer in brain, plasma, urinary sediment, cultured skin fibroblasts, and most viscera in these patients.

Brady et al. (60) demonstrated the enzymatic defect was absence of α-galactosidase A, which can be assayed for in plasma, urinary sediment, cultured skin fibroblasts, and cultured amniotic fluid. The disease has an incidence of 1 in 40,000.

The disease is inherited in an X-linked recessive manner. This mode of transmission is supported by the absence of parental consanguinity, absence of male-to-male transmission, occurrence of female-to-male transmission, measurable linkage between the α-galactosidase loci and the X_g^a blood-group antigen, the absence of any sign of the disease in more than 35 known sons of affected fathers, and the presence of three pedigrees in which two affected sons were born to the same mother by different fathers.

Clinical Features

Male hemizygote

The clinical manifestations are periodic episodes of fever and severe distal extremity pain, with associated vascular lesions of the skin, conjunctiva, and oral mucosa, and crystalline deposits in the conjunctiva. The onset is from childhood to adolescence.

Pain is often the initial symptom and may have an excruciating burning or lightning character. The pain most commonly involves the fingers and toes and is accompanied by paresthesias; with time it spreads proximally. Fever, changes in environmental temperature, and physical exercise may all initiate the painful episodes. Since many of the painful episodes are associated with fever and an elevated erythrocyte sedimentation rate, the children are often erroneously diagnosed as having rheumatic fever.

Telangiectasis (angiokeratomas) may be one of the initial signs and are classically clusters of dark red angiectasias in the superficial layers of the skin (Fig. 32). The skin lesions are usually bilaterally symmetrical in their placement and show a predilection for the hips, buttocks, back, thighs, penis, and scrotum. The oral mucosa and conjunctiva are also commonly involved. With progressive accumulation of glycosphingolipids in the kidneys, progressive renal failure is manifested by azotemia.

Diffuse deposits of glycosphingolipids in the vascular system and myocardium may manifest as hypertension, cardiomegaly, myocardial ischemia or infarction, and brain signs and symptoms of ischemia and/or infarction. The brain manifes-

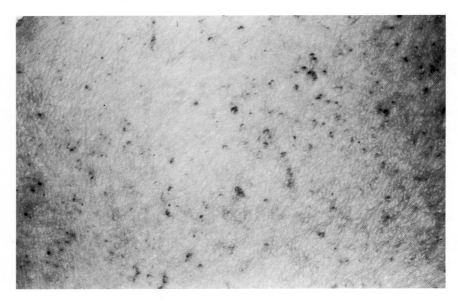

FIG. 32. Telangiectasia (angiokeratomas) on a patient with Fabry's disease. (From ref. 505, with permission.)

tations may be seizures, motor or sensory impairment, aphasia, various brainstem syndromes, or intracranial mass lesions secondary to intracranial hemorrhage. The characteristic ocular lesions are aneurysmal dilation of veins in the conjunctiva and retina. Corneal opacities are also commonly found. Progressive vascular disease of the brain, heart, and kidneys usually leads to death in the fourth or fifth decades of life.

Female heterozygote

In general, all the clinical manifestations found in the hemizygous male are also found in the heterozygous female but are less severe and have a later onset in the heterozygote. However, the disease becomes more severe in middle life in the heterozygous female, and death can usually be attributed to renal or cardiac complications of the disease.

The diagnosis is based on the clinical presentation of widespread small-vessel pathology and confirmed by the absence of activity of α-galactosidase A in plasma, leukocytes, fibroblasts, and tissues of these patients. The diagnosis may also be made *in utero* from enzymatic analysis of amniotic fluid cells.

Genetics and Biochemistry

The disease is inherited as an X-linked recessive disorder, and the pathology results from an accumulation of cerebroside trihexoside caused by α-galactosidase deficiency. Affected hemizygous individuals have 10 to 25% of the normal α-galactosidase A activity. The enzyme deficiency in hemizygous individuals appears to be limited to the thermally labile α-galactosidase A, whereas any residual α-galactosidase activity appears to be caused by α-galactosidase B. Most heterozygous females have intermediate levels of α-galactosidase A activity.

This circulating cerebroside trihexoside is thought to gain access to vascular endothelial cells and to endothelial and adjacent epithelial cells in the renal glomeruli by receptor-mediated uptake. This accumulation within blood vessels gives rise to narrowing, dilatation, instability, and motor unresponsiveness of the blood vessels. These are major physiologic features of the disorder (129).

Therapy

Fabry's disease is characterized by a chronic debilitating course that extends over many years. The single most debilitating aspect is the excruciating pain.

Various drugs have been tried for relief of the pain, including the α-adrenergic blocking agent phenoxybenzamine to increase peripheral vascular flow. In one patient phenoxybenzamine did appear to provide pain relief on several occasions, but epistasis and priapism were early complications in two other patients. Recently a report of a hemizygous patient indicated the combination of diphenylhydantoin and carbamazepine significantly reduced the pain.

Because renal insufficiency is a very common late complication, chronic hemodialysis and renal transplantation may be life-saving. So far, the use of renal allografts to alter the progression of the disease remains controversial.

In the future enzyme replacement therapy may hold promise in this disorder. Studies of fibroblasts in tissue culture from hemizygous subjects have shown that α-galactosidase A exogenously supplied to the media is capable of gaining access to fibroblasts and catabolizing the accumulated Gal-Gal-Gluc-Cer. Furthermore, it was demonstrated that less than 5% of exogenous enzyme was capable of causing substantial substrate metabolism.

Brady (65) administered α-galactosidase purified from human placenta to two hemizygous individuals. It was shown that the enzyme was rapidly cleared from the blood, taken up by the liver, and caused a decrease in the circulating level of Gal-Gal-Gluc-Cer.

Other Hereditary Leukodystrophies

Canavan's Disease

Megalocephaly in infancy, mental retardation, seizures, cortical blindness, flaccidity, and failure of neurologic development because of abnormal cerebral edema inherited as an autosomal recessive constitute the syndrome. It is sometimes referred to as spongy sclerosis. There is extensive demyelination and astrocytic edema throughout the white matter (Fig. 33). The life span of affected children is usually less than 5 years. There is no specific therapy.

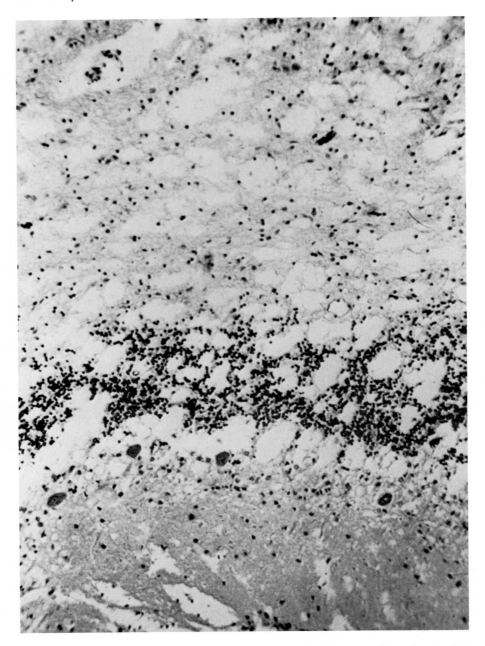

FIG. 33. Megalocephaly in Canavan's disease is associated with large, swollen astrocytes that are illustrated in this brain biopsy. (Courtesy of Dr. M. E. Blaw, University of Texas Health Science Center at Dallas.)

Alexander's Disease

Megalocephaly in the first year of life, failure of neurologic development, spasticity, and decerebration are the features of this poorly characterized disorder. Impaired myelination, presence of Rosenthal fibers within astrocytes, and eosinophilic hyaline bodies are the characteristic features. The mode of inheritance is not clear, as most cases are sporadic. There is no specific therapy and patients live only a few years.

Pelizaeus-Merzbacher Disease

This is a rare disorder characterized by spasticity, ataxia, coarse ocular nystagmus, optic atrophy, and head tremor. It is thought to be X-linked when it presents in early childhood and autosomal dominant when it presents in early adulthood. There is moderate to severe demyelination of central white matter with an impairment in the formation of compact myelin.

Hereditary Adult Onset Leukodystrophy Simulating Chronic Progressive Multiple Sclerosis

Eldridge et al. reported in 1984 (156) a large kindred with a chronic progressive neurologic disorder affecting 10 men and 11 women in four generations in an autosomal dominant pattern of inheritance. In examining an individual patient without access to family history or CT findings, one would conclude the disease process was multiple sclerosis. Patients present in the fourth or fifth decades with progressive cerebellar, pyramidal, and autonomic abnormalities. The CT scan shows symmetrical reductions in white matter density involving all cerebral lobes as well as cerebellar white matter. The white matter on pathologic examination shows severe degeneration with microscopic vacuolation, preserved subcortical U fibers, and no inflammatory changes or reactive gliosis. The primary genetic defect is unknown and there is no specific therapy.

Disorders of Mucopolysaccharide Metabolism

The mucopolysaccharides are a diverse set of compounds containing polysaccharide, alternating amino sugars, and uronic acids (Table 3). Dermatan sulfate and heparan sulfate are two major mucopolysaccharides that increase, are stored, and are excreted in the mucopolysaccharidoses (MPS). The compounds are sequentially degraded by specific lysosomal enzymes—exoglycosidases or exosulfatases—and an enzyme deficiency results in an increased degree of cellular lysosomal storage of mucopolysaccharide.

The first clinical description of Hurler's syndrome was probably provided by John Thompson in 1900 from the Royal Infirmary, Edinburgh. Hunter's (292) syndrome was recorded in 1917 in two brothers, and in 1920 Hurler (293) reported

TABLE 3. *Mucopolysaccharides of connective tissue*

Name	Amino sugar	Uronic acid	Sulfate	Amino substitution	Linkage Uronide hexosaminidic	Linkage to protein	Occurrence
Dermatan sulfate	D-GalN	L-IdUA D-GlcUA	O-SO$_4$	N-Ac	α1 → 3β1 → 4	Gal-Gal-Xyl-Ser	Skin, lung
Heparan sulfate	D-GlcN	D-GlcUA L-IdUA	N-SO$_4$ O-SO$_4$	N-Ac N-SO$_4$	β1 → 4 α1 → 4α1 → 4	Gal-Gal-Zyl-Ser	Lung, spleen, liver, muscle
Keratin sulfate I (cornea)	D-GlcN	Gal(mann)	O-SO$_4$	N-Ac	β1 → 4β1 → 3	GalNAc-AspNH$_2$	Cornea, nucleus pulposus, cartilage
Keratin sulfate II (skeletal)	D-GlcN D-GalN	Gal(mann)	O-SO$_4$	N-Ac	β1 → 4β1 → 3	GalNAc-Ser GalNAc-Thr	

From ref. 505, with permission.

two boys having the stigmata of the disorder associated with that eponym. The first organized nosologic classification was provided in 1952 by Brante (68), who used the term mucopolysaccharidosis for the first time. Excessive urinary excretion of these compounds was reported by Dorfman and Lorinez (142), Brown (75), and Meyer et al. (399). The concept of an MPS caused by an enzyme defect resulting in a lysosomal storage disorder was put forth initially in 1964 by van Hoff and Hers (614), and the *in vitro* accumulation of mucopolysaccharide by fibroblasts in culture was reported by Danes and Bearn (115) using cells from MPS patients. The McKusick classification of MPS was published in 1965 (387).

It was Elizabeth Neufeld who made a brilliant series of enzymatic observations in the early 1970s showing that the MPS were caused by specific catabolic enzyme defects resulting in accumulation of substrate and not by increased synthetic rates (430). She and her colleagues demonstrated that [^{35}S]mucopolysaccharide accumulated in fibroblasts from MPS patients in cell culture and that a corrective factor, which later was shown to be normal lysosomal enzyme, could prevent [^{35}S]mucopolysaccharide storage and led to the identification of the enzyme defects involved. Fratantoni et al. (199–201) demonstrated that cocultured fibroblasts from Hurler and Hunter patients did cross-correct and prevented [^{35}S]mucopolysaccharide storage. This corrective effect was due to complementary enzymatic replacement by the MPS cell line from the Hurler patient on the Hunter patient cells and vice versa. These disorders have been reviewed recently by McKusick and Neufeld (384a).

α-L-IDURONIDASE DEFICIENCY

This enzyme deficiency has been associated with Hurler's syndrome (MPS I H), Scheie's syndrome (MPS I S), and a genetic compound form, Hurler-Scheie syndrome (MPS I H/S).

HURLER'S SYNDROME (MPS I H)

This is an autosomal recessive disorder described in 1920 by Gertrud Hurler (293) that has an incidence of approximately 1 in 100,000 and an estimated carrier rate of 1 in 150.

Clinical Features

Children develop an unrelenting, progressive syndrome caused by mucopolysaccharide storage in the CNS, cornea, bone, heart, liver, and spleen. Severe mental retardation, corneal clouding, hepatosplenomegaly, and skeletal deformities progressively occur, with death occurring before the first decade of life. Characteristic facial coarsening occurs associated with hypertelorism, hirsutism, shallow orbits producing proptosis, and scaphocephaly caused by early sagittal suture closing. Other skeletal defects include a J-shaped sella turcica, joint malformations, chest defects, lumbar lordosis, a widened medial end of the clavicle, vertebral hypoplasia with a hooked appearance to the apical dorsal vertebrae, iliac wing flaring, claw hand deformities, hip flexion, contractures, and dwarfism.

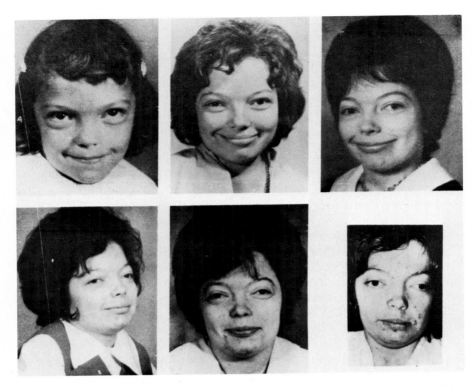

FIG. 34. Serial photographs illustrating the change in facial features with development of Hurler-Scheie syndrome. The **top** row shows the patient at ages 5, 13, and 18 years and the **bottom** row at ages 20, 24, and 25 years. The initial presence of hypertelorism, saddle nose, and short neck is noted in the picture at age 5 years. Subsequent photographs indicate the coarsening of facial features and a left ocular exotropia consistent with a mucopolysaccharide disorder. (From ref. 641, with permission.)

The clinical diagnosis is established by the increased urinary excretion of dermatan and heparan sulfate (2:1), in association with the typical skeletal deformities, mental retardation, corneal clouding, and hepatosplenomegaly. The enzyme defect is α-L-iduronidase, which can be measured in fibroblast cultures (379).

Therapy

Enzyme replacement therapy has not been useful, and at present there is no specific therapy (110).

SCHEIE'S SYNDROME (MPS I S)

This is an autosomal recessive disorder described by Scheie et al. in 1962 (529) that has an estimated incidence of 1 in 500,000.

Clinical Features

These patients present in adulthood with hirsutism, joint stiffening, claw hand, genu valgum, pes cavus, aortic valve disease, and prominent corneal clouding. The syndrome resembles a mild, incomplete presentation of Hurler's syndrome. It is an allelic disorder of Hurler's syndrome, as it is caused by a milder degree of deficiency of α-L-iduronidase.

Therapy

Corneal transplantation and the surgical repair of nerve entrapments are the principal forms of therapy. There is no specific therapy for the underlying disease.

HURLER-SCHEIE GENETIC COMPOUND (MPS I H/S)

Since McKusick's report in 1972 (385), a series of patients have been reported who are deficient in α-L-iduronidase and who phenotypically are intermediate between Hurler and Scheie patients. We also have reported one such interesting genetic compound patient (641) (Figs. 34–36). These patients have 50% of their enzyme inherited from one parent, which represents the Hurler allelic defect, and the other 50% from the other patient, which represents the Scheie allelic defect.

Clinical Features

These patients develop in early adulthood progressive mental retardation, skeletal defects, and cardiac and hepatic disease. Associated corneal clouding, joint stiffening, and cardiac valvular disease occur.

Our report described for the first time the storage of mucopolysaccharide material in neurons of the brain and spinal cord, with their characteristic lysosomal storage pattern on electron microscopy (641).

Therapy

No specific therapy is available.

HUNTER'S SYNDROME (IDURONATE SULFATASE DEFICIENCY, MPS II)

This is an X-linked recessive disorder with an unknown incidence. Hunter (292) first described the syndrome, and Wolff (644) and Njaa (432) suggested the X-linked mode of inheritance.

Clinical Features

The disease presents with a spectrum of severity, which may be caused by allelic defects at the iduronate sulfatase locus on the X chromosome.

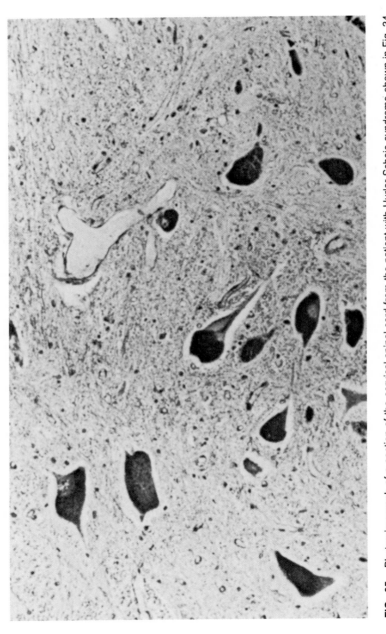

FIG. 35. Photomicrograph of a section of the cervical spinal cord from the patient with Hurler-Scheie syndrome shown in Fig. 34 stained with luxol fast blue. The cytoplasm of the anterior horn cells is distended by lipid-containing granules. Original magnification ×600. (From ref. 641, with permission.)

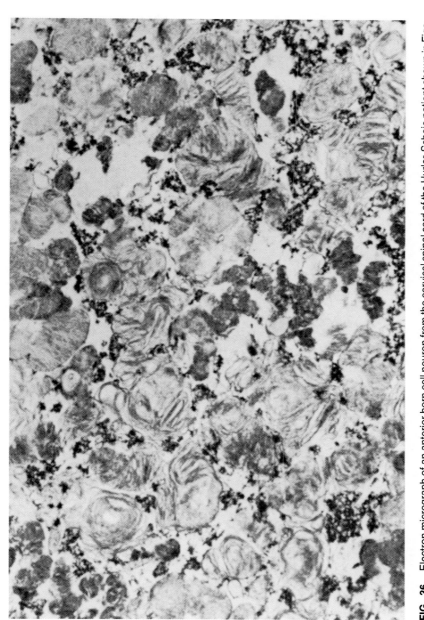

FIG. 36. Electron micrograph of an anterior horn cell neuron from the cervical spinal cord of the Hurler-Scheie patient shown in Figs. 34 and 35. Cytoplasmic granules consist of concentric and lamellar arrays of membrane indicative of mucopolysaccharide. Original magnification, ×6100. (From ref. 641, with permission.)

It bears a strong resemblance to MPS IH but is separated clinically from MPS IH by the absence of corneal clouding, perhaps a more placid personality, and a longer life span. Patients are identified by the typical clinical phenotype, the excretion of equal amounts of dermatan sulfate and heparan sulfate, and a deficiency of iduronate sulfatase in serum and cultured fibroblasts.

Therapy

There is no specific therapy.

SANFILIPPO'S SYNDROME (HEPARAN SULFATASE DEFICIENCY, MPS III TYPE A; N-ACETYL-α-GLUCOSAMINIDASE DEFICIENCY, MPS III TYPE B; ACETYL-COA:α-GLUCOSAMINIDE N-ACETYLTRANSFERASE DEFICIENCY, MPS III TYPE C; N-ACETYLGLUCOSAMINE-6-SULFATE SULFATASE DEFICIENCY, MPS III TYPE D)

Sanfilippo's syndrome (522) is inherited as an autosomal recessive disorder, and the different enzyme defects are indistinguishable clinically. It was Harris (263) who first described this new form of MPS, which subsequently turned out to be type B disease (143). Type A disease was shown to be caused by a deficiency of heparan sulfatase (332,380).

Clinical Features

Patients develop in childhood a severe form of mental retardation with minimal skeletal defects and hepatosplenomegaly. Corneal clouding does not occur. Epilepsy may occur. The diagnosis is established by the increased excretion of heparan sulfate and a deficiency of heparan sulfatase or N-acetyl-α-glucosaminidase in cultured fibroblasts or amniotic fluid cells for types A and B, respectively. Types C and D are identified by finding a deficiency in the two enzymes reported for them as listed in the beginning of this section.

Therapy

There is no specific therapy.

MORQUIO'S SYNDROME (GALACTOSAMINE-6-SULFATASE DEFICIENCY TYPE A; β-GALACTOSIDASE DEFICIENCY, TYPE B) (MPS IV)

This is an autosomal recessive disorder described initially in 1935 by Morquio (408), who described the disorder in four children of Swedish parents who were first cousins.

Clinical Features

Patients have serious skeletal defects and coarsening of facial features but normal intelligence. Chest deformities with a pectus carinatum occur. The odontoid process of the axis is malformed, hypoplastic, or absent, which results in atlantoaxial subluxation and cervical cord compression in many patients (328). Joint instability, deafness, and corneal clouding occur.

The diagnosis is based on the severe, characteristic skeletal defects, normal intelligence, and increased excretion of keratan sulfate. Deficiency of one of the two enzymes mentioned firmly establishes the type, as types A and B are clinically indistinguishable.

Therapy

The one form of therapy that must be emphasized is identification and correction of the unstable atlantoaxial joint, which may produce cervical cord compression and thus significant morbidity.

MAROTEAUX-LAMY SYNDROME (ARYLSULFATASE B OR GALACTOSAMINE-4-SULFATASE DEFICIENCY) (MPS VI)

This is an autosomal recessive disorder described initially by Maroteaux and Lamy (372,373) as a Hurler's variant in which intellect is preserved and there is increased urinary excretion of dermatan sulfate.

Clinical Features

This is a highly variable disorder with a spectrum of severity resembling Hurler's at one end and Scheie's disorder at the other. As McKusick points out, these patients are uniformly short, whereas Scheie's syndrome patients (MPS IS) are in the normal range for height, and this feature has differentiating value. Intelligence is preserved, which is also an important separating point.

Patients excrete high levels of dermatan sulfate exclusively, and assays of leukocytes, fibroblasts, and amniotic cells in culture show very low levels of arylsulfatase B (N-acetylgalactosamine-4-sulfatase) activity.

This enzyme has been mapped to a locus on chromosome 5.

Therapy

An encouraging report in 1984 by Gasper et al. (215) demonstrated that a bone marrow transplant corrected the hereditary enzyme deficiency in a 2-year-old male siamese cat with advanced MPS VI. Leukocyte arylsulfatase B activity increased 30-fold by 232 days after transplantation. Corneal clouding, mobility, and demeanor all improved, suggesting that similar therapy for a child with this syndrome might be useful. In fact, in 1984 Krivit et al. (333) reported a 13-year-old girl with a severe form of Maroteaux-Lamy syndrome who underwent a successful bone marrow transplant. Arylsulfatase B activity increased to normal levels in peripheral lymphocytes and granulocytes, and increased from 3 to 16% of the mean normal level at 680 days posttransplant in a liver biopsy sample. Hepatosplenomegaly was substantially decreased, and cardiopulmonary function was normal. Visual acuity and joint mobility also improved, and she returned to school. Thus a bone marrow transplant did provide a source of enzymatically normal cells, which significantly improved this single patient. This therapy will be attempted in future children because of this very positive, exciting result. Clearing of the corneal opacity after perforating keratoplasty was reported in 1985 by Naumann (425).

SLY SYNDROME (β-GLUCURONIDASE DEFICIENCY, MPS VII)

This is an autosomal recessive disorder with considerable clinical variation between reported patients. It was described by Sly et al. in 1973 (566), and Hall et al. (256) described β-glucuronidase in patient fibroblast cultures as being deficient. It was mapped to a locus on chromosome 7 in 1975 with somatic cell hybrid techniques by Grzeschik (242) and by Lalley et al. (339).

Clinical Features

Patients may develop severe skeletal defects and progressive mental retardation. Sly et al. reported in their index case a child who at 7 weeks had dysmorphic facies, hepatosplenomegaly, umbilical hernia, a thoracolumbar gibbus, and puffy hands and feet. Later an anterior chest defect developed, and bilateral inguinal hernias required surgical reduction. By age 3 years there was obvious mental retardation.

The diagnosis is made on the basis of this clinical phenotype along with minimal increases of dermatan and heparan sulfate in urine. It is confirmed by finding reduced activity of β-glucuronidase in cultured patient fibroblasts or in leukocytes or serum.

Therapy

There is no specific therapy.

DIFERRANTE'S SYNDROME (MPS VIII, GLUCOSAMINE-6-SULFATE SULFATASE DEFICIENCY)

This is a rare entity that resembles both clinically and biochemically Morquio's and Sanfilippo's syndromes. The one reported patient was a boy of 5 years who was mentally retarded, of short stature, and had hepatomegaly, mild dysostosis multiplex, odontoid hypoplasia, and a clear cornea (388). He excreted keratan and heparan sulfate. The enzyme glucosamine-6-sulfate sulfatase was deficient in the patient and partially so in both parents, thus showing it was inherited as an autosomal recessive disorder (388).

MUCOLIPIDOSES

There are three principal mucolipidoses, designated types I, II, and III, with a spectrum of clinical forms. Their characteristic feature is the storage of mucopolysaccharide but without mucopolysacchariduria. Multiple catabolic, degradative mucopolysaccharide enzymes are deficient within their normal lysosomal site in types II and III because of a loss of a lysosomal recognition signal by lysosomal enzymes, but there is a significant increase in the activity of these enzymes in extracellular fluid spaces (serum). They are inherited as autosomal recessive disorders.

Clinical Features

Mucolipidosis I (Lipomucopolysaccharidosis)

The disorder is characterized by mild Hurler features, with moderate mental retardation without mucopolysacchariduria, and with fibroblast inclusions. Levels of fibroblast lysosomal enzymes are normal rather than the low values reported in mucolipidosis II. Patients develop moderate dwarfism, coarse facies, pectus carinatum, thoracic kyphosis, mental retardation, muscle atrophy, hypotonia, choreoathetosis, inability to walk at puberty, and death in early adulthood.

Mucolipidosis II (I Cell Disease)

This has a similar phenotype to classic MPS I H, Hurler's disease, but differs from it by an earlier age of onset (in fact, it can be present at birth), by the absence of corneal clouding, and by the lack of mucopolysacchariduria. There develops a severe psychomotor retardation, and patients usually die by age 6 years.

N-Acetylglucosamine-1-phosphotransferase is absent in type II patient fibroblast lysosomal fractions and reduced in type III patients. It is an enzyme that phosphorylates mannose residues of glycoprotein-lysosomal enzymes and in so doing provides a needed signal to recognize binding sites on the lysosome. Absence or deficiency of it would explain the low lysosomal enzyme activities and high serum levels simply as a result of lack of lysosomal uptake of these degradative enzymes. Apparently types II and III mucolipidoses are allelic disorders. Fibroblast inclusions are seen by electron microscopy to be dilated lysosomes that are filled with mucopolysaccharide and membrane because the lysosomes lack the enzymes needed to degrade mucopolysaccharide.

Mucolipidosis III (Pseudo-Hurler's Polydystrophy)

This is similar in most respects to mucolipidosis II but is less aggressive and less severe in its manifestations.

Patients manifest disease between 2 to 4 years of age with stiffness of hands and shoulders suggestive of juvenile rheumatoid arthritis. Subsequently, a claw hand, dwarfism, facial coarsening, corneal clouding, and aortic or mitral valve lesions with valve murmurs occur. Progressive mental retardation develops in the early elementary school years. There are characteristic roentgenographic changes of the hips. The disorder is similar to MPS I S or mild forms of MPS VI.

The disorder exhibits the clinical features of an MPS, no mucopolysacchariduria, increased levels of activity of lysosomal enzyme hydrolases in extracellular fluid spaces (serum), with deficiencies of these same enzymes in lysosomal fractions of fibroblasts in cultures. A partial deficiency in *N*-acetylglucosamine-1-phosphotransferase is present in cellular lysosomal fractions, resulting in storage of mucopolysaccharide, as explained under mucolipidosis type II. It has been suggested by McKusick that types II and III represent homozygosity for different mutant genes at the same locus, one that is responsible for a lysosomal recognition marker or receptor for multiple lysosomal enzyme uptake.

Lysosomal enzymes that are reduced within the lysosome and increased in serum include α-L-iduronidase, iduronidate sulfatase, β-glucuronidase, *N*-acetyl-β-hexosaminidase, arylsulfatase A, β-galactosidase, α-mannosidase, and α-L-fucosidase. Activities of acid phosphatase and β-glucosidase are normal. It has been suggested that a two- or threefold increase of *N*-acetyl-β-hexosaminidase or arylsulfatase-A activity in serum is a useful screening procedure for both mucolipidosis II and III.

Fibroblasts from mucolipidosis I and II patients contain inclusions which on electron microscopy appear to be enlarged lysosomes containing mucopolysaccharide and membranous whorls.

Therapy

There is no specific therapy. Orthopedic correction of skeletal defects may be useful in selected patients.

FUCOSIDOSIS

The fucosidoses are a group of disorders caused by a defect in the lysosomal enzyme α-L-fucosidase resulting in the storage of glycolipids, glycoproteins, and mucopolysaccharides containing fucose. These disorders are inherited as autosomal recessives, and at least three forms are described clinically. Type I disease begins in early infancy and produces severe mental retardation, occasional hepatosplenomegaly, and a rapidly fatal course. Type II disease begins in the late infantile period and produces mental and motor retardation, skeletal malformations typical of gargoylism, and prominent skin lesions of angiokeratoma corporis diffusum. Type III disease is less aggressive and can continue into adulthood. Severe mental retardation with spasticity and skeletal defects was present in three young adult patients reported by Ikeda et al. in 1984 (296). Rectal biopsy has been used to show neuronal storage material, which is rather specific for the fucosidoses.

α-L-Fucosidase (EC 3.2.1.51) is encoded by a single locus on the short arm of chromosome 1 (1p34). In 1985 it was reported that a cDNA was obtained that coded for at least 80% of the mature enzyme (207).

Muscle Diseases

Genetic muscle diseases or the muscular dystrophies have been a vigorous area of investigation in recent years. The biochemical genetics of many specific disorders have been solved and a meaningful start into the molecular genetics of these disorders using recombinant DNA methods has already begun.

DISORDERS OF GLYCOGEN METABOLISM

The major disorders of glycogen metabolism have already been described in the section on Glycogen Storage Diseases.

DISORDERS OF LIPID METABOLISM

Carnitine Palmityltransferase Deficiency

DiMauro and DiMauro (137) and DiMauro (134) initially described this syndrome in 1973 in a patient with a familial syndrome of recurrent myoglobinuria. Carnitine palmityltransferase (CPT) deficiency was documented by them in patient muscle. Bank described two brothers in 1975 (29) who had recurrent myoglobinuria and absence of CPT activity in muscle samples. Subsequently it has been described in about 17 patients, of which 16 were men, suggesting either an autosomal or an X-linked recessive disorder. These patients present predominantly with myoglobinuria with muscle cramps that can be precipitated by extended exercise or dietary fasting. It is of note that the creatine kinase, which is normal at rest, will increase quickly during episodes of myoglobinuria (91). Usually the muscle biopsy is normal histologically. Although muscle lipid metabolism is defective in both carnitine and CPT deficiencies, it has not been resolved why there is no lipid accumulation in CPT deficiency and why the two clinical phenotypes are so divergent. It is also not clear why this syndrome is limited to muscle, as the enzyme defect is also present in leukocytes, platelets, fibroblasts, and liver. Some patients develop an improved exercise tolerance on a low-fat, high-carbohydrate diet.

The basis for the pathogenesis of disease is the absence of CPT activity, a key enzyme for lipid oxidation in muscle that is located on the inner mitochondrial membrane. It is established that short-chain fatty acids can be readily transported from the cytosol into the mitochondrion, but that long-chain fatty acids, such as oleic and palmitic, require a carnitine-based carrier system. Carnitine is synthesized in liver and is transported to muscle by a specific active transport system. Free fatty acids are activated to fatty acyl-CoA and then are joined with carnitine by CPT I to form fatty acyl-carnitine, which is then transported into the mitochondrion. Within the mitochondrion CPT II reforms fatty acyl-CoA, which then proceeds to be β-oxidized by the tricarboxylic acid cycle (91).

Carnitine Deficiency

Engel and Siekert described in 1972 (170) a young female with generalized weakness that continued to progress, requiring ventilation assistance. Lipid storage in type 1 muscle fibers was described. In 1973 Engel and Angelini (167) determined that this lipid storage was associated with carnitine deficiency. Subsequently, carnitine deficiency has been described in a restricted myopathic form, type 1, and a generalized type, type 2, in which carnitine deficiency is systemic and is associated with an acute encephalopathy. In the myopathic form muscle carnitine is significantly and selectively reduced to 10% of normal. In this case lipid accumulates in muscle as long-chain fatty acids cannot be transported into the mitochondrion and are shunted to triglyceride synthesis. Serum carnitine in the myopathic type of disease is normal, thus indicating that an active carnitine transport from blood to muscle is defective. The mode of inheritance is autosomal recessive, based on supportive evidence that there is a reduced carnitine concentration in muscle or relatives of patients (91). Therapy with corticosteroid or carnitine administration has been effective (138).

The systemic form was described initially in 1975 by Karpati (313) in a young boy with generalized weakness and undefined hepatic encephalopathy. Although muscle showed a lipid storage disorder in type 1 fibers, carnitine was not only absent in muscle but significantly reduced in liver and plasma as well. In the systemic type carnitine is reduced in muscle, liver, and heart, suggesting a primary hepatic defect in its synthesis. One patient reported by Karpati did show improvement in liver function on serum carnitine replacement therapy. Secondary carnitine deficiency may result in the organic acidemias. A clinically significant response to carnitine was found in propionic acidemia and methylmalonic acidemia (581,582).

Lipid Neuropathy with Normal Carnitine

Askanas et al. (21) reported a unique family with autosomal dominant muscle weakness and intolerance of fatty food. A histochemical analysis of muscle from three affected patients demonstrated increased lipids in type 1 muscle fibers. Electron micrographs of muscle showed increased lipids, abnormal mitochondria, and increased lipofuscin granules. Electron micrographs of sural nerve showed abnormal inclusions in most Schwann cells, with lipid inclusions, zebra bodies, and abnormal mitochondria. Of importance to distinguish this syndrome from other lipid myopathies was the fact that carnitine and carnitine palmityltransferase levels were normal in serum and muscle. These patients responded with a marked improvement on a diet free of long-chain fatty acids.

Myoadenylate Deaminase Deficiency

A syndrome of weakness and muscle cramps in five male patients was initially described in 1978 (192). The essential biochemical defect was a lack of muscle adenylate deaminase. An additional observation may be the failure of ammonia to rise in patients after vigorous exercise. The syndrome is inherited as an X-linked recessive disorder (278).

Malignant Hyperthermia

In this autosomal dominant syndrome severe autonomic abnormalities abruptly occur, including tachycardia, cardiac arrhythmias, hypotension, cyanotic skin changes, and muscle rigidity in association with hyperthermia that can attain 43°C. The syndrome is induced in susceptible persons by the anesthetics halothane and suc-cinylcholine and by ketamine or depolarizing relaxants. It carries a mortality of 60%. The primary defect is unknown, but it is significant that it has been described with two genetic disorders of muscle, Duchenne's muscular dystrophy and central core disease (91,126). Recognition of a susceptible patient prior to general anes-thesia is crucial, and a positive family history and an elevated creatine kinase level in serum are strong indicators that the patient is indeed at risk. An *in vitro* study using the patient's biopsied muscle has been suggested as a predictive test, but its reliability is questioned. Therapy for a patient in the throes of an attack should include stopping the anesthetic, intravenous use of dantrolene as the primary means to control muscle rigidity, vigorous cooling of the patient, bicarbonate to reverse tissue acidosis, diuretics to maintain urine formation and counteract renal tubular necrosis, and 100% oxygen administration (91,239).

CONGENITAL MYOPATHIES

Several congenital disorders of muscle development, including central core dis-ease, nemaline myopathy, myotubular myopathy, and congenital fiber type dispro-portion, have been described in recent years. In general, patients have a delay in motor development because of weakness, hypotonia, and associated skeletal mal-formations, but gradually patients stabilize and improve. Central core disease, so named because of abnormal fibrillary muscle bundles in the central region of most fibers, is inherited as an autosomal dominant disorder or occurs sporadically. Nemaline myopathy takes its name from the Greek, meaning nema or thread, as there are threadlike structures occupying the entire length of about half the medium-sized fibers. It is inherited as an autosomal dominant or autosomal recessive disorder. It is of interest that central core disease and nemaline myopathy have been reported in one family. Myotubular myopathy presents with congenital weak-ness along with ptosis, ophthalmoparesis, and facial and neck muscle paresis. Muscle biopsy indicates central nuclei with a halo devoid of myofibrils. The disorder has considerable variation in severity and is inherited as an autosomal dominant, autosomal recessive, or X-linked recessive trait. Congenital fiber type disproportion is so called because there is an increased number of small type 1 fibers and a reduced number of enlarged type 2 fibers (73,91,552,553,577).

PERIODIC PARALYSIS

The inherited paralytic syndromes referred to here are a group of disorders inherited as autosomal dominant traits in which defects in serum potassium con-centration or potassium flux occur.

Hypokalemic Periodic Paralysis

Although dominantly inherited, this disorder affects males three to four times more frequently than females, in whom apparently the gene has a reduced degree of penetrance. Attacks of paralysis can be severe, involving even muscles required for respiration. Attacks occur in the morning after a night's sleep. Exertion followed by rest, carbohydrates, exposure to cold, or alcohol can also precipitate an episode. The hallmark of the condition is a low serum potassium concentration, usually in the 2 to 3 mEq/liter range, but sometimes potassium concentration is normal. A diagnostic provocative test can be given if the diagnosis is in doubt by administering 2 g glucose/kg body weight orally with 20 U insulin subcutaneously. Treatment of an acute attack is with 5 to 10 g KCl orally. To prevent episodes, avoidance of a high-carbohydrate diet and of intense physical activity is recommended. Acetazolamide in a dose up to 150 mg daily may be highly effective for avoiding future attacks. By the Nernst-Goldman equation it is assumed that the resting membrane potential should be hyperpolarized during an attack; however, direct measurements with microelectrodes have shown that the membrane potential is hypopolarized. Weakness results because the hypopolarized membrane cannot repolarize and again depolarize to generate a propagated impulse throughout the T-tube system of muscle (91,166,236).

In 1985 Buruma et al. (82) reported a 50-year follow-up of a large family showing two new cases in the third generation and 12 in the fourth generation, bringing the pedigree up to 28 affected persons in four generations. A linkage study could not localize the gene on the human genome.

Hyperkalemic Periodic Paralysis

This disorder is also inherited as an autosomal dominant and consists of increased serum potassium associated with mild attacks of weakness beginning in the daytime and lasting less than an hour. Attacks of weakness can be precipitated by fasting, resting after strenuous exercise, and cold. Clinical myotonia may present in some persons. The serum potassium during an episode can become elevated to values as high as 7 to 8 mEq/liter. Patients can be challenged by an oral provocative dose of 0.05 to 0.5 g/kg body weight of KCl if the diagnosis is not established. If the patient is having a severe episode, therapy consisting of 100 g glucose by mouth and 20 U insulin subcutaneously can be administered. Acetazolamide is effective in preventing attacks. Paramyotonia congenita refers to attacks of weakness precipitated by cold associated with clinical myotonia and hyperkalemia. This disorder bears many similarities to hyperkalemic periodic paralysis and is probably the same entity. Normokalemic periodic paralysis has been described in persons and families with clinical and laboratory findings similar to those of hyperkalemic periodic paralysis, but with a normal serum potassium concentration during an episode. Perhaps they are in reality the same disorder (91,166,236).

MYOTONIC MUSCULAR DYSTROPHY

This classic dominantly inherited muscle disorder described by Steinert has a multifaceted clinical presentation. In the United States it has a frequency of about 3.3 per 100,000 population.

Clinical Features

Muscle atrophy and weakness occur symmetrically and insidiously in childhood and the early adult period. The distribution of weakness may be more distal than proximal, and it is associated with exercise-induced or percussion myotonia. A "hatchet-shaped facies" may occur because of muscle loss involving temporalis, masseter, sternocleidomastoid, and anterior compartment neck muscles. A protruded upper lip is common (Fig. 37). In addition, other organs and tissues may be affected, producing frontal baldness, cataracts, mental dulling, testicular atrophy, infertility, amenorrhea, cardiac conduction defects, glucose intolerance, hyperinsulinemia, and hypercatabolism of serum IgG producing low serum values.

A severe neonatal form of disease usually inherited from the mother has a high mortality because of severe problems in feeding, swallowing, and breathing. Mental retardation is common. It is not clear why the neonatal form occurs almost exclusively when the mother is affected, but presumably a maternal factor, perhaps on the X chromosome and perhaps involving a mitochondrial function, is responsible.

Electromyography will demonstrate the characteristic myotonic response.

Genetics

This autosomal dominant disorder with variable penetrance and expressivity has been mapped to chromosome 19 and linked near the gene for the third component of complement (C_3). It also shows linkage with both Lutheran and Lewis blood groups. It was subsequently shown to be closely linked with the secretor locus (262) on chromosome 19. A. D. Roses (Duke University) is attempting to obtain a DNA probe that will distinguish those with the disorder from persons in the same family who are not at risk. He is constructing a genomic library of DNA obtained from chromosome fractions enriched in DNA from chromosomes 19 and 20. Unique DNA sequences from chromosome 19 are being screened for and isolated. RFLPs that are unique and nonrepetitive obtained from chromosome 19 will be isolated and used as DNA probes to hybridize against genomic material from patients. It is hoped that in this way a genetic linkage map of chromosome 19 will be obtained leading to a probe that will be informative for diagnostic purposes and that will permit elimination of disease with appropriate genetic counseling. This is one major dominantly inherited disease for which recombinant DNA approaches will be effective, it is believed, in the near future to reduce the incidence of the disease and provide a means to isolate and clone the mutant gene (A. D. Roses, *personal communication*).

Treatment

No therapy is available to address the primary genetic defect, but the use of quinine, procainamide, and dilantin has been effective to reduce the myotonia, which can be very incapacitating.

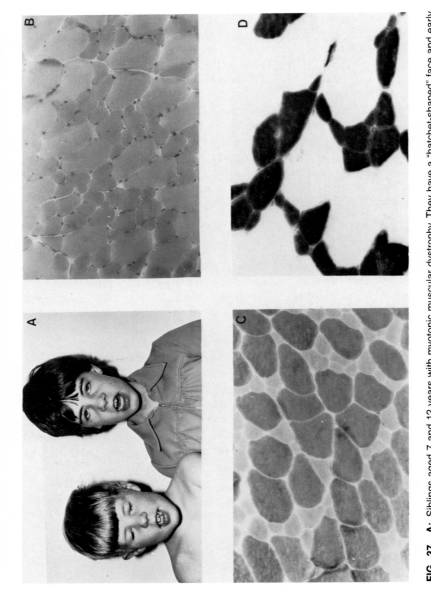

FIG. 37. **A:** Siblings aged 7 and 12 years with myotonic muscular dystrophy. They have a "hatchet-shaped" face and early ocular ptosis. **B:** trichrome stain showing individual fiber loss. **C:** ATPase stain at pH 9.4 showing dark type 2 fibers that are large in size. **D:** ATPase stain at pH 4.3 showing atrophied dark type 1 fibers (×15). (Courtesy of Dr. Jay D. Cook, University of Texas Health Science Center at Dallas.)

THOMSEN'S MYOTONIA CONGENITA

This is an autosomal dominant disorder characterized by mild myotonia present at birth and benign in presentation. There is associated muscle hypertrophy (Herculean physique), which is retained, but the myotonia resolves (Fig. 38). It is also reported as an autosomal recessive in which the onset is later in childhood and myotonia is pronounced.

SCHWARTZ-JAMPEL SYNDROME

This rare, unique syndrome, inherited as an autosomal recessive, has as its clinical features muscle hypertrophy, blepharospasm, myotonia, short stature, progressive joint contractures, bone dysplasia, a nasal speech, muscle stiffness, and an unusual facial appearance (541). No metabolic defect has been identified, but the finding of increased and diffusely distributed acetylcholinesterase activity over muscle fibers suggested a failure of localization of this enzyme to the endplate regions (262).

X-LINKED MUSCULAR DYSTROPHY (DUCHENNE'S FORM OF DYSTROPHY)

This form of progressive weakness begins in the early childhood years between ages 2 and 6 years. It is one of the most common and serious forms of human X-linked disorders. It occurs at a frequency of up to 1 in 5,000 newborn males.

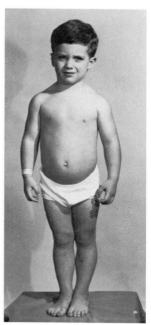

FIG. 38. A 6-year-old boy with muscle hypertrophy typical of Thomsen's myotonia congenita. (Courtesy of Dr. M. E. Blaw, University of Texas Health Science Center at Dallas.)

Clumsiness of gait and difficulty in climbing stairs are common features. Calf muscle enlargement is a common feature and a distinctive one. By the time patients are in their twenties, there are severe generalized muscle weakness and atrophy, sparing the bulbar muscles. It is of interest to note that about 25% of affected boys have an IQ of less than 75. This form of dystrophy has been reported rarely in girls, but only if they have abnormal karyotypes, as in Turner's syndrome (XO), or if the X chromosome is structurally abnormal (118).

The serum creatine phosphokinase is elevated, sometimes strikingly so. The electromyogram and muscle biopsy findings are myopathic and diagnostic of this disease (91).

Genetics

It has been estimated that one-third of the incidence of Duchenne's dystrophy is due to a spontaneous mutation and two-thirds to a carrier mother, who on the average will pass the mutant X chromosome to one-half of her sons. It was J. B. S. Haldane, the great English geneticist, who in 1935 (255) stated that for an X-linked recessive lethal disease like Duchenne's dystrophy, one-third of the cases in a generation would be the result of a new mutation. By analysis of a pedigree it can be readily determined that the mother in question is a definite carrier by the fact that one son and a male relative are affected; she is a probable carrier when two or more sons are affected and a possible carrier when only one son is affected. The measurement of serum creatine phosphokinase has also been useful to describe a carrier status, as it is elevated in 70% of carriers (91).

In 1982 and 1983 Williamson and his colleagues (122,421) reported on two cloned DNA sequences flanking the Duchenne's dystrophy locus on the short arm of the X chromosome. One sequence was loosely linked to the Duchenne locus at a distance of approximately 10 centimorgans (cM) as determined by studies on nine informative families. Their probe, λ RC8, was localized to the Xp21-Xp223 region of the human X chromosome, which is the site of the mutation, by the use of a panel of rodent-human cell hybrids. Their probe identifies a site loosely linked to the Duchenne locus and not tight enough to be used for genetic counseling purposes. For example, in one of their families a crossing-over between the two loci using their probe was identified. However, they are working to find a probe 1 or 2 cM away from the disease locus that will be clinically useful. Bakker et al. (27) reported on 11 informative restriction fragment length polymorphism (RFLP)-markers presently available on the short arm of the X chromosome that are useful in making a diagnosis because they bridge the Duchenne locus between 3 and 20 cM. Griggs and Fischbeck, and Ar-Rushdi are also trying to find a DNA polymorphism with the appropriate probe that will be clinically applicable to reduce the incidence of this disease and provide a means to isolate and clone the mutant gene (122,191,237,421). Once the gene has been cloned and its product identified, it will be possible to determine what the normal gene encodes for, which in turn might lead to effective therapy for patients with this devastating disease.

Treatment

Therapy is supportive and is directed at providing proper bracing and orthopedic surgical procedures to maintain good ambulation for as long as possible.

EMERY-DREIFUSS SYNDROME

In 1966 Emery and Dreifuss (165) described an X-linked recessive form of benign muscular dystrophy associated with a cardiomyopathy, joint contractures, and absence of muscle hypertrophy. Subsequently, a similar syndrome has been reported inherited as an autosomal dominant (186) and an autosomal recessive trait (282).

BECKER'S MUSCULAR DYSTROPHY

Becker and Kiener (41) described an X-linked form of dystrophy with onset in the adolescent years with a mild progression and minimal disability. According to Zatz (654), linkage data indicated that the Duchenne and Becker forms of muscular dystrophy are not allelic.

OTHER MUSCULAR DYSTROPHY SYNDROMES

Syndromes that are far rarer in incidence include ocular myopathy, oculopharyngeal dystrophy, limb-girdle muscular dystrophy, scapuloperoneal dystrophy, and fascioscapulohumeral dystrophy. They are named for the muscle groups involved and in general are adult onset, slowly progressive syndromes, with the named muscles undergoing atrophy over an extended period. These syndromes are inherited usually as autosomal dominant disorders but sometimes as autosomal recessives.

Mitochondrial Encephalomyopathies

Rowland (509), Rowland et al. (510), Pavlakis et al. (451), DiMauro et al. (139), and DiMauro et al. (136) have reviewed a controversial, complex, and recently emerging literature and have defined several new inherited syndromes associated with mitochondrial metabolic defects (Table 4).

MITOCHONDRIAL ENCEPHALOMYOPATHY WITH LACTIC ACIDOSIS AND STROKE (MELA SYNDROME)

At least 11 patients with a syndrome consisting of normal development in early life with symptoms starting between ages 3 and 11 years were described by Rowland et al. (510) and Pavlakis et al. (451). These patients were short and had seizures. All patients except one had a stroke-like illness with hemiparesis, hemianopia, or cortical blindness. Nine had hemiparesis or hemianopsia and six had episodes of cortical blindness. Nine patients developed dementia. Vomiting and sensory neural

TABLE 4. *Inherited mitochondrial encephalomyopathies*

Alper's syndrome (cerebral poliodystrophy)
Canavan's disease (spongy degeneration of white matter)
Carnitine deficiency syndrome or carnitine palmityltransferase deficiency
　(long-chain fatty acid oxidation defect)
Kearns-Sayre syndrome (ophthalmoplegia-plus; ragged red fibers)
Leigh's disease (subacute necrotizing encephalopathy)
Mitochondrial encephalomyopathy with lactic acidosis (MELA syndrome)
Myoclonus epilepsy with ragged red fibers (Ramsay Hunt syndrome
　variant) (MERRF syndrome or Fukuhara syndrome)
Menkes's kinky hair disease (trichopoliodystrophy)
Refsum's disease (lipid α-oxidase defect)
Zellweger syndrome (cerebrohepatorenal syndrome)

---

hearing loss were present in several. Two pairs of siblings were affected. Prominent in their absence were cerebellar deficits, interictal myoclonus, heart block, ophthalmoplegia, and retinal changes. This clinical complex is referred to by the acronym MELA syndrome. NADH-CoQ reductase (complex 1) deficiency has been found in one patient with this syndrome. Oxygen uptake by isolated mitochondria with NAD-linked substrate such as pyruvate is low, whereas flavin-linked substrates such as succinate and ascrobate support normal respiration (406).

MYOCLONUS EPILEPSY WITH RAGGED RED FIBERS (MERRF SYNDROME)

Fukuhara et al. (205,206) described a different syndrome from the MELA complex of Rowland et al. (510), but there are similarities. At least 16 patients have now been described with normal early development, myoclonus, and a cerebellar syndrome. Eleven patients had seizures, 11 became demented, and six had hearing loss. Ten of the 16 patients had a positive family history. All patients had myoclonus and ataxia, and none had hemiparesis, hemianopia, or cortical blindness, as did MELA patients. Twelve patients had an intention tremor. Optic nerve atrophy was present in eight patients. No patient in this group had ophthalmoplegia, pigmentary retinal degeneration, or heart block. The acronym MERRF (myoclonus epilepsy with ragged red fibers) was applied to this group of patients. It bears a resemblance to the syndrome described by Ramsay Hunt (291) of dyssynergia cerebellaris myoclonica with myoclonus, tremor, and a cerebellar syndrome. A deficiency of the enzyme CoQ-cytochrome *c* reductase (complex III) was reported in a single patient with proximal weakness, ataxia, myoclonus, and dementia, presumably a MERRF syndrome patient. The patient had a low oxygen uptake with NADH and flavin-linked substrates and normal oxygen uptake with ascorbate (319). In 1985 Rosing et al. (507) described a family with familial myoclonic epilepsy associated with a mitochondrial myopathy. The disorder followed a maternal inheritance pattern consistent with a mitochondrial DNA mutation.

In several cases a muscle biopsy has shown ragged red fibers on light microscopy and the presence of mitochondrial proliferation of cristae with paracrystalline inclusions on electron microscopy (206). Feit et al. (184) reported a patient with progressive myoclonus, ataxia, mild mental retardation, abnormal muscle mitochondria, and exquisite hypersensitivity to anticonvulsant medication with respiratory insufficiency. Both hypoventilation and myoclonus responded favorably to L-5-hydroxytryptophan for a limited period.

KEARNS-SAYRE SYNDROME

This entity is usually an acquired disorder, although a positive family history was reported twice (451). Clinical features include ragged red fibers on muscle biopsy, ophthalmoplegia, pigmentary retinal degeneration, heart conductive block elevated CSF protein (>100 mg/dl), and a cerebellar syndrome.

As pointed out by Rowland et al. (510), all three syndromes—MELA, MERRF, and Kearns-Sayre syndrome—have spongy degeneration of the brain, giving them some basis of neuropathologic commonality.

The cause of these syndromes is not clear. Nonmendelian maternal inheritance or an X-linked recessive mendelian trait may be the mode of heredity. All have abnormal ragged red fibers, morphologic mitochondrial abnormalities, and an elevated blood lactate concentration. Thus major biochemical defects in muscle and brain mitochondria are postulated. Several biochemical abnormalities have been associated with ragged red fibers and mitochondrial morphologic defects, including defects in cytochrome c oxidase, cytochrome b and aa_3, cytochrome b, NADH-CoQ reductase complex, or ATPase and loose coupling of oxidative phosphorylation. A defect in succinate-cytochrome c reductase was found in two siblings with the MERRF syndrome, and one patient with the MELA complex had deficiencies of cytochrome c oxidase and pyruvate dehydrogenase (451).

Both X-linked and nonmendelian maternal modes of inheritance may be present in the MELA syndrome, as both sets of twins reported with it may have had a mother partially affected with the syndrome. One mother is said to have had neurosensory hearing loss and diabetes mellitus, and the other night blindness and an abnormal electrocardiogram. Mendelian inheritance involves the transmission to successive generations of DNA contained in genes in the nucleus, but DNA is also contained in mitochondria, where it is believed to be responsible for the encoding of certain mitochondrial enzymes (154). As almost all mitochondrial DNA is maternally transmitted, a nonmendelian pattern of inheritance is possible in a mitochondrial disorder. These disorders may include a structural membrane mitochondrial defect or an enzyme defect that is coded in the nucleus or by mitochondrial DNA. The latter is becoming better understood as evidence has emerged recently that subunits of respiratory enzyme complexes are encoded solely by mitochondrial DNA (154).

Additional comprehensive papers on the subject include those of Shapira et al. (548) and Morgan-Hughes et al. (407).

ALPER'S SYNDROME (CEREBRAL POLIODYSTROPHY)

This is a syndrome in children associated with seizures, myoclonus, optic atrophy, and motor and mental retardation with spasticity. There is severe brain atrophy with impressive cortical neuronal loss. There is also neuronal loss in thalamus, basal ganglia, brainstem, and cerebellum (5).

Hemispheric demyelination is prominent, and there may be a spongiform change in white matter because of glial vacuolation. Lactic acid may be elevated in concentration in the CSF and serum. Serum pyruvate dehydrogenase has been reported to be low in brain in some patients (472,547). The presence of large mitochondria in neurons of some patients provides linkage of this syndrome with other described mitochondrial encephalopathies. The mode of inheritance is not clear and could be X-linked recessive or nonmendelian maternal inheritance for the mitochondrial genome. No effective therapy is available and the syndrome inexorably progresses.

LEIGH'S DISEASE (NECROTIZING ENCEPHALOMYELOPATHY AND LACTIC ACIDOSIS)

The clinical features are those of an acute encephalopathy in infants or young children, with loss of mental and motor development, extraocular muscle palsies, nystagmus, ataxia, hypotonia and quadriparesis, seizures, and feeding and breathing difficulties. Acute attacks or the insidious development of the above symptom complex may occur. The spectrum of these features has been widened in recent years to include older children and even adults (183,230,350,560). A hallmark of the syndrome is an elevated lactate and pyruvate in CSF and serum, indicating a defect in pyruvate metabolism. The CT brain scan sometimes shows lucent areas in the basal ganglia or thalamus. The neuropathology resembles Wernicke's disease, with necrosis present in the periaqueductal regions of the midbrain, pons, and periventricular regions of the pons and medulla. Neuronal loss, necrosis, demyelination, and blood vessel proliferation are prominent in the brainstem with sparing of the hypothalamus and mamillary bodies, which distinguishes it from Wernicke's disease in which necrosis is prominent in hypothalamus and mamillary bodies.

Defects in the enzymes pyruvate carboxylase, succinate-cytochrome c reductase and cytochrome c oxidase (complex IV) have been reported in some patients (70). An inhibitor of the enzyme ATP-thiamine triphosphate transferase has been reported in some Leigh's disease patients, and low levels of thiamine triphosphate in patient brain but not liver have been found. The precise defect or family of oxidative disorders for pyruvate metabolism has not been completely described for each of the clinical forms of this syndrome. It is probably inherited as an autosomal recessive disorder and may overlap with other mitochondrial encephalopathies such as Alper's disease, Kearns-Sayre syndrome, and the MELA and MERRF syndromes (49,50,130,131,138,462,465,483).

DYSTONIA, OPTIC ATROPHY, PUTAMINAL ATROPHY, AND MATERNAL INHERITANCE SYNDROME

Recently Novotny et al. (435) described a kindred with features of dystonia, mild mental retardation, short stature, optic atrophy, and myopathic findings. CT brain scans showed putaminal atrophy. The mode of inheritance was compatible with maternal transmission or cytoplasmic inheritance. Preliminary DNA polymorphism studies of mitochondrial DNA indicated that segregation of patterns on Southern blots was appropriate for those affected.

MENKES'S DISEASE

In 1962 Menkes et al. (392) first recognized and characterized this disease. Danks in 1972 (116) demonstrated that these patients were unable to absorb copper, leading to a severe copper deficiency state.

The incidence has been estimated by Danks to be as high as 1 in 35,000. This disorder is inherited in an X-linked recessive fashion.

Clinical Features

Many patients are premature, with a birth weight appropriate for gestational age. As neonates they demonstrate poor feeding, poor weight gain, transient jaundice, and instability of body temperature. Seizures, usually myoclonic, develop early, and a progressive delay in psychomotor development occurs (Fig. 39A).

The hair is normal at birth, but the secondary hair growth lacks luster, is somewhat depigmented, and breaks off easily. Microscopic examination reveals pili torti (trichopoliodystrophy) (Fig. 39B).

Arteriography reveals the vessels to be elongated and tortuous with irregularity of the lumen and sometimes arterial occlusion. Radiologic examination reveals spurs on the metaphyses of long bones and subperiosteal calcifications. Wormian bones appear in the posterior sagittal and lambdoidal sutures. The clinical course is one of progressive neurologic deterioration, with death usually between 6 months and 3 years of age.

The diagnosis is suspected on the basis of the clinical findings and confirmed by the demonstration of low total serum copper and even lower liver copper. Cytochrome oxidase deficiency has been reported in a few patients. This is a copper-dependent enzyme, and reduced activity may be secondary to the copper transport defect.

Pathology

It appears the absorptive defect is not in the uptake of copper by mucosal cells, but rather in the mucosal intracellular transport or transport of copper across the mucosal cell serosal membrane.

The main pathologic findings are in the brain and consist of extensive neuronal degeneration and gliosis. The arteries are fragmented, with splitting of the internal

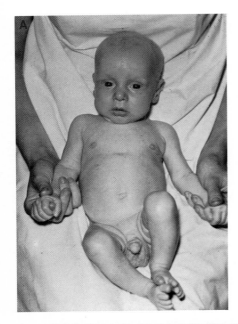

FIG. 39.   A: A 2-month-old child with Menkes's kinky hair disease.   B: The abnormal pili torti pattern of hair strands. (Courtesy of Dr. John H. Menkes, Beverly Hills, CA.)

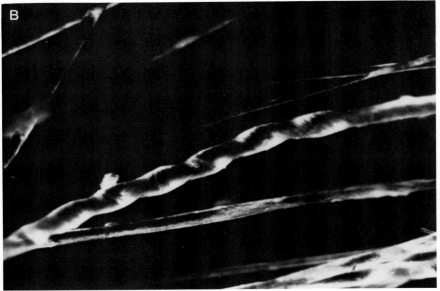

elastic lamina and intimal proliferation, with narrowing and occlusion. Structurally abnormal mitochondria are found on muscle biopsy as well as decreased activity of cytochromes a and a_3 in brain, muscle, and liver. The disease is thus a member of the mitochondrial encephalomyopathies related here to copper metabolism.

Therapy

The present treatment regimen is parenteral copper administration, which must be started early to prevent organ damage. Although this may help the nonneurologic aspects of the disease, it is not clear if the neurologic findings are altered.

Multifactorial Genetic Bases for Neurologic Disorders

Epilepsy, brain tumors, migraine, aneurysms, myasthenia gravis, and multiple sclerosis represent neurologic conditions in which no clear mendelian pattern can be determined to be responsible for their expression. Rather, multifactorial genetic factors are involved that interact in a complex and poorly characterized manner to predispose patients to disease.

EPILEPSY

In general, it is stated that between 1 and 3% of persons with an epileptic parent or sibling will have epilepsy. Epilepsy, of course, is a symptom and not a disease, and so the causes of it are extremely broad and the finding of families with primary epilepsy are rare and usually not well studied. In one good study (397,398) 10% of children who had a sibling with a history of any form of epilepsy had seizures, compared with 3.4% of normal children. The 3 per second spike-and-wave abnormality or centrencephalic epilepsy in siblings and offspring was found in the same study to be 8 and 10%, respectively.

Febrile convulsions also have a familial occurrence, and those with a positive family history are more likely to go on and have epilepsy. A positive family history is found in about 30% of patients with febrile convulsions. About 11% of siblings of an affected child will develop them, compared with an incidence of 2% in the control population. The incidence is higher in monozygotic than in dizygotic twins, supporting a genetic predisposition.

Ounsted (447) and Frantzen et al. (198) put forth evidence suggesting that familial febrile convulsions are inherited as an autosomal dominant with variable penetrance, but this issue is not yet resolved.

Partial complex seizures caused by temporal lobe epileptiform activity also have been shown to have a familial tendency. Falconer (178) reported that there was a positive family history in 13% of patients with mesial temporal lobe sclerosis.

Other forms of epilepsy that have an increased familial incidence include reading epilepsy, akinetic seizures, hypsarrhythmia, photoconvulsive seizures, pyridoxine-dependent epilepsy, benign familial neonatal epilepsy, and familial paroxysmal choreoathetosis. Eldridge et al. (160) described autosomal recessive myoclonus epilepsy that responded to valproate and worsened with phenytoin. It has been suggested by White (634) that "epilepsy genes" might be found by obtaining DNA polymorphisms that are associated with such genes in informative families. Such a postulated gene would predispose persons to an epileptiform process.

BRAIN TUMORS

Meningiomas may have a familial occurrence, although the mode of inheritance is not clear. Meningiomas occurred in two members of the same family (209) and in mother and daughter (312) without other evidence of neurofibromatosis. Loss of an acrocentric chromosome, usually number 22, has been associated with a high percentage of meningiomas (652,653); the production of the tumor cell is thought to result from this chromosome loss rather than from cellular transformation. In 1985 Bolger et al. (54) described a family in which a father and three of his offspring had meningiomas with clinical onset at ages 35 to 65 years. A fourth child died of multiple neoplasms arising at 29 years. The three siblings had a constitutional robertsonian translocation, t(14;22)(14qter-cen-22qter), in peripheral blood leukocytes.

GLIOMAS

Familial examples of gliomas are rare but have been reported. Von Motz et al. (620) reported three sisters with astrocytomas; Kaufman and Brisman (314) reported two brothers with glioblastoma multiforme. Other examples could be cited, but it is sufficient to state that familial gliomas, including astrocytoma, glioblastoma multiforme, oligodendroglioma, cerebral sarcoma, and medulloblastoma, have been described.

CEREBROVASCULAR DISEASE

Migraine Headaches

Migraine headaches represent a syndrome with a variety of causes, including aneurysms, arteriovenous malformations, and an abnormality in the metabolism of serotonin affecting its role as a neurotransmitter at synapses innervating cerebral vessels. There is a wide variation in the incidence of familial migraine, but all agree there is a multifactorial genetic predisposition to its presence. Lucas (361) reported a 26% percent concordance rate for dizygotic twins. Zeigler et al. (658) reported a concordance rate of 29% for monozygotic and 17% for dizygotic twins. More complex forms of migraine, including basilar migraine and hemiplegic migraine, also can be familial because of multifactorial genetic traits.

Aneurysms

The familial presentation of cerebral aneurysm is rare indeed, but it has been associated with another, more well-established genetic syndrome, Ehlers-Danlos syndrome, and with polycystic renal disease. Families have been reported in which more than one member was affected (266). Aneurysms in twins have also been described (177). Most interesting was a family reported by Edelsohn et al. (152) in which a father and four of his 10 children had aneurysms. It is clear that this vascular anomaly has a multifactorial genetic predisposition.

Other Vascular Syndromes

Multifactorial genetic predispositions for carotid artery hypoplasia, stroke due to mitral valve prolapse, and moya-moya disease have all been recorded (24,322,482).

MYASTHENIA GRAVIS

About 4% of myasthenia gravis patients have an affected relative and about 40% of familial occurrences develop before age 2 years. The infantile form of myasthenia gravis in siblings was reported by Greer and Schotland (235) and by Conomy et al. (100). Recently Gieron and Korthals (219) described three siblings with familial myasthenia gravis and emphasized the aggressiveness of its natural history and the poor response to thymectomy and steroid therapy. The prevalence of myasthenia gravis in close relatives of probands of the juvenile and adult types is about 2% (80). Pirskanen (463) estimated that the risk of a child developing the disease when one parent is affected is 0.6%, which is also the risk of having another affected sibling. This is an exceedingly low risk, but still it is about 100 times higher than the risk for the general population.

The higher frequency of the HLA-B8 haplotype in myasthenic patients than in the general population has been noted several times. It has been noted especially in females with an onset of disease before age 35 years and in patients with thymic hyperplasia (463).

MULTIPLE SCLEROSIS

Familial multiple sclerosis varies widely in prevalence in different geographic locales. The incidence is higher in cold climates and lower in warm climates, paralleling the incidence of all cases of multiple sclerosis. Kuwert (336) estimated that about 6% of probands have a close relative who also has disease and that females are more frequently affected than males. It has been estimated in other studies that the prevalence of multiple sclerosis in first degree relatives of probands is 10 to 20 times higher than the prevalence of disease in the general population (146,336).

There is an increased incidence of HLA-A and HLA-DW$_2$ histocompatibility haplotypes in multiple sclerosis patients in general and also in familial cases. Eldridge et al. (159) reported their HLA findings in seven families of their own and from published data of 28 other families. They did not find a consistent association with a specific haplotype among these families, and within a family there was not a good correlation for the presence or absence of disease with the same haplotype.

In a recent careful study, Visscher et al. (618) reported 13 families with multiple sclerosis, of which four had more than one generation affected and the remainder had siblings affected. In each family all patients with disease had a common HLA haplotype. Weak linkage between the HLA complex and a multiple sclerosis gene (20 cM) was reported by Haile et al. (253). Thus multiple sclerosis can be familial, with a clear increased risk for first degree relations of an affected individual. Further, it is suggested that individuals having haplotypes HLA-A$_3$, HLA-B$_7$, and HLA-DW$_2$ have a much higher risk for multiple sclerosis than does the general population, suggesting a possible association between the HLA complex and a multiple sclerosis gene (303,336).

Comings (96) reported a potentially important brain protein polymorphism detected on two-dimensional gels that was associated with patients having multiple sclerosis. This protein, Pcl, was a common variant of a human brain specific protein, and it is present in one-third of the control population with a gene frequency of 0.17. Comings found it to be associated with multiple sclerosis and also with similar diseases such as subacute sclerosing panencephalitis (SSPE) and even ALS, all disorders in which a viral etiology has been suggested (ALS, multiple sclerosis) or demonstrated (SSPE).

Chromosomal Abnormalities

Major advances in the identification of structural chromosomal defects have been achieved in recent years as a result of improved specific staining and banding techniques. The human karyotype consists of 22 pairs of autosomes and two sex chromosomes, XX for the female and XY for the male (Fig. 40). Increases or decreases in the number of autosomal or sex chromosomes result in important and common neurogenetic syndromes and are emphasized here. Balanced reciprocal translocations also occur, as shown in Fig. 41A, in which a portion of the short arm of chromosome 6 has been translocated to the long arm of 17. Such rearrangements do not cause an increase or decrease in chromosome number or content and usually do not affect the phenotype of the balanced carrier, but they do predispose such a carrier to an increased risk of having spontaneous abortions or abnormal children with neural defects. An example of such an abnormality in a child of a balanced carrier father is seen in Fig. 41B. She is missing a normal chromosome 17, which is replaced by the derivative chromosome 17, causing her to have three copies of 6p21 to pter, the terminal end of 17. The child had multiple congenital anomalies and died at age 4 days. Examination of her pons showed selective neuronal necrosis with neurons having eosinophilic shrunken cytoplasm and pyknotic nuclei.

Normal persons with balanced inversions are also encountered (Fig. 42). Such rearrangements do not affect the phenotype of the balanced inversion carrier, but they do lead to an increased risk of abnormal children or spontaneous abortions. The fragile X syndrome in boys is also quite important, as it is the most common

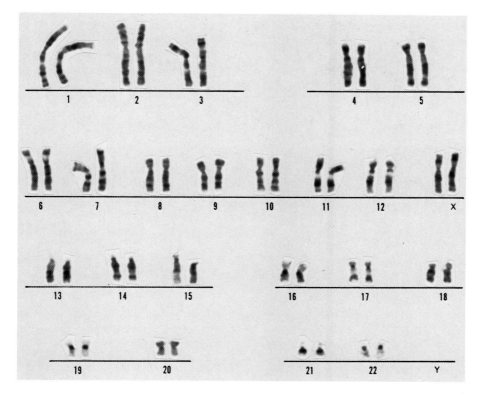

FIG. 40. A normal female karyotype (46,XX) for purposes of comparison with other syndromes. (Courtesy of Dr. P. Howard-Peebles, University of Texas Health Science Center at Dallas.)

form of inherited mental retardation among institutionalized boys in the United States, and its characteristic clinical and karyotypic features are included in this section. Chromosomal defects and their neurologic consequences have been reviewed previously by Rosenberg and Pettegrew (505) and are revised, amplified, and updated here.

AUTOSOME INCREASE SYNDROMES

Chromosome 21 Trisomy (47,XY, + 21; Down's Syndrome)

Down in 1866 (144) described the clinical phenotype that now eponymically recognizes him. Lejeune and colleagues demonstrated that the clinical entity was associated with a chromosomal aberration consisting of an extra, small, acrocentric chromosome (171). Down's syndrome is the most common chromosomal syndrome, occurring in approximately 1 in every 660 live births. The genetics of Down's syndrome may be one of three types: nondisjunction, translocation, or mosaicism.

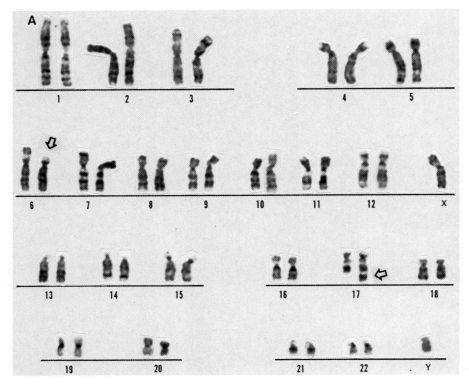

FIG. 41. A: Translocation syndrome. A normal male with a balanced reciprocal translocation (between the short arm of 6 and the long arm of 17) [46,XY,t(6;17)(p21;q25)]. Such rearrangements do not usually affect the phenotype of the balanced carrier but predispose such a carrier to an increased risk of having spontaneous abortions and/or abnormal children. The actual risk depends on the chromosomes involved and the location of the break points. (Courtesy of Dr. P. Howard-Peebles, University of Texas Health Science Center at Dallas.) *(Continued.)*

Between 92 and 94% of patients have trisomy 21, in which the small, acrocentric chromosome 21 is in triplicate. The extra chromosome 21 is a result of defective separation of the chromosomes (nondisjunction) in the meiotic phase of cellular division during ovum formation. This form of Down's syndrome is maternal age dependent and increases in frequency from 1 in 2,400 for the maternal age group 15 to 19 years to 1 in 40 for the maternal age group 45 to 49 years. In families with one trisomy 21 child, these risks are tripled: the 15-to-19-year maternal age group has a risk of 1 in 800 and the 45-to-49-year age group has a risk of 1 in 10.

The translocation group comprises 4 to 5% of Down's cases. This group is considered maternal age independent, and translocation of chromosomal material from the long arm of chromosome 21 to chromosomes 2, 4, 10, 11, 13, 14, 15, 19, 21, or 22 has been reported. Although the total chromosome number is 46, there still is extra chromosome 21 material, as in trisomy 21. More than 1% of the

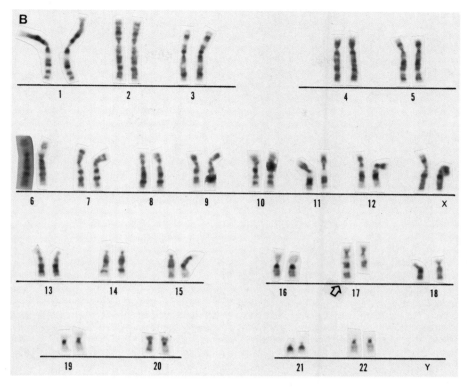

FIG. 41. *(Continued.)* **B:** Partial duplication of chromosome 17. Karyotype of an abnormal female who is the offspring of a balanced carrier father. She is missing a normal 17, which is replaced by the derivative 17, making her have three copies (instead of two) of 6p21 to pter (terminal) [46,XX, − 17, + der(17),t(6;17)(p21;q25)pat]. She had multiple congenital abnormalities including intrauterine growth retardation, abnormal facies, low-set, malformed ears, severe congenital heart anomalies, and bilateral renal hypoplasia. (Courtesy of Dr. P. Howard-Peebles, University of Texas Health Science Center at Dallas.)

translocation cases are inherited from one parent who has 45 chromosomes but a normal chromosomal mass because of a balanced translocation, and who has a normal phenotype. The risk factors for the various translocations are as follows: t(13,21), unknown at this time; t(14,21) maternal carrier, 1 in 10; t(14,21) paternal carrier, 1 in 20; t(21,22) maternal carrier, 1 in 6; t(21,22) paternal carrier, 1 in 12. It is of interest that for maternal carriers the known risk is twice that for paternal carriers.

Mosaic cases (46/47, + 21) comprise 2 to 3 percent of Down's syndrome patients. The percentage of trisomic cells varies from 11 to 70%, and accordingly, the clinical picture varies from practically a normal phenotype to a typical Down's phenotype. On the basis of meiotic studies in germinal tissue, if the mosaic parents have 50% abnormal cells, about 25% of the children will be affected.

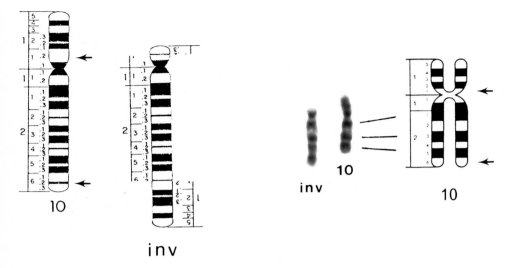

FIG. 42. Inversion of chromosome 10. A normal female with a balanced pericentric inversion of chromosome 10 [46,XX,inv(10)(p11q26)]. Such rearrangements do not usually affect the phenotype of the balanced carrier, but predispose such carriers to an increased risk of having abnormal children or spontaneous abortions. The actual risk of having abnormal children or abortions is directly proportional to the size of the inverted segment. (Courtesy of Dr. P. Howard-Peebles, University of Texas Health Science Center at Dallas.)

Chromosomal banding studies have allowed more precise analysis of chromosome 21, and the evidence at present reveals that the terminal portion of band q22 of chromosome 21 contains determinants for the general Down's syndrome. Specifically, the following conclusions seem reasonable: (a) trisomy of 21q22 causes the specific anomalies of Down's sydnrome; (b) trisomy of 21pter→21q21 may cause nonspecific features such as mild mental deficiency, low posterior hairline, and fleshy external ears; and (c) deficiency of 21pter→21q21 may be a determinant of mental retardation.

Clinical Features

The head is usually round in the newborn and becomes more brachycephalic with age, developing a shortened anterior-posterior diameter, flat occiput, and flattened nasal bridge. The palpebral fissures are narrowed and slanted upward, and epicanthal folds become more prominent as the child grows older. Brushfield's spots, which are tiny white spots in the midzone of the iris, are seen in 85% of Down's patients but also in 25% of normal patients. There may be hypoplasia of the periphery of the iris, and refractive errors are common. In the newborn the ocular fundus contains an increased number of retinal vessels arranged in a spoke-like pattern. The mouth is small and held open with a protruding tongue, which is usually fissured or furrowed in the adult patient. The hard palate is high-arched;

the ears are low-set with small auricles, folded helices, and small or absent lobes. The neck is short and, in the neonate, contains loose skin posteriorly.

The hands are short and broad with clinodactyly of the fifth finger secondary to hypoplasia of the middle phalanx. There is only one flexion crease of the fifth finger instead of the normal two, and the thumb is proximally placed. A simian crease is present unilaterally or bilaterally, and there is increased distance between the first and second toes.

Dermatoglyphics often demonstrate ulnar loops on all 10 fingers. The palmar triradius, which is normally found between the thenar and hypothenar areas, and the flexion crease at the wrist are distally placed to the center of the palm. Therefore, the acute angle formed by lines drawn from the triradius at the base of the fifth finger to the palmar triradius is greater than the normal 45° angle. A tibial arch on the hallucal areas of the sole, which is seen in only 1% of the normal population, is highly typical of Down's patients, and a distal loop in the fourth interdigital area of the foot is seen twice as often as in normal individuals.

The patients are hypotonic at birth and may lack a normal Moro reflex. The joints are also hypermobile. Muscle tone does improve with age but it does not become normal.

In the newborn the skin is characterized by acrocyanosis and cutis marmorata; thereafter it becomes pale, pasty, and waxy. Older patients have rough, dry, and prematurely wrinkled skin. The hair is fine and sparse.

Most patients are small for gestational age, and postnatal growth is slow with delayed skeletal maturation. The ultimate height is usually attained by age 15.

Mental retardation is a prominent feature, with a spectrum of severity ranging from educationally retarded to severely retarded. The distribution of IQ is as follows: 30%, less than 20; 45%, from 20 to 35; 20%, from 35 to 50; and 5%, from 50 to 65. There does not appear to be a direct correlation between the severity of the phenotypic stigmata and the severity of mental retardation. The developmental deterioration can be diagnosed before the age of 6 months in the severely affected infant, with a progressive lag becoming apparent thereafter. Trisomy 21 patients usually exhibit poor articulation and limited vocabulary. Fewer than 5% can read and even fewer can write. Most of the patients have a pleasant, docile personality; but some may have emotional problems and exhibit outbursts of anger and hyperactivity. A recent study comparing the mental development of age- and sex-matched mosaic and trisomy 21 Down's patients revealed that the mosaic group had significantly higher intellectual potential, better verbal facility, and fewer visual perceptual difficulties than the trisomy 21 group.

Roentgenographic findings include narrowing of the cervical canal and subluxation of the atlantoaxial process, which can lead to medullary and cervical cord compression. The acetabulum is flattened, with lateral flaring of the iliac wings, and the acetabular and iliac angles are narrowed. One-third of the patients have 11 ribs, and multiple centers of ossification in the manubrium of the sternum are characteristic. Basal ganglia calcifications have been noted in about one-half of 33 patients, all over 1 year of age, examined neuropathologically (590).

The immaturity of the CNS is documented by neurophysiologic studies. Sleep electroencephalograms (EEGs) and sensory evoked potentials demonstrate, respectively, a large amount of rapid eye movement and absence of a decremental response with repetitive stimulation. Both of these findings are characteristic of the immature nervous system.

The two most significant major somatic malformations involve the heart and the gastrointestinal (GI) tract, with tetralogy of Fallot, duodenal atresia, and annular pancreas being the most common.

The diagnosis of Down's syndrome is made on the basis of the constellation of clinical features and confirmed by chromosomal karyotyping using banding techniques. It is important that at least 50 cells be karyotyped before a mosaic condition can be safely ruled out.

Neuropathology

Grossly, the brain is reduced in size and weight, involving the frontal lobes, brainstem, and especially the cerebellum. The weight of the fully developed trisomy 21 brain rarely exceeds 1,200 g, and it is usually closer to 1,000 g. The brain is abnormally rounded and short, with a flattened, vertical occipital area. The convolutional pattern is usually grossly normal except for a narrow superior temporal gyrus and an exposed insula secondary to lack of development of the third frontal gyrus. There is also a reduction in the development of secondary sulci.

One of the clinical findings in Down's syndrome is premature senility demonstrable even in the presence of mental retardation. In keeping with this clinical finding is the pathologic finding of senile plaques and neurofibrillary tangles ultrastructurally identical with those seen in typical cases of Alzheimer's disease. Recently, Wisniewski et al. (642) reported 7 Down's syndrome patients above age 40. The occurrence of dementia in these patients was of the type seen in Alzheimer's disease. A morphometric analysis of the brains of these 7 patients showed a high incidence of plaques and tangles, and 5 of the 7 had amyloid angiopathy.

A number of neurochemical abnormalities have been reported, including a decreased amount of encephalogenic basic protein, abnormal tryptophan metabolism with normal central monoamine turnover, hyperuricemia, hyperreactivity to atropine, low serum calcium, minor changes in immunoglobuin and lipoproteins, and elevated CSF dicarboxylic acids.

Therapy

There is no specific treatment for this condition, but supportive care and treatment of associated conditions, such as cardiac and GI anomalies, are indicated. Approximately one-third of the patients die in infancy and 50% during the first 5 years from cardiac complications and respiratory infections. There is also a greater incidence of acute leukemia than in the general population. A leukemoid reaction may occur that is secondary to bone marrow dysfunction and that mimics acute myelocytic leukemia. It usually disappears spontaneously over weeks or months.

Chromosome 22 Trisomy (47,XY, + 22)

Trisomy 22 is much rarer than trisomy 21. Since the early 1960s a number of clinical cases with small, extra acrocentric and metacentric chromosomes but without Down's syndrome have been recognized. Certain phenotypic characteristics are common to trisomy 22, confirmed by recent banding studies. Further reports have attempted to call attention to partial trisomy 22 in variant forms. Since it is highly probable that nonmosaic complete trisomy 22 is lethal, no good figures are available for its true incidence. Up to the fall of 1974, only 50 cases of trisomy of the nonmongoloid G chromosome had been reported. At this time there is no clear delineation of trisomy 22 cytogenetics. The question of partial trisomy 22 translocation and mosaic forms awaits the development of more refined karyotype banding procedures.

Clinical Features

Classic trisomy 22 is characterized by cleft palate as a cardinal sign. More variable findings are growth failure, mental retardation, periauricular appendages and/or sinuses, large and low-set ears, antimongoloid slant of the palpebral fissures, micrognathia, and, in rare instances, myopia, deafness, congenital dislocation of the hip, aplasia of one kidney, atresia of the external auditory canal, and fingerlike thumb (Fig. 43A).

The cat's eye syndrome has as its cardinal features iris coloboma, imperforate anus, or both. Variable findings are very similar to those for the classic trisomy 22 cases.

Recently a "partial trisomy 22" group was reported that had the features of mental retardation, congenital heart disease, usually coarctation of the aorta, minor skeletal anomalies (especially extra ribs), antimongoloid slant of the palpebral fissures, periauricular tags and sinuses, and large or low-set ears. Cleft palate and micrognathia were not prominent, in contrast to the classic trisomy 22 cases. The diagnosis at this time is entirely based on the karyotype banding of chromosomes, the clinical features being of some help in characterizing the classic and variant forms (Fig. 43B).

Therapy

Supportive care and treatment are all that is available at this time. The majority of patients with classic trisomy 22 die in infancy or early childhood, whereas the patients with cat's eye syndrome have a longer survival.

Chromosome 18 Trisomy (47,XY, + 18; Edwards's Syndrome)

Almost simultaneously in 1960, Edwards et al. (153) and Patau et al. (449) described a new clinical entity associated with an extra autosome. Trisomy 18 syndrome is the second most common multiple malformation syndrome, having an incidence of approximately 0.3 per 1,000 newborn infants and a 3-to-1 preponder-

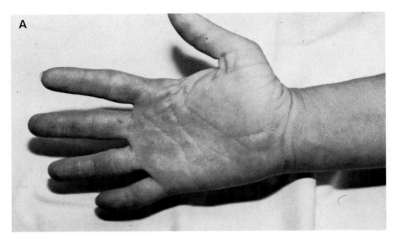

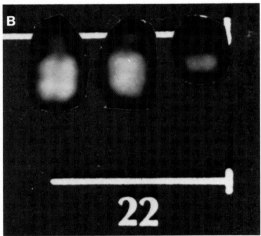

FIG. 43. Partial trisomy of chromosome 22. The patient is a 32-year-old woman evaluated for mental retardation. She has delayed motor and mental development and an IQ of 53. She has down-slanting palpebral fissures and low-set ears.   **A:** Her hands appear short, with total hand length of 16 cm (third percentile). She has short fingers, a proximally placed thumb, and fifth finger clinodactyly bilaterally.   **B:** Karyotype indicating partial trisomy of chromosome 22. (Courtesy of Dr. C. B. Mankinen and Dr. L. Russell, Texas Department of Mental Health and Mental Retardation.)

ance of females to males. The great majority of cases are trisomic for the entire chromosome 18, which is thought to be secondary to nondisjunction in the first or second meiotic division in the formation of the ovum. This anomaly is accordingly found in the older maternal population, the mean maternal age being 32 years.

Translocation cases should be considered and carefully looked for by banding techniques, especially in the younger maternal age groups. If a translocation case is found, parental karyotyping is indicated to rule out a balanced translocation in one of the parents.

Partial trisomy and mosaic cases should also be considered, but at this time little information is available concerning them.

Clinical Features

The clinical findings can be subdivided into those occurring in 50% or more of patients, 10 to 50% of patients, or less than 10% of patients. Only those findings occurring in 50% or more of patients will be given here.

The general findings in the fetus and the newborn include the following: feeble fetal activity and altered gestational timing, with one-third of the patients being premature and one-third postmature; hydramnios; a small placenta with a single umbilical artery; hypotonia and weak cry in the newborn, with the hypotonia being converted to hypertonia over a period of weeks to months; growth deficiency, with a mean birth weight of 2,340 g; hypoplasia of muscle, adipose, and subcutaneous tissue; diminished response to sound; and a global psychomotor retardation.

The occiput is prominent, with a narrow bifrontal diameter. The ears are low-set with malformed auricles. The eyes are almond-shaped and the palpebral fissures are small. The oral opening is small, with micrognathia, and the palate is narrow. The upper lip is long with a flat philtrum (Fig. 44A). The hands are held clenched with overlapping of the second finger over the third and the fifth finger over the fourth. Also noted is a low-arch dermal pattern on six or more fingertips, with absence of the distal crease on the fifth finger. The hallux is short and frequently dorsiflexed, with hypoplasia of the nails, especially on the fifth fingers and toes.

The sternum is short with a reduced number of ossification centers, and the nipples are small.

Inguinal and umbilical hernias as well as diastasis recti are common. The pelvis is small with limitation of hip abduction, and the males usually have cryptorchidism.

Redundancy of skin, mild hirsutism of the forehead and back, and prominent cutis marmorata are seen.

Cardiac malformations include ventricular septal defect, atrial septal defect, and patent ductus arteriosus.

The diagnosis is based on the constellation of physical findings and confirmed by Giemsa and fluorescent banding techniques (Fig. 44B).

Neuropathology

The most consistent neuropathologic findings are various anomalies in gyral and lobar patterns; dysplasias of the hippocampus, lateral geniculate body, and inferior olivary nuclei; and a hypoplastic basis pontis.

The gyral anomalies include variations in the volume or discernibility of specific gyri, including the superior temporal gyrus, gyrus rectus, precentral, and postcentral gyri. There are also anomalies in the volume of the temporal, parietal, and occipital lobes and the hippocampi.

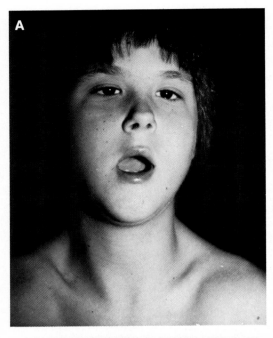

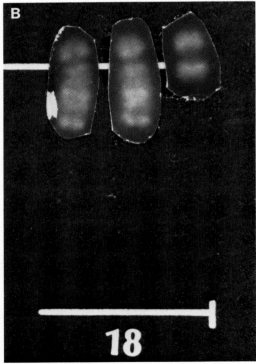

FIG. 44. Trisomy 18 [47,XY + i(18p)]. **A:** The patient is a 16-year-old boy. He is short for his age and has a head circumference of 51.5 cm (second percentile). He has mild mental retardation, an awkward gait, and low-set ears. **B:** Karyotype indicating trisomy of chromosome 18. (Courtesy of Dr. C. B. Mankinen and Dr. M. V. R. Freeman, Texas Department of Mental Health and Mental Retardation.)

Therapy

There is no specific treatment available. Thirty percent of these infants die within the first month and 50% by 2 months. Only 10% survive the first year and they are severely retarded.

Chromosome 13 Trisomy (47,XY, + 13; Patau's Syndrome)

The trisomic etiology of this syndrome was discovered in 1960 by Patau et al. (449).

Recent estimates indicate the incidence to be approximately 1 in 7,000, with a female preponderance.

Chromosome 13 trisomy (Fig. 45) is usually the result of nondisjunction in meiosis, and as such is more common in the older maternal age groups. Translocation may also result in this syndrome, and in fact the frequency of translocation is greater than in trisomy 21. The translocation is usually D/D because of centric

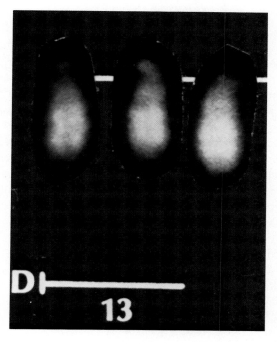

FIG. 45. Trisomy 13. The patient is a newborn boy who has multiple dysmorphic features, including bachycephaly, small palpebral fissures, micophthalmia, low-set ears, depressed nasal bridge, and a cleft lip and palate. He has a harsh grade 3/6 precordial murmur, a micropenis with distended scrotum, and a nubbin of an extra digit on the fifth fingers. There is radial deviation of the distal portion of the index fingers. Mild flexion contracture of all digits is present. Toenails are hypoplastic and the great toe is extremely broad, giving them an almost triangular appearance. A karyotype showed trisomy 13. (Courtesy of Dr. C. B. Mankinen and Dr. M. V. R. Freeman, Texas Department of Mental Health and Mental Retardation.)

or near-centric fusion, to which chromosome 13 seems particularly susceptible. The translocation cases tend to occur in the younger maternal age groups, and when found, a parental balance carrier must be carefully ruled out. Mosaicism also appears to be more common in trisomy 13 than in trisomy 21, and again, sufficient cells (at least 50) should be karyotyped before a mosaic condition can be ruled out.

Clinical Features

The cardinal clinical features are multiple congenital anomalies, including severe retardation; holoprosencephaly; major ocular anomalies such as anophthalmia, microphthalmia, or colobomas; clefts of lip and palate; polydactyly; congenital heart disease; and cutaneous defects of the scalp.

Newborn infants with trisomy 13 have a somewhat low birth weight for gestational age, and this continues as severe postnatal growth retardation. They have a weak cry and fail to respond to sound. Studies of the temporal bone have revealed bony and membranous anomalies of the internal ear.

In the neonatal period jitteriness and episodes of apnea are common. Minor motor seizures occur in approximately 66% of cases, with associated prominent EEG abnormalities.

Dermatoglyphic analysis reveals distal axial triradii. Arch patterns on the fingertips are increased, and there is an S-shaped modification of the hallucal arch.

Congenital heart disease is a prominent feature of this syndrome, and the most common cardiac defects are ventricular septal defect, patent ductus arteriosus, and atrial septal defect. GI anomalies include malrotations and Meckel's diverticulum.

Female patients often have bicornuate uteri and abnormal fallopian tubes or hypoplastic ovaries, and the male patients frequently have cryptorchidism. Cystic kidneys or unilateral renal agenesis may also be seen. Inguinal and umbilical hernias as well as accessory spleens and ectopic spleens are also common.

There is polydactyly on the ulnar and fibular sides of the extremities, and flexion contractures of the fingers are prominent, as well as a so-called "trigger thumb" in which, on passive extension, clicks are palpable at the metacarpalphalangeal joint. The thumb and index finger have a tendency to overlap the third finger, and the fifth finger may overlap the fourth. There may also be a marked posterior prominence of the heels, although not as frequently as in trisomy 18, and talipes equinovarus.

Roentgenographic features of this syndrome are not unique, but the occurrence of hypotelorism and small, poorly formed orbits with a sloping forehead, cleft palate, and polydactyly usually is diagnostic. The skull is poorly ossified and the ribs may be ribbonlike.

Hematologic abnormalities include persistent or unusually high levels of fetal and embryonic hemoglobins.

Neuropathology

The most characteristic neuropathologic finding in trisomy 13 is holoprosencephaly. There is invariably incomplete development of forebrain, often with absence of the olfactory nerve and corpus callosum. Fusion of the frontal lobes and a central ventricle is suggestive of cyclopia. Varying degrees of holoprosencephaly are found in about 80% of patients with trisomy 13. Defects in the corpus callosum are found in 21.8% and hydrocephalus in 12.4%.

Cerebellar anomalies occur in 28% of the patients and consist of exceptionally large nests of matrix cells in the dentate nucleus, nests of heterotopic neurons in the subcortical white matter, dysplasias of the dentate nucleus, and focal disorganization of the cerebellar cortex, particularly the vermis.

Therapy

There is no specific treatment for this abnormality. The average life span is under 9 months, with fewer than 18% of these infants reaching their first birthday.

Chromosome 12 Partial Duplication (12q24-qter)

See Fig. 46.

Chromosome 8 Trisomy (47,XY, + 8)

Trisomy 8 was the first syndrome to be described in humans that involved trisomy of a large autosome. Karyotype banding techniques reveal a total of 47 chromosomes with an extra chromosome 8. The majority of the cases that have

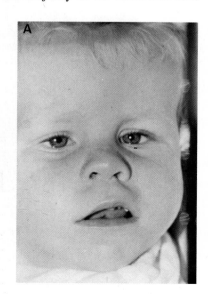

FIG. 46. Partial duplication of chromosome 12 (12q24-qter). **A:** The patient is a 3-year-boy with a head circumference at birth of 35.5 cm (50th percentile). Irritability, hypertonia, and depressed primitive reflexes were evaluated by CT scan of the head, which showed a posterior fossa cyst communicating with the fourth ventricle, indicative of a Dandy-Walker cyst. *(Continued)*.

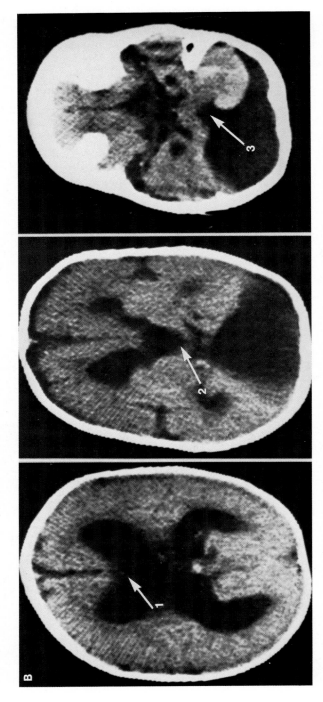

FIG. 46. *(Continued.)* **B:** *Arrow 1* indicates upward extension of the third ventricle, *arrow 2*, the third ventricle, and *arrow 3*, communication between the fourth ventricle and the posterior fossa cyst. *(Continued.)*

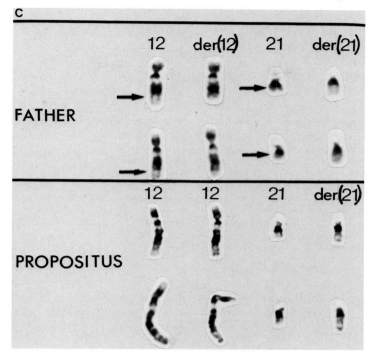

FIG. 46. *(Continued.)* **C:** Karyotypes of chromosomes 12 and 21 of the father and child show at the *arrows* the breakpoints of the translocation. One chromosome 21 had extra material at the distal end of the long arm in the child. The father also had 46 chromosomes, but a translocation between the long arm of chromosome 12 and the long arm of chromosome 21 was found. The breakpoint on chromosome 12 is most likely at q24.1 and that on chromosome 21 at q22.1. His karyotype is described as 46,XY,rcp(12:21)(q24.1;q22.1). The chromosomal constitution of the propositus can be described as 46,XY,der(21)t(12;21)(q24.1;q22.1)pat. The der(21)pat chromosome can be described as 21pter-21q22.1::12q24.1,12qter. Both paternal grandparents had normal karyotypes, indicating the father has a *de novo* translocation. This patient has additional clinical features that include abnormal skull shape, epicanthal folds, prominent nose tip, downturned corners of mouth, micrognathia, undescended testes, renal malformation, psychomotor retardation, hypertonia, and hip dislocations. (From ref. 364, with permission.)

been reported, however, have been mosaics (46,XY/47,XY, + 8). An increased paternal age has been noted in some cases.

Clinical Features

There is a wide variation in the phenotype of these patients. The most usual defects include spinal dysrhaphia and hypertonia.

Therapy

As there is no specific treatment for this disorder, supportive measures are indicated. The prognosis for life is good. However, the prognosis for a normal existence is guarded because of the associated musculoskeletal defects.

AUTOSOME DECREASE SYNDROMES

Chromosome 4 (Deletion of the Short Arm; 46,XX,4p − ; Wolfe's Syndrome)

These children have mental retardation and severe facial anomalies, including cleft palate and lip, a broad nasal bridge, a beaked or deformed nose, hypertelorism, epicanthic folds, a carp-shaped mouth, ptosis, and a hypoplastic chin. The ears are low-set. Males have hypospadias and often cryptorchidism. Congenital heart disease, often with atrial septal defects, occurs. Death often results in the first few months of life from congestive heart failure with associated pneumonia. Deletion of the short arm of chromosome 4 establishes the diagnosis. No reported patient has had a familial unbalanced translocation, in contrast to the presence of this finding in families in which the 5p − syndrome has occurred. These patients do not make a sound like the cry of a cat, as do 5p − patients.

Chromosome 5 Partial Monosome (46,XY,5p − ; Cri du Chat Syndrome)

This chromosomal abnormality was first described in 1963 and later found to involve a deletion in the short arm of chromosome 5 arising *de novo* (351). Although 30 cases have been reported, the true incidence and prevalence of this disorder are unknown. It may well be a relatively common cause of mental retardation. A balanced translocation parent with an increased risk for recurrence has been found in 10 to 15% of cases.

Clinical Features

The characteristic clinical features are the following: a weak meowing cry, often reminiscent of a kitten, among the newborn infants; low birth weight and subsequent failure to thrive; hypertelorism; antimongoloid slant of the palpebral fissures; micrognathia; prominent epicanthal folds; a round face; microcephaly; simian crease; and hypoplastic thumbs (Fig. 47). The striking cry and prominent epicanthal folds disappear with age, and the moonlike face becomes thin and asymmetrical in the majority of patients. Older patients show signs of upper motor neuron disease, and seizures are common.

Therapy

There is no specific treatment for this disorder, and supportive care is indicated.

Partial Deletion of Chromosome 8

See Fig. 48.

Partial Deletion of Chromosome 13 (13q −)

Patients have severe mental retardation and microcephaly. Hypertelorism, narrow palpebral fissures, a prominent nasal bridge, epicanthal folds, ptosis, a small chin,

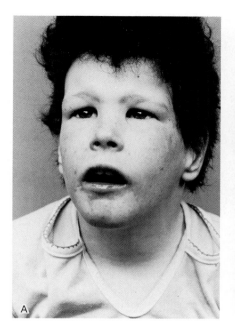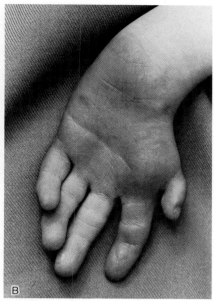

FIG. 47. A 6-year-old child with the cri du chat syndrome. **A:** Hypertelorism, the antimongoloid slant of the eyes, epicanthal folds, and microcephaly are present. **B:** The hypoplastic thumb, incurvation of the fifth digit, malformation of the hand, and simian crease are present and characteristic of the syndrome. (From ref. 505, with permission.)

and facial asymmetry are typical features (Fig. 49A). In addition, microphthalmos, colobomas, cataract, and retinoblastoma may occur. Boys may have cryptorchidism and hypospadias. A high percentage of patients have absence or hypoplasia of the thumb. Patients are short of stature. Two patients have been reported to have arhinencephaly. The diagnosis is made by these characteristic features and a karyotype showing a 13q− deletion (Fig. 49B).

Prader-Willi Syndrome (Deletion of 15q12)

This syndrome is usually sporadic, but autosomal recessive, multifactorial inheritance and autosomal dominant inheritance have been reported. About 50% of patients have a deletion of 15q12, and the other 50% have intact karyotypes. It is a common disorder, occurring in 1 in 25,000 to 50,000 newborns. Initially patients are hypotonic, areflexic, and generally unresponsive to external stimuli. Boys have a hypoplastic scrotum and a small penis, and girls have hypoplastic or absent labia minora. Older children become obese because of excessive appetite (Fig. 50A). They often show emotional lability, and most children are mentally retarded. Amenorrhea and infertility are common features. The primary genetic defect that explains the clinical features is not known. This may be a heterogeneous disorder

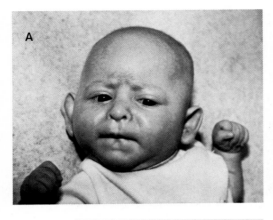

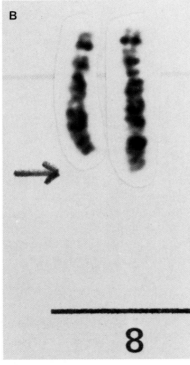

8

FIG. 48. Partial deletion of chromosome 8 [46,XX,del(8)(pter to q22.3::q24 to ter]. **A:** The patient is a 12-day-old girl with multiple dysmorphic features. She has short downslanting palpebral fissures, a thickened midportion of her nose, and a small anteverted tip. The philtrum is long with a midline groove. The right ear is prominent and cup-shaped. The fingers are long and thin with small, short hypoplastic nails. There is interdigital webbing of the fingers. The legs have tibial torsion and bilateral equinovarus deformity. (Courtesy of Dr. C. B. Mankinen and Dr. M. K. Kukolich, Texas Department of Mental Health and Mental Retardation.) **B:** Partial deletion of chromosome 8 between bands 8q22.3 and 8q24.12. Patients with a deletion of this region have been reported to develop Langer-Giedion syndrome with significant exostoses by the age of 4 years. (Courtesy Dr. C. B. Mankinen and Dr. M. K. Kukolich, Texas Department of Mental Health and Mental Retardation.)

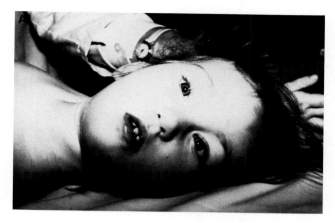

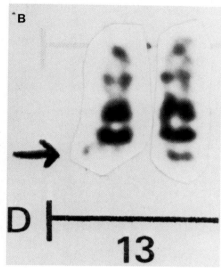

FIG. 49. Partial deletion of chromosome 13. **A:** The patient is a 23-month-old girl who is severely retarded and nonambulatory. She is less than the fifth percentile in height, weight, and head circumference. She has up-slanting palpebral fissures and an "ironed-out" left ear. She has evidence of lower extremity spasticity. **B:** A karyotype showed a partial deletion of one chromosome 13 (46,XX,13q −). (Courtesy of Dr. C. B. Mankinen and Dr. R. Roberts, Texas Department of Mental Health and Mental Retardation.)

caused by a variety of genetic defects, including the deletion of 15q11-q13 (Fig. 50B). However, Prader-Willi children may not have the 15q deletion, and children with this deletion may not express this syndrome. The H_3O rule has been applied as a mnemonic device, referring to hypomentia, hypotonia, hypogonadism, and obesity (Russel Snyder, *personal communication*).

Chromosome 18 Deletion of Long Arm (46,XX,18q −)

Patients show a rather consistent picture of microcephaly, retardation, and deafness. The midportion of the face appears underdeveloped. The eyes have an anti-mongoloid slant and are deeply set. The external genitalia are underdeveloped and

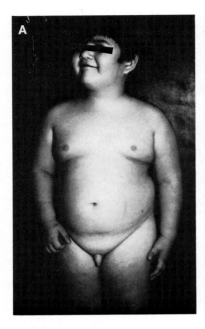
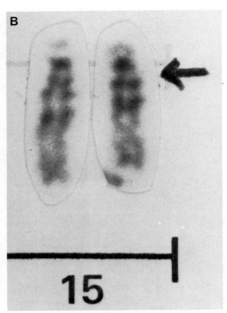

FIG. 50. Prader-Willi syndrome (chromosome 15q11-q13 deletion). **A:** The patient is a 6-year-old boy who at birth was hypotonic and had a poor suck and failure to gain weight. He was slow to develop his normal motor and mental milestones. He became moderately obese, and at 6 years he weighed 73 lb (95th percentile) and was 42 inches tall (10–25th percentile). The penis is of normal size and he has cryptorchidism. There is hyperextension of the hands at the proximal interphalangeal joints and there is mild syndactyly. The fourth and fifth fingers have clinodactyly. He has hyperextensible joints and genu valgum. His gait is broad based and waddling. Based on mental retardation, hypotonia, hypogonadism, and obesity it was felt he had the Prader-Willi syndrome. **B:** A karyotype showed deletion of bands 15q12 and 15q13 [46,XY,del(15)(q11-q13)] on one chromosome 15. (Courtesy of Dr. C. B. Mankinen and Dr. R. Redheendran, Texas Department of Mental Health and Mental Retardation.)

the testes are undescended. The diagnosis is established by finding a deletion of the long arm of chromosome 18. Patients having a deletion of the short arm of chromosome 18 (46,XX,18p−) are also retarded, of short stature, microcephalic, and brachycephalic. They also have webbing of the neck and a shieldlike chest.

SEX CHROMOSOME INCREASE SYNDROMES

X Chromosome Increase Syndromes

Klinefelter's Syndrome

This syndrome is associated with a karyotype of XXY (Fig. 51). Clinical features include hypogonadism, gynecomastia, acne, tall stature, limited forearm pronation-supination, and mental retardation or behavioral abnormalities. The presence of a

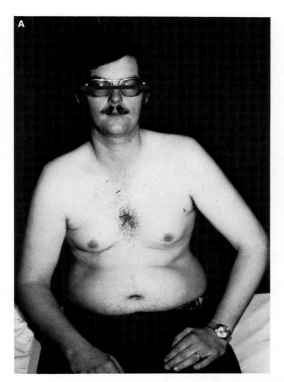

FIG. 51. XXY syndrome. Klinefelter's syndrome is illustrated in this 30-year-old man **(A)** with a 47,XXY karyotype **(B)**. He was referred for medical evaluation of azoospermia. (Courtesy of Dr. C. B. Mankinen and Dr. M. V. R. Freeman, Texas Department of Mental Health and Mental Retardation.)

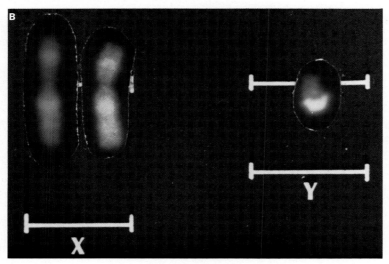

male phenotype with a positive Barr body from a buccal smear, indicating the presence of two X chromosomes genotypically, is most suggestive of a diagnosis of Klinefelter's syndrome prior to obtaining a formal karyotype. Additional karyotypic abnormalities include XXYY and XXXY patterns. There is a correlation between additional sex chromosomes and an increased dysmorphic state or mental retardation. The syndrome has an incidence of 1 in 1,000 in newborns.

Trisomy X Syndrome

Patients present with mild mental retardation and delayed menarche but no other specific phenotypic features. The three X chromosomes are illustrated in Fig. 52. Girls with four X chromosomes are also mildly retarded. Five X chromosomes have been reported about four times, and these girls are severely retarded, microcephalic, hyperteloric, and have mild scoliosis.

Y Chromosome Increase Syndromes

XYY Syndrome

These patients may have a normal appearance (Fig. 53A), but most patients have an increased height noted at birth, which is maintained through the second decade of life. Patients have mild mental retardation, with an average IQ of 90. These XYY males (Fig. 53B) may have acne, have more difficulty in school, and are said to be more immature and more impulsive. It is reported that minor criminal acts may occur slightly more commonly in this group, but this point is controversial.

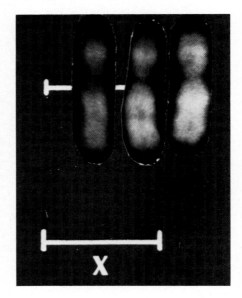

FIG. 52. Trisomy X syndrome. The patient is a 15-year-old girl who sought medical evaluation for lack of secondary sexual development. She had minimal breast development and minimal suprapubic hair. Her neurologic functions were normal. A karyotype showed trisomy X syndrome. (Courtesy of Dr. C. B. Mankinen and Dr. M. V. R. Freeman, Texas Department of Mental Health and Mental Retardation.)

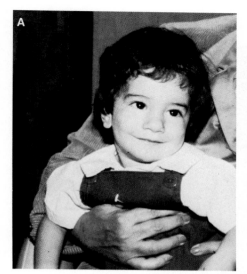

FIG. 53. XYY syndrome. **A:** The patient is a 4-year-old boy who appears thin and small for his age. He is in the fifth percentile for age for height, weight, and head circumference. His development has been normal. His ears are somewhat low-set with pointed helices bilaterally. The upper lip is rather long and there is a chin dimple. He was evaluated for his small size and multiple minor dysmorphic features. **B:** A karyotype showed an XYY pattern. Thus this chromosome abnormality can result in early impairment of growth but with normal neurologic development. (Courtesy of Dr. C. B. Mankinen and Dr. M. V. R. Freeman, Texas Department of Mental Health and Mental Retardation.)

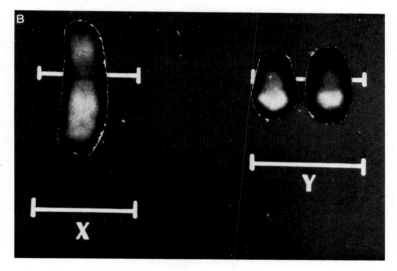

Pregnancies produced by XYY males have a high incidence of spontaneous abortions associated with neural tube defects and chromosome defects including trisomy 21, XYY or XYYq −, or a mosaic pattern of X/XX or X/XY. Boys may have abnormal seminiferous epithelia on testicular biopsy, and spermatogenesis may be impaired to the point of infertility. The P-R interval on an EKG may be excessively prolonged. The incidence is about 1.3 per 1,000 males born. An XXYY syndrome has also been reported (48,XXYY), and these patients have severe retardation, skeletal abnormalities, and genital anomalies.

SEX CRHOMOSOME DECREASE SYNDROME

X Chromosome Decrease

Turner's syndrome is associated with the 44XO karyotype, and clinical features include short stature, webbed neck, coarctation of the aorta, wide carrying angle of the forearms, amenorrhea. and infertility. It has an incidence of 1 in 10,000 newborns.

FRAGILE X CHROMOSOME SYNDROME

Mental retardation can be inherited in an X-linked manner (608). In about 30% of families, affected males have the X-chromosomal marker fra(x) (q27) for the "fragile site" in cultured lymphocytes (Fig. 54) (419). Macroorchidism is present

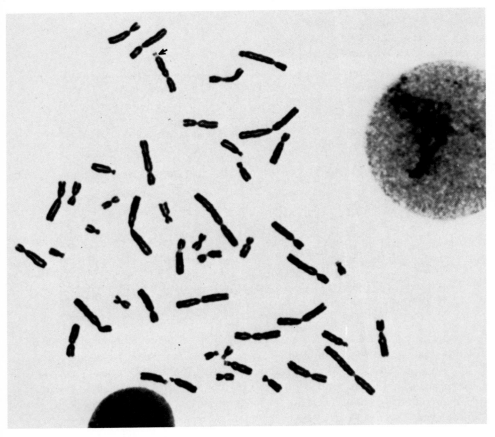

FIG. 54. A chromosomal preparation from a white blood cell from a male with marker X chromosome. The fragile site, a constricted area, in the long arm of the X is indicated by the *arrow*. (Courtesy of Dr. R. Rodney Howell, University of Texas Health Science Center at Houston.)

in affected males, and occasionally females who are carriers of this syndrome may be mildly retarded. Abruzzo et al. (2) tested the effects of 5-azacytidine and methionine on fragile X expression in lymphocytes. 5-Azacytidine inhibited fragile X formation in both males and females, but only at a high concentration. Turner et al. concluded that the rate of DNA methylation is likely to be secondary, the primary effect being due to thymidylate depletion. A review of the clinical features in 17 patients was recently published by Finelli et al. (188).

RING CHROMOSOME 22 SYNDROME

A ring 22 chromosome (r22) in a retarded person was described by Weleber et al. (629). Reeve et al. (475) reported a 28-year-old mentally retarded man with r22 with deterioration of mood and behavior, decreased speech, and bradykinesia. Treatment with methylphenidate hydrochloride produced a rapid improvement of mood, behavior, and motor abilities. On the basis of these pharmacologic observations, the authors suggest that genes mapped to chromosome 22 may have a direct effect on dopamine metabolism. In addition to having moderately severe mental retardation, patients are short of stature. The diagnosis is based on finding a ring 22 chromosome on a karyotype (Fig. 55). Other autosome ring chromosomes have been described, and an additional illustration is seen in Fig. 56 of a ring 4 chromosome. These rings are caused by loss of short and long arms on opposite sides of a centromere with joining of the ends of the remaining two opposite short and long arms.

Other Developmental Defects

ALSTRÖM-HALLGREN SYNDROME

This is a rare syndrome inherited as an autosomal recessive that is separated from Laurence-Moon-Biedl syndrome because polydactyly and mental retardation are not present. The two syndromes are similar, as both express obesity, hypogonadism, and retinitis pigmentosa. Nerve deafness and diabetes mellitus are also seen in this syndrome.

BIEMOND SYNDROME

This is also a very rare syndrome probably inherited as an autosomal recessive disorder. Clinical features include obesity, mental retardation, coloboma of the iris, polydactyly, and hypogonadotropic hypogonadism.

BÖRJESON-FORSSMANN-LEHMANN SYNDROME

This is a very rare syndrome probably inherited as an autosomal recessive. Clinical features include mental retardation, microcephaly, short stature, dys-

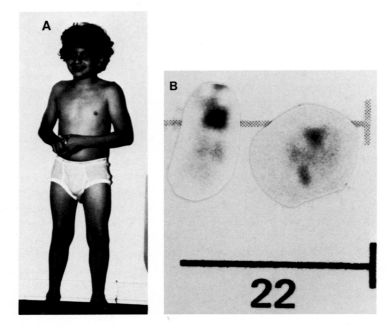

FIG. 55. Ring chromosome 22. **A:** The patient is a mentally retarded 12-year-old boy. He had delays in both motor and mental milestones. Head circumference was 55 cm (50th percentile). **B:** A karyotype showed a ring chromosome 22. (Courtesy of Dr. C. B. Mankinen and Dr. M. V. R. Freeman, Texas Department of Mental Health and Mental Retardation.)

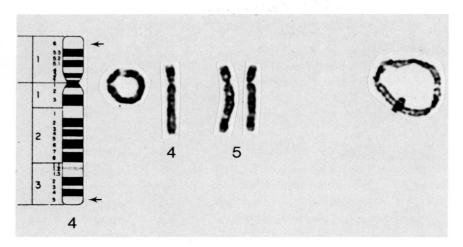

FIG. 56. Ring chromosome 4. A short and a long arm from one chromosome 4 are lost and the remaining linear structure fuses at the tips of the remaining short and long arms. (Courtesy of Dr. P. Howard-Peebles, University of Texas Health Science Center at Dallas.)

morphic facies, truncal obesity, gynecomastia, and hypogonadism. It bears a resemblance to Prader-Willi syndrome.

COFFIN-LOWRY SYNDROME

This is a very rare syndrome probably inherited as an X-linked dominant disorder. Clinical features include mental retardation, facial dysgenesis, large hands, and dysgenesis of the digits and vertebrae.

CORNELIA DELANGE SYNDROME

This is a rare syndrome in which the mode of inheritance is not clear. Clinical features include mental retardation, seizures, short stature, short neck, microcephaly, brachycephaly, hirsutism, congenital heart disease, cleft palate, hypospadias, undescended testes, and facial dysgenesis. Life expectancy is limited to childhood.

CORPUS CALLOSUM AGENESIS (AICARDI'S SYNDROME)

Abnormalities of the formation and structure of the corpus callosum with defects in the hippocampus and anterior commissures of the brain are associated with an extra ring chromosome with mosaicism. Aicardi's syndrome includes agenesis of the corpus callosum, mental retardation, seizures, and retinal dysgenesis. Other complications in these patients include hydrocephalus, meningomyelocele, cerebellar malformations, and architectonic abnormalities of brain histology such as microgyri and gray matter heterotopias.

LAURENCE-MOON-BIEDL SYNDROME

This is a rare syndrome inherited as an autosomal recessive. Clinical features include obesity, hypogonadism, small penis, polydactyly, mental retardation, and retinitis pigmentosa.

OROFACIALDIGITAL SYNDROME

This is a rare entity inherited as an X-linked dominant. Only girls have been reported; it is lethal in hemizygous boys. Clinical features include mental retardation, cleft palate, hamartoma of the tongue, and skeletal abnormalities of the maxilla and fingers.

NOONAN-EHMKE SYNDROME

This is an autosomal dominant inherited disorder that bears a resemblance to Turner's syndrome, including such clinical features as short stature, coarse facies, neck webbing, antimongoloid eye slant, epicanthal folds, low-set ears, and low hairline of the neck. Most patients are mentally retarded, in contrast to those with Turner's syndrome. Also in contrast to Turner's syndrome, these patients have a high incidence of right heart and pulmonary vessel anomalies. Some patients also have genitourinary anomalies. These patients also have a normal karyotype and both sexes are affected equally.

OSTEOPOROSIS WITH RENAL TUBULAR ACIDOSIS AND CEREBRAL CALCIFICATION

Osteoporosis is a rare syndrome in which two genetic forms have been described: an autosomal dominant form that is a benign disorder and a severe autosomal recessive type. A common feature to these forms is a failure of bone resorption. A subtype of this syndrome complex includes renal tubular acidosis and cerebral calcification, which is inherited as an autosomal recessive trait. A severe deficiency of carbonic anhydrase II has been described in patient erythrocytes and intermediate values in erythrocytes of their parents. Clinical features of the syndrome may include failure to thrive in infancy, developmental delay, short stature, apathy, muscle weakness, hypotonia, mental retardation, anemia, cranial nerve deficits, acidosis, skeletal fractures, and cerebral calcification (565,567).

RETT'S SYNDROME

Rett described a syndrome in female infants presumably inherited as an X-linked dominant that results in a developmental arrest. The arms and hands characteristically become useless for any purposeful movement. An autistic behavioral regression results, with associated seizures in some patients. Corticospinal deficits eventually occur in the teenage years. Although Rett in his reports cited the occurrence of hyperammonemia as part of the syndrome (479,480), subsequent reports have not found it to be a characteristic feature (250).

RUBINSTEIN-TAYBI SYNDROME

This is a rare syndrome whose mode of inheritance is unknown. Clinical features include mental retardation and broad terminal phalanges of the thumbs and great toes. Facial dysgenesis, scoliosis, kyphosis, pectus excavatum, and malformations of the heart and genitourinary systems may occur.

SJÖGREN-LARSSON SYNDROME

This is a rare autosomal recessive syndrome characterized by congenital ichthyosis, spastic paresis, and mental retardation. It is grouped on occasion as one of the neuroectodermal dysplasias. In 1985 Avigan et al. (26) reported that there was no significant effect of the disease on the composition of polyunsaturated fatty acids or on the rate of linoleic acid desaturation in cultured fibroblasts from two patients compared with control fibroblasts in culture. Thus there is no evidence from their report for a desaturase deficiency, and thus the previously reported defects in the fatty acid composition of sera from patients do not seem to be caused by a radical enzymatic defect.

WAARDENBURG SYNDROME

This is a rare syndrome inherited as an autosomal dominant with varying degrees of penetrance and expressivity. It has an estimated incidence of 1 in 40,000. Its features include partial albinism of the hair appearing as a white or gray forelock, heterochromia of the iris, and unilateral or bilateral congenital nerve deafness in about one-third of cases. Patients also have lateral displacement of the medial canthi of the eyes producing an appearance of hypertelorism. A broad and prominent bridge of the nose may occur. Mutism sometimes is the result of early total deafness.

WILLIAMS SYNDROME

This is a rare disorder whose mode of inheritance is not known. The clinical characteristics include mild mental retardation, short stature, destructive behavior, and facial dysgenesis (elfin facies). In addition most children have blue eyes, a stellate pattern to the iris, micrognathia, aortic stenosis, digit dysgenesis, and hypercalcemia. Recently Garabedian et al. (210) reported elevated plasma levels of 1,25-dihydroxyvitamin D during the hypercalcemic phase of the disease when the children were 5 to 9 months old, which they decreased thereafter.

NEURAL TUBE DEFECTS

These comprise a class of embryologic disorders that result in failure of the neural tube to close during the fourth week of development. The spectrum of involvement includes anencephaly, encephalocele, spinal rachischisis (open spinal column), and spina bifida with varying myelocele or myelomeningocele. An Arnold-Chiari malformation may be associated with these defects and contributes to the production of hydrocephalus. In the United Kingdom the incidence of neural tube defects is between 2 and 8 in 1,000 births and in Europe in general is about 2 in 1,000 births. These disorders tend to be slightly more common in females and are presumably inherited in a multifactorial genetic manner in which environmental factors are significantly involved.

Neural tube defects are diagnosable prenatally by measuring amniotic fluid α-fetoprotein. With open neural tube defects, including anencephaly and open myelomeningocele, it is possible to detect elevated α-fetoprotein levels in the amniotic fluid in the second trimester.

Levels of α-fetoprotein may reach up to 60 to 100 mg/liter (normal levels are up to 40 mg/liter) in patients with anencephaly. Ultrasound examination of the uterus may indicate the presence of anencephaly or a severe spina bifida deformity with a large myelomeningocele sac (343).

Specific Treatment of Genetic Neurologic Diseases

DIETARY THERAPY

Specific treatment of these diseases is currently limited but new strategies are constantly being developed. Dietary management and megavitamin therapy have been the main approaches employed. Phenylketonuria caused by phenylalanine hydroxylase deficiency is the classic example in which dietary restriction of the precursor amino acid, phenylalanine, results in striking clinical improvement. Similarly, dietary restriction of methionine in patients with homocystinuria caused by cystathionine synthase deficiency results in a significant clinical improvement in mental functioning. The use of a ketogenic diet in conjunction with anticonvulsants has been helpful in the treatment of intractable seizures in patients with maple syrup urine disease and various gangliosidoses, particularly Tay-Sachs disease, GM_1 gangliosidosis, and Gaucher's disease.

Recently lecithin has been used in high doses to treat various progressive inherited ataxias, with some improvement in selected patients. A more comprehensive experience will be required before its value can be accurately determined. Refsum's disease is one lipid storage disorder that responds favorably to a low-phytol, low-phytanic acid diet. Foods high in phytol, such as green leafy vegetables, meat, milk, butter, and cheese, are eliminated and replaced by a liquid formula diet containing skim milk, corn oil, sugar, salt, and vitamin and iron supplements. This dietary therapy has resulted in meaningful clinical improvement.

VITAMIN-RESPONSIVE THERAPY

Leon Rosenberg and Charles Scriver have pioneered the identification of various inborn errors of metabolism that are amenable to megavitamin therapy. In 1969 Scriver (544) showed that early diagnosis and treatment of pyridoxine-dependent seizures was compatible with normal mental development. As of 1976 Rosenberg (494) has been able to identify 25 different vitamin-responsive inherited metabolic diseases. Fourteen of these vitamin-responsive disorders, involving six different water-soluble vitamins, produce neurologic abnormalities. These vitamin-responsive neurologic disorders produce a variety of diverse neurologic features. Early onset clinical manifestations include lethargy and coma in the branched-chain ketoacidurias, methylmalonic acidemia, and propionic acidemia. As in the pyridoxine-dependent state, seizures in early life are noted in pyruvic acidemia. Conversely, late onset neurologic findings are documented by cerebellar ataxia in pyruvic acidemia and in Hartnup disease, and by mental retardation in xanthurenic aciduria and in biotin-responsive carboxylase deficiency. Psychotic behavior may also be a late presentation in pyridoxine-responsive homocystinuria with hypomethioninemia. Although these are rare disorders, L. E. Rosenberg (494) emphasizes the point that they are treatable by megavitamin administration provided early diagnosis is established.

In summary, the major and important vitamin-responsive inherited disorders affecting the nervous system include the following categories (494):

1. B_1-Responsive disorders: branched-chain ketoaciduria caused by branched-chain ketoacid decarboxylase deficiency, lactic acidosis caused by pyruvate carboxylase deficiency, and pyruvic acidemia caused by pyruvate dehydrogenase deficiency.

2. B_6-Responsive disorders: homocystinuria caused by cystathionine synthase deficiency, infantile convulsions caused by glutamic acid decarboxylase deficiency, and xanthurenic aciduria caused by kynureninase deficiency.
3. B_{12}-Responsive disorders: methylmalonic acidemia caused by adenosylcobalamin synthesis defect, methylmalonic aciduria with homocystinuria and hypomethioninemia caused by adenosylcobalamin and methylcobalamin synthesis defects.
4. Folic acid-responsive disorders: homocystinuria and hypomethioninemia caused by N^5,N^{10}-methylene-tetrahydrofolate reductase.
5. Nicotinamide-responsive disorder: Hartnup disease caused by the intestinal malabsorption of tryptophan.

It is clear that specific and effective dietary or vitamin therapy exists for these disorders, but that new approaches are needed for the gangliosidoses, leukodystrophies, and mucopolysaccharidoses.

ENZYME REPLACEMENT THERAPY

The lipidoses have been classified, the storage products identified, and the biochemical-enzymatic defects largely determined. These major achievements have been due largely to a brilliant series of investigations by Roscoe O. Brady and colleagues at the National Institutes of Health during the 1960s and 1970s (58,59). However, specific treatment of these disorders has been more elusive, but attempts are currently under way by Brady and his colleagues (63).

Enzyme replacement therapy was theoretically considered soon after the intial enzymatic defects had been documented in the lipidoses. Human urine and placenta were employed as source materials, as it was believed that enzymes from human sources would be less likely to sensitize the recipient.

Initially studies were undertaken with hexosaminidase A, the enzyme that is deficient in Tay-Sachs disease, as obtained from human urine and placenta. More recently clinical trials have been conducted using fresh human placental tissue for the isolation of enzymes for several lipidoses. Ceramidetrihexosidase for the therapy of Fabry's disease and glucocerebrosidase for treatment of Gaucher's disease (63) have been purified by Brady and colleagues and administered intravenously to patients.

In 1973 Johnson and colleagues (308), working in Brady's laboratory, gave hexosaminidase A intravenously to a patient with the Sandhoff form of Tay-Sachs disease. Unfortunately, because of the presence of the blood-brain barrier, none of the injected enzyme entered the brain, but there was a reduction in the level of serum globoside by 43% 4 hr after infusion.

Infusion of ceramidetrihexosidase in patients with Fabry's disease did reduce the elevated serum levels of ceramidetrihexoside to normal, but only for 3 days. Brady and colleagues had more encouraging results in two patients with Gaucher's disease in whom purified placental enzyme caused a 26% reduction of hepatic glucocerebroside and a prolonged decrease of glucocerebroside in the circulation.

By modifying glucocerebrosidase Brady is attempting to target enzyme to the hepatic Kupffer cell, where substrate is excessively stored, to improve mobilization further.

Barranger is now attempting to open the blood-brain endothelial-glial-epithelial barrier with osmotic agents to allow infused enzymes to enter brain tissue (33). In experimental animals it has been possible to show increased enzyme transfer of the enzyme hexosaminidase A and to show that neurons have high-affinity receptors for this enzyme on their surface. These highly encouraging preliminary results suggest that enough purified enzyme in patients with a lipid storage disorder can be obtained, infused, and delivered to the impaired neuron where the storage material is located. Limiting factors for success would include obtaining enough starting material for enzyme purification, frequency of enzyme infusion, antigenicity of enzyme with possible autoimmunity, and delivery of the enzyme into the neuronal lysosome. With the advent of recombinant DNA technology it may be feasible in the near future to introduce the human gene for each of the necessary enzymes into bacterial hosts and generate easily the necessary amounts of these enzymes for clinical studies and long-term maintenance of patients. More specifically and elegantly, with the use of retroviruses and proper promoters, it will be possible to perform somatic cell gene therapy by transfecting patient bone marrow cells with virus containing the normal human gene insert for the mutant gene of the patient. As discussed by Rosenberg in 1984 (499), reinfusion of the genetically engineered cells would allow synthesis of the gene product needed by the patient and curing of the genetic disease.

PLASMAPHERESIS

The use of plasmapheresis can benefit certain patients with a lipid storage disorder. To date good results have been obtained in Refsum's disease patients, mainly because the stored lipid, phytanic acid, is derived from the diet and is in great excess in plasma accessible to plasmapheresis for exchange. Patients with Fabry's disease or Gaucher's disease (type I, extraneural, adult form) can have their plasma lipid levels reduced with inconsistent improvement in the symptoms of peripheral neuropathy in Fabry's patients. Thus this technique at present is limited in its application, but it may be useful to collect large amounts of donor enzyme-competent plasma with continuous flow instrumentation for infusion in enzyme-deficient patients. Plasma as a source of enzyme is of limited value, but there are exceptions such as in Hunter's disease.

REFERENCES

1. Abramov, A., Schorr, S., and Wolman, M. (1956): Generalized xanthomatosis with calcified adrenals. *Am. J. Dis. Child.*, 91:282.
2. Abruzzo, M., Mayer, M., and Jacobs, P. (1985): The effect of methionine and 5-azacytidine on fragile x expression. *Am. J. Hum. Genet.*, 37:193–198.
3. Aguilar, M. J., et al. (1968): Pathological observations in ataxia-telangiectasia. *J. Neuropathol. Exp. Neurol.*, 27:659–676.
4. Allan, J., Cusworth, D., Dent, C., and Wilson, V. (1958): A disease, probably hereditary,

characterized by severe mental deficiency and a constant gross abnormality of amino acid metabolism. *Lancet*, 1:182.

5. Alpers, B. (1960): Progressive cerebral degeneration in infancy. *J. Nerv. Ment. Dis.*, 130:442–448.

6. Alpers, B. J., and Conroe, B. I. (1931): Syringomyelia with choked disc. *J. Nerv. Ment. Dis.*, 73:557–586.

7. Alzheimer, A. (1910): Beitrage zu Kenntnis der pathologischen Neuroglia und iher Beziehung zu den Abbauvorgangen im Nervengewebe nissle. *Alzheimers Histol. Histopathol. Arb.*, 3:493.

8. Ammann, M. D., et al. (1969): Immunoglobin E deficiency in ataxia telangiectasia. *N. Engl. J. Med.*, 281:469–472.

9. Anderson, B. (1965): Marinesco-Sjogren syndrome, spinocerebellar ataxia, congenital cataract, somatic and mental retardation. *Dev. Med. Child Neurol.*, 7:249–257.

10. Anderson, D. H. (1956): Familial cirrhosis of the liver with storage of abnormal glycogen. *Lab. Invest.*, 5:11–20.

11. Anderson, E. P., Kalckar, H. M., Kurahashi, K., and Isselbacher, K. J. (1957): A specific enzymatic assay for the diagnosis of congenital galactosemia. *J. Lab. Clin. Med.*, 50:469–477.

12. Anderson, W. (1898): A case of angiokeratoma. *Br. J. Dermatol.*, 10:113.

13. Andrade, C. (1952): A peculiar form of peripheral neuropathy: Familial atypical generalized amyloidosis with special involvement of peripheral nerves. *Brain*, 75:408–427.

14. Angelini, C. (1975): Carnitine deficiency. *Lancet*, 2:554.

15. Angelini, C., Engel, A., and Titus, J. (1972): Adult acid maltase deficiency abnormalities in fibroblasts from patients. *N. Engl. J. Med.*, 287:948–951.

16. Appel, L., and van Bogaert, L. (1951): Etudes sur la paraplegie spasmodique famille Ameil: Formes tres precoces et congenitales; contribution histopathologique. *Acta Neurol. Psychiatr. Belg.*, 51:129.

17. Arnason, A. (1935): Apoplexie und ihre Vererbung. *Acta Psychiatr. Neurol.*, (suppl.) 7:1–180.

18. Arnold, A., Edgren, D. C., Palladino, V. S. (1953): Amyotrophic lateral sclerosis. *J. Nerv. Ment. Dis.*, 117:135–139.

19. Aronson, S. M., and Volk, B. S., eds. (1967): Inborn disorders of sphingolipid metabolism. *Proceedings of the Third International Symposium on the Cerebral Sphingolipidoses.* Pergamon, New York.

20. Asbury, A. K., Gale, M. K., Cox, S. C., et al. (1972): Giant axonal neuropathy: A unique case with segmental neurofilamentous masses. *Acta Neuropathol.*, 20:237–247.

21. Askanas, V., Engel, W. K., Kwan, H. A., Reddy, N. B., et al. (1985): Autosomal dominant syndrome of lipid neuromyopathy with normal carnitine: Successful treatment with long-chain fatty-acid-free diet. *Neurology*, 35:66–72.

22. Austin, J. H. (1956): Observations on the syndrome of hypertrophic neuritis. *Medicine*, 35:187–237.

23. Austin, J. H. (1959): Metachromatic sulfatides in cerebral white matter and kidney. *Proc. Soc. Exp. Biol. Med.*, 100:361–364.

24. Austin, J. H., and Stears, J. C. (1971): Familial hypoplasia of both internal carotid arteries. *Arch. Neurol.*, 24:1–16.

25. Austin, J. H., Armstrong, D., and Shearer, L. (1965): Metachromatic form of diffuse cerebral sclerosis. V. Nature and significance of low sulfatase activity: A controlled study of brain, liver, and kidney in four patients with metachromatic leukodystrophy (MLD). *Arch. Neurol.*, 13:593–614.

26. Avigan, J., Campbell, B., Yost, D., et al. (1985): Sjögren-Larsson syndrome, delta 5 and delta 6 fatty acid desaturases in skin fibroblasts. *Neurology*, 35:401–403.

27. Bakker, E., Goor, M., Wrogemann, K., Kunkel, L., et al. (1985): Prenatal diagnosis and carrier detection of Duchenne muscular dystrophy with closely linked RFLP's. *Lancet*, 1:655–658.

28. Ball, M. J., Hachinski, V., Fox, A., Kirshen, A. J., Fisman, M., Blume, W., Kral, V. A., and Fox, H. (1985): A new definition of Alzheimer's Disease: A hippocampal dementia. *Lancet*, 1:14–16.

29. Bank, W. J., DiMauro, S., Bonilla, E., et al. (1975): A disorder of muscle lipid metabolism and myoglobinuria. *N. Engl. J. Med.*, 292:443–449.

30. Barbeau, A., Roy, M., Cunha, L., DeVincente, A. N., Rosenberg, R. N., Nyhan, W. L., MacLeod, P. L., Chazot, G., Langston, L. B., Dawson, D. M., and Coutinho, P. (1984): The natural history of Machado-Joseph disease. *Can. J. Neurol. Sci.*, 11:510–525.

31. Baron, D. N., Rent, C. E., Harris, H., Hart, E. W., and Jepson, J. B. (1956): Hereditary pellagra-like skin rash with temporary cerebellar ataxia. Constant renal amino-aciduria, and other bizarre biochemical features. *Lancet*, 2:421–428.
32. Barranger, J. A., Pentchev, P. G., Rapoport, S. I., and Brady, R. O. (1977): Augmentation of a brain lysosomal enzyme activity following enzyme infusion with concomitant alteration of the blood-brain barrier. *Trans. Am. Neurol. Assoc.*, 102:10–12.
33. Barranger, J., Rapoport, S., Frederick, W., et al. (1979): Modification of the blood-brain-barrier: Increased concentration and fate of enzymes entering the brain. *Proc. Natl. Acad. Sci. USA*, 76:481–485.
34. Barranquer-Ferre, L., and Barraquer-Bordas, L. (1951): Contribution a la connaissance de l'etiologie de la sclerose laterale amyotrophique. *Acta Neurol. Psychiatr. Belg.*, 51:264.
35. Bassen, F. A., and Kornzweig, A. L. (1950): Malformation of erythrocytes in a case of atypical retinitis pigmentosa. *Blood*, 5:381–387.
36. Bassoe, P. (1920): The coincidence of cervical ribs and syringomyelia. *Arch. Neurol. Psychiatr.*, 4:542.
37. Batten, F. E. (1903): Cerebral degeneration with symmetrical changes in the macula in two members of a family. *Trans. Ophthalmol. Soc. UK*, 23:386.
38. Bearn, A. G. (1972): Wilson's disease. In: *The Metabolic Basis of Inherited Disease*, 3rd ed., edited by J. B. Stanbury, J. B. Wyngaarden, and D. S. Fredrickson, pp. 1033–1050. McGraw-Hill, New York.
39. Bearn, A. G., and Kunkel, H. G. (1952): Biochemical abnormalities in Wilson's disease (Abstr.). *J. Clin. Invest.*, 31:616.
40. Beaudet, A. L., Su, T.-S., Bock, H.-G., D'Eustachio, P., Ruddle, F. H., and O'Brien, W. E. (1981): Use of a cloned cDNA to study human argininosuccinate synthetase (Abstr.). *Am. J. Hum. Genet.*, 33:364.
41. Becker, P. E., and Kiener, F. (1955): Eine neue X-chromosomale Muskel dystrophie. *Arch. Psychiatr. Nervenkr.*, 193:427.
42. Bergeron, J. A., and Singer, M. (1958): Metachromasia: An experimental and theoretical reevaluation. *J. Biophys. Biochem. Cytol.*, 4:433.
43. Berginer, V. M., Salen, G., and Shefer, S. (1984): Long term treatment of cerebrotendinous xanthomatosis with chenodeoxycholic acid. *N. Engl. J. Med.*, 311:1649–1652.
44. Bermann, E. J. (1927): Die Syringomyelie in Kindesalter. *Monatsschr. Kinderheilkd.*, 37:1.
45. Bernheimer, H., and Seitelberger, F. (1968): Uber das Verhalten der Ganglioside im Gehirn bie 2 Fallen von spatinfantiler amaurotischer Idiotie. *Wien Klin. Wochenschr.*, 80:163.
46. Bernsohn, J., and Grossman, H. J., eds. (1971): *Lipid Storage Diseases: Enzymatic Defect and Clinical Implications*. Academic Press, New York.
47. Bicherstaff, E. R. (1950): Hereditary spastic paraplegia. *J. Neurol. Neurosurg. Psychiatry*, 13:134–145.
48. Bickel, H., Gerrard, J., and Hickmans, E. (1954): Influence of phenylalanine intake on the chemistry and behavior of a phenylketonuric child. *Acta Pediatr.*, 43:64.
49. Blass, J. P. (1979): Disorders of pyruvate metabolism. *Neurology*, 29:280–286.
50. Blass, J. P., Kark, R. A. P., and Menon, N. K. (1976): Low activities of the pyruvate and oxoglutarate dehydrogenase complexes in five patients with Friedreich's ataxia. *N. Engl. J. Med.*, 295:62–76.
51. Blaw, M. E. (1970): Melanodermic type of leukodystrophy (adrenoleukodystrophy). In: *Handbook of Clinical Neurology*, edited by P. J. Vinken and G. W. Bruyn, Vol. 10, pp. 128–133. North Holland, Amsterdam.
52. Bobowick, A. R., and Brody, J. A. (1973): Epidemiology of motor neuron diseases. *N. Engl. J. Med.*, 288:1047–1055.
53. Bockman, J. M., Kingsbury, D. T., McKinley, M. P., Bendheim, P. E., and Prusiner, S. B. (1985): Creutzfeldt-Jakob disease prion proteins in human brains. *N. Engl. J. Med.*, 312:73–78.
54. Bolger, G., Stamberg, J., and Kirsch, I. (1985): Chromosome translocation t(14;22) and oncogene variant in a pedigree with familial meningioma. *N. Engl. J. Med.*, 312:564–567.
55. Bowman, K., and Meurman, T. (1967): Prognosis of amyotrophic lateral sclerosis. *Acta Neurol. Scand.*, 43:489.
56. Boyer, S. H., Chisholm, A. W., and McKusick, V. A. (1962): Cardiac aspects of Friedreich's ataxia. *Circulation*, 25:493–305.

163. Elizan, T. S., et al. (1966): Amyotrophic lateral sclerosis and Parkinsonism dementia complex of Guam. *Arch. Neurol.*, 14:356–368.
164. Ellenberger, C., Jr., Campa, J. F., and Netsky, M. D. (1968): Opsoclonus and parenchymatous degeneration of cerebellum. *Neurology (Minneap.)*, 18:1041–1046.
165. Emery, A. E. H., and Dreifuss, F. E. (1966): Unusual type of benign X-linked muscular dystrophy. *J. Neurol. Neurosurg. Psychiatry*, 29:338–342.
166. Engel, A. G. (1977): Hypokalemia and hyperkalemia periodic paralyses. In: *Scientific Approaches to Clinical Neurology*, edited by E. S. Goldensohn and S. H. Appel, pp. 1742–1765. Lea and Febiger, Philadelphia.
167. Engel, A. G., and Angelini, C. (1973): Carnitine deficiency of human skeletal muscle with associated lipid storage myopathy: A new syndrome. *Science*, 179:899–902.
168. Engel, A. G., Lambert, E. H., and Gomez, M. R. (1977): A new myasthenic syndrome with end plate acetylcholinesterase deficiency, small nerve terminals and reduced acetylcholine release. *Ann. Neurol.*, 1:315–330.
169. Engel, A. G., Lambert, E. H., Mulder, D. M., Torres, C. F., Sahashi, K., Bertorini, T. E., and Whitaker, J. N. (1982): A newly recognized congenital myasthenic syndrome attributed to a prolonged open time of the acetylcholine induced ion channel. *Ann. Neurol.*, 11:553–569.
170. Engel, A. G., and Siekert, R. G. (1972): Lipid storage myopathy responsive to prednisone. *Arch. Neurol.*, 27:174–181.
171. Engel, E. (1972): The chromosome basis of human heredity. In: *The Metabolic Basis of Inherited Disease*. 3rd ed., edited by J. Stanbury, J. Wyngaarden, and D. Fredrickson, pp. 52–79. McGraw-Hill, New York.
172. Engel, G. L., and Aring, C. D. (1945): Hypothalamic attacks with thalamic lesions. *Arch. Neurol. Psychiatry*, 54:37–43.
173. Engel, W. K., Dorman, J. D., Levy, R. I., and Fredrickson, D. S. (1967): Neuropathy in Tangier disease. *Arch. Neurol.*, 17:1–9.
174. Enna, S., Bird, E., Bennett, J., Jr., Bylund, D., Yanamura, H., Iversen, L., and Synder, S. (1976): Huntington's chorea: Changes in neurotransmitter receptors in brain. *N. Engl. J. Med.*, 294:1305–1309.
175. Fabricant, R., Todaro, G., and Eldridge, R. (1979): Increased levels of a nerve-growth factor cross-reacting protein in "central" neurofibromatosis. *Lancet*, 1:4–6.
176. Fabry, J. (1898): Ein Beitrag zur Kenntnis der Purpura hemorrhagica nodularis (Purpura papulosa hemorrhagica Hebrae). *Arch. Dermatol. Syphilol.*, 43:187.
177. Fairburn, B. (1973): Twin intracranial aneurysms causing subarachnoid hemorrhage in identical twins. *Br. Med. J.*, 210–211.
178. Falconer, M. A. (1971): Genetic and related etiological factors in temporal lobe epilepsy. *Epilepsia*, 12:13–31.
179. Farrell, D. F., and MacMartin, M. P. (1981): GMI gangliosidosis: Enzymatic variation in a single family. *Ann. Neurol.*, 9:232–236.
180. Farrell, D., MacMartin, M., and Clark, A. (1979): Multiple molecular forms of arylsulfatase A in different forms of metachromatic leukodystrophy. *Neurology*, 29:16–20.
181. Farrell, D. F., and Ochs, U. (1981): GMI gangliosidosis: Phenotypic variation in a single family. *Ann. Neurol.*, 9:225–231.
182. Farrell, D. F., and Sumi, M. (1977): Skin punch biopsy in the diagnosis of juvenile neuronal ceroid-lipofuscinoses. *Arch. Neurol.*, 34:39–44.
183. Feigin, I., and Wolf, A. (1954): A disease in infants resembling chronic Wernicke's encephalopathy. *J. Pediatr.*, 45:243–263.
184. Feit, H., Kirkpatrick, J., Van Worert, M. H., Pandian, G., et al. (1983): Myoclonus, ataxia, and hypoventilation: Response to L-5-hydroxytryptophan. *Neurology*, 33:109–112.
185. Feldman, R. G., Chandler, K., Levy, L., and Glaser, G. (1963): Familial Alzheimer's disease. *Neurology*, 13:811–824.
186. Fenichel, G. M., Sul, Y. C., Kilroy, A. W., et al. (1982): An autosomal-dominant dystrophy with humeropelvic distribution and cardiomyopathy. *Neurology*, 32:1399–1404.
187. Fialkow, P., Sagebiel, R., Gartler, S., and Rimoin, D. (1971): Multiple cell origin of hereditary neurofibromas. *N. Engl. J. Med.*, 284:298–300.
188. Finelli, P., Pueschel, S., Padre-Mendoza, T., and O'Brien, M. (1985): Neurological findings in patients with the fragile X syndrome. *J. Neurol. Neurosurg. Psychiatry*, 48:150–153.

189. Finocchiaro, G., Taroni, F., and DiDonato, S. (1985): Glutamate dehydrogenase activity in leukocytes and muscle mitochondria in olivopontocerebellar atrophies. *Neurology (Suppl.* 1), 35:193.

190. Fiorilli, M., Carbonari, M., Crescenzi, M., Russo, G., and Aiuti, F. (1985): T cell receptor genes and ataxia telangiectasia. *Nature*, 313:186.

191. Fischbeck, K. H., and Ar-Rushdi, N. (1985): Duchenne carrier detection with DNA probes. *Neurology (Suppl.* 1), 35:260.

192. Fishbein, W. N., Armbrustmacher, V. W., and Griffin, J. L. (1978): Myoadenylate deaminase deficiency. *Science*, 200:545–548.

193. Fleischer, B. (1903): Zwei weitere Falle von grunlicher Verfarbung der Kornea. *Klin. Monatsbl. Augenheilkd.*, 41:489–491.

194. Folch-Pi, J., and Bauer, H., eds. (1963): *Brain Lipids and Lipoproteins and the Leukodystrophies.* Elsevier, Amsterdam.

195. Folling, A. (1934): Uber Ausscheidung von Phenylbrenztraubenaure in den Harn als Stoffwechselanomalie in Verbindung mit Imbezzillitat. *Z. Physiol. Chem.*, 227:169.

195a.Folstein, S., Phillips, J., Meyers, D., Chase, G., Abbott, M., Franz, M., Waber, P., Kazazian, H., Conneally, P., Hobbs, W., Tanzio, R., Faryniary, A., Gibbons, K., and Gusella, J. (1985): Huntington's disease: Two families with different clinical features show linkage to the G8 probe. *Science*, 229:776–779.

196. Forster, F. M., Borkowski, W. J., and Alpers, B. J. (1946): Effects of denervation on fasciculations in human muscle: Relation of fibrillations to fasciculations. *Neurol. Psychiatry*, 56:276.

197. Francois, J., and Descamps, L. (1951): Heredo-ataxie par degenerescence spinopontocerebelleuse avec manifestations tapetoretiniennes et cochleovestibulaires. *Monatsschr. Psychiatr. Neurol.*, 121:23.

198. Frantzen, E., Lennox-Buchthal, M., Nygaard, A., and Stene, J. (1970): A genetic study of febrile convulsions. *Neurology*, 20:909–917.

199. Fratantoni, J. C., Hall, C. W., and Neufeld, E. F. (1968): The defect in Hurler's and Hunter's syndromes: Faulty degradation of mucopolysaccharide. *Proc. Natl. Acad. Sci. USA*, 60:699–706.

200. Fratantoni, J. C., Hall, C. W., and Neufeld, E. F. (1968): Hurler and Hunter's syndromes; mutual correction of the defect in cultured fibroblasts. *Science*, 162:570–572.

201. Fratantoni, J. C., Hall, C. W., and Neufeld, E. F. (1969): The defect in Hurler and Hunter syndromes. II. Deficiency of specific factors involved in mucopolysaccharide degradation. *Proc. Natl. Acad. Sci. USA*, 64:360–366.

202. Freeman, J. M., Nicholson, J. F., Masland, W. S., Rowland, L. P., and Carter, S. (1964): Ammonia intoxication due to a congenital defect in urea synthesis. *J. Pediatr.*, 65:1039–1040.

203. Friedman, A. P., and Freedman, D. (1950): Amyotrophic lateral sclerosis. *J. Nerv. Ment. Dis.*, 111:1.

204. Frydman, M., Bonne-Tamir, B., Farrer, L., Conneally, P., et al. (1985): Assignment of the gene for Wilson disease to chromosome 13: Linkage to the esterase D locus. *Proc. Natl. Acad. Sci. USA*, 82:1819–1821.

205. Fukuhara, N. (1983): Myoclonus epilepsy and mitochondrial myopathy. In: *Mitochondrial Pathology in Muscle Disease*, edited by C. Cerri and G. Scarlato, pp. 87–111. Piccin, Padua.

206. Fukuhara, N., Tokiguchi, S., Shirakawa, K., and Tsubaki, T. (1980): Myoclonus epilepsy associated with ragged-red fibers disease entity in a syndrome. *J. Neurol. Sci.*, 47:117–133.

207. Fukushima, H., deWet, J., and O'Brien, J. (1985): Molecular cloning of a cDNA for human alpha-L-fucosidase. *Proc. Natl. Acad. Sci. USA*, 82:1262–1265.

208. Furukawa, T., et al. (1969): Neurogenic muscular atrophy simulating fascioscapulohumeral muscular dystrophy. *J. Neurol. Sci.*, 9:389–397.

209. Gaist, G., and Piazza, G. (1959): Meningiomas in two members of the same family. *Neurosurgery*, 16:110–113.

210. Garabedian, M., Jacqz, E., Guillozo, H., Grimberg, R., et al. (1985): Elevated plasma 1,25 dihydroxyvitamin D concentrations in infants with hypercalcemia and an elfin facies. *N. Engl. J. Med.*, 312:948–952.

211. Gardner, W. J. (1965): Hydrodynamic mechanism of syringomyelia: Its relationship to myelocoel. *J. Neurol. Neurosurg. Psychiatry*, 28:247–259.

212. Gardner-Medwin, D., et al. (1967): Benign spinal muscular atrophy arising in childhood and adolescence. *J. Neurol. Sci.*, 5:121–158.

213. Garland, H. G., and Astley, C. D. (1950): Hereditary spastic paraplegia with amyotrophy and pes cavus. *J. Neurol. Neurosurg. Psychiatry*, 13:130–133.

214. Garrod, A. E. (1906): Peculiar pigmentation of the skin in an infant. *Trans. Clin. Soc. Lond.*, 39:216.

215. Gasper, P. W., Thrall, M. A., Wenger, D. A., Macy, D. W., Ham, L., Dornsife, R. E., McBiles, K., Quackenbush, S. L., Kesel, M. L., Gillette, E. L., and Hoover, E. A. (1984): Correction of feline arylsulphatase B deficiency (mucopolysaccharidosis VI) by bone marrow transplantation. *Nature*, 312:467–469.
216. Gaucher, P. C. E. (1882): De l'épithéliome primitif de la rate. Thèse de Paris.
217. Geary, J. F., Earle, K. M., and Rose, A. S. (1956): Olivopontocerebellar atrophy. *Neurology (Minneap.)*, 6:218–224.
218. Giannelli, F. (1980): DNA repair in human diseases. *Clin. Exp. Dermatol.*, 5:119–138.
219. Gieron, M. A., and Korthals, J. K. (1985): Familial infantile myasthenia gravis. *Arch. Neurol.*, 42:143–144.
220. Gilroy, J., et al. (1966): Chemical, biochemical, and neurophysiological studies of chronic interstitial hypertrophic polyneuropathy. *Am. J. Med.*, 40:368–383.
221. Glazebrook, A. J. (1945): Wilson's disease. *Edinb. Med. J.*, 52:83–87.
222. Glick, N., Snodgrass, P., and Schafer, I. (1976): Neonatal argininosuccinic aciduria with normal brain and kidney but absent liver argininosuccinate lyase activity. *Am. J. Hum. Genet.*, 28:22–30.
223. Goldberg, M. F., Payne, J. W., and Brunt, P. W. (1968): Ophthalmologic studies of familial dysautonomia. *Arch. Ophthalmol.*, 80:732–743.
224. Goldfischer, S., Collins, J., Rapin, I., et al. (1985): Peroxisomal defects in neonatal-onset and X-linked adrenoleukodystrophies. *Science*, 227:67–70.
225. Goldstein-Nieviazhski, C., and Wallis, K. (1966): Riley-Day syndrome: Survey of 27 cases. *Ann. Pediatr.*, 206:188.
226. Gomez, M., Clermont, V., and Bernstein, J. (1962): Progressive bulbar paralysis in childhood (Fazio-Londe's disease). *Arch. Neurol.*, 6:317–323.
227. Gompertz, D., Draffan, G., Watts, J., and Hull, D. (1971): Biotin-responsive β-methyl-crotonylglycinuria. *Lancet*, 2:22–24.
228. Goodman, S. (1973): Antenatal diagnosis of argininosuccinic aciduria. *Clin. Genet.*, 4:236–240.
229. Gottlieb, R. P., Koppel, M. M., Nyhan, W. L., Bakay, B., Nissinen, E., Borden, M., and Page, T. (1982): Hyperuricemia and choreoathetosis in a child without mental retardation or self-mutilation—A new HGPRT variant. *J. Inher. Metab. Dis.*, 5:183–186.
230. Gray, F., Louarn, F., Gherardi, R., Eizenbaum, J., and Marsault, C. (1984): Adult form of Leigh's disease: A clinical-pathological case with CT scan examination. *J. Neurol. Neurosurg. Psychiatry*, 47:1211–1215.
231. Gray, R., and Kumar, D. (1985): Mitochondrial malic enzyme in Friedreich's ataxia: Failure to demonstrate reduced activity in cultured fibroblasts. *J. Neurol. Neurosurg. Psychiatry*, 48:70–74.
232. Greenfield, J. G. (1954): *The Spino-Cerebellar Degenerations*. Charles C Thomas, Springfield, IL.
233. Greenfield, J. G. (1963): Syringomyelia and syringobulbia. In: *Greenfield's Neuropathology*, 2nd ed., edited by W. Blackwood et al., pp. 331–335. Williams and Wilkins, Co., London.
234. Greenfield, J. G., and Stern, R. O. (1973): The anatomical identity of the Werdnig-Hoffman and Oppenheim forms of infantile muscular atrophy. *Brain*, 50:652–686.
235. Greer, M., and Schotland, M. (1960): Myasthenia gravis in the newborn. *Pediatrics*, 26:101–108.
236. Griggs, R. C. (1977): The myotonic disorders and the periodic paralyses. In: *Advances in Neurology, Vol. 17*, edited by R. C. Griggs and R. T. Moxley, pp. 143–159. Raven Press, New York.
237. Griggs, R. C., Doherty, R. A., Mendell, J. R., et al. (1985): Combined use of serum creatine kinase and pyruvate kinase and genetic linkage for carrier detection in Duchenne dystrophy. *Neurology (Suppl. 1)*, 35:260.
238. Griggs, R., Moxley, R., LaFrance, R., et al. (1978): Hereditary paroxysmal ataxia: Response to acetazolamide. *Neurology*, 28:1259–1264.
239. Gronert, G. A. (1980): Malignant hyperthermia. *Anesthesiology*, 53:395–423.
240. Grubb, A., Jensson, O., Gudmundsson, G., Arnason, A., Lofberg, H., and Malm, J. (1984): Abnormal metabolism of gamma trace alkaline microprotein. *N. Engl. J. Med.*, 311:1547–1549.
241. Grundy, S. M. (1984): Cerebrotendinous xanthomatosis. *N. Engl. J. Med.*, 311:1694–1695.
242. Grzeschik, K.-H. (1975): Assignment of human genes: β-Glucuronidase to chromosome 7, adenylate kinase-1 to 9, a second enzyme with enolase activity to 12, and mitochondrial IDH to 15. *Gene Mapping Conference, Baltimore*, 3:142–148.
243. Gusella, J. F. (1984): Genetic linkage of the Huntington's disease gene to a DNA marker. *Can. J. Neurol. Sci.*, 11:421–425.
244. Gusella, J. F., Wexler, N. S., Conneally, P. M., Naylor, S. L., Anderson, M. A., Tanzi, R. E., Watkins, P. C., Ottina, K., Wallace, M. R., Sakaguchi, A. Y., Young, A. B., Shoulson, I., Bonilla,

E., and Martin, J. B. (1983): A polymorphic DNA marker genetically linked to Huntington's disease. *Nature*, 306:234–238.

245. Gustavson, K.-H., and Hagberg, B. (1971): The incidence and genetics of metachromatic leukodystrophy in northern Sweden. *Acta Paediatr. Scand.*, 60:585–590.

246. Guthrie, R., and Susi, A. (1963): A simple phenylalanine method for detecting phenylketonuria in large populations of newborn infants. *Pediatrics*, 32:338–343.

247. Haas, J. E., Johnson, E. S., and Farrell, D. L. (1982): Neonatal-onset adrenoleukodystrophy in a girl. *Ann. Neurol.*, 12:449–457.

248. Haase, F. R., and Shy, M. (1960): Pathological changes in muscle biopsies from patients with peroneal muscular atrophy. *Brain*, 83:631–637.

249. Hagberg, B. (1963): Clinical symptoms, signs and tests in metachromatic leucodystrophy. In: *Brain Lipids and Lipoproteins and the Leukodystrophies*, edited by J. Folch-Pi and H. Bauer, pp. 134–146. Elsevier, Amsterdam.

250. Hagberg, B., Aicardi, J., Dias, K., and Ramos, O. (1983): A progressive syndrome of autism, dementia, ataxia, and loss of purposeful hand use in girls of Rett's syndrome. *Ann. Neurol.*, 14:471–479.

251. Hagberg, B., Kollberg, H., Sourander, P., and Akesson, H. O. (1970): Infantile globoid cell leucodystrophy (Krabbe's disease). A clinical and genetic study of 32 Swedish cases 1953–1967. *Neuropadiatrie*, 1:74.

252. Hagen, P. B., Noad, K. B., and Latham, O. (1951): Syndrome of lamellar cerebellar degeneration associated with retinitis pigmentosa, heterotopias, and mental deficiency. *Med. J. Aust.*, 1:217–223.

253. Haile, R. W., Hodge, S. E., Visscher, R., Spence, M. A., Detels, R., McAuliffe, T. L., Park, M. S., and Dudley, J. P. (1980): Genetic susceptibility to multiple sclerosis: A linkage analysis with age of onset corrections. *Clin. Genet.*, 18:160–167.

254. Haines, J., Schut, L., Weitkam, P. L., and Thayer, M. (1984): Spinocerebellar ataxia in a large kindred: Age at onset, reproduction and genetics linkage studies. *Neurology*, 34:1542–1548.

255. Haldane, J. B. S. (1935): Rate of spontaneous mutation of human gene. *J. Genet.*, 31:317–326.

256. Hall, C. W., Cantz, M., and Neufeld, E. F. (1973): A beta-glucuronidase deficiency mucopolysaccharidosis: Studies in cultured fibroblasts. *Arch. Biochem. Biophys.*, 155:32–38.

257. Harbaugh, R. E., Roberts, D. W., Coombs, D. W., Saunders, R. L., and Reeder, T. M. (1984): Preliminary report: Intracranial cholinergic drug infusion in patients with Alzheimer's disease. *Neurosurgery*, 15:514–518.

258. Harding, A. E., Diengdoh, J. V., and Lees, A. J. (1984): Autosomal recessive late onset multisystem disorder with cerebellar cortical atrophy at necropsy: Report of a family. *J. Neurol. Neurosurg. Psychiatry*, 47:853–856.

259. Harding, A. E., and Thomas, P. K. (1980): The clinical features of hereditary motor and sensory neuropathy; Type I and II. *Brain*, 103:259–280.

260. Harding, A. E., and Thomas, P. K. (1984): Peroneal muscular atrophy with pyramidal features. *J. Neurol. Neurosurg. Psychiatry*, 47:168–172.

261. Harley, R. D., et al. (1967): Ataxia telangiectasia: Report of seven cases. *Arch. Ophthalmol.*, 77:582–592.

262. Harper, P. (1983): Myotonic dystrophy and related disorders. In: *Principles and Practice of Medical Genetics*, edited by A. Emergy and D. Rimoin, pp. 426–441. Churchill-Livingstone, New York.

263. Harris, R. C. (1961): Mucopolysaccharide disorder: A possible new genotype of Hurler's syndrome (Abstr.). *Am. J. Dis. Child.*, 102:741.

264. Hart, R., Kwentus, J., Leshner, R., and Frazier, R. (1985): Information processing speed in Friedreich's ataxia. *Ann. Neurol.*, 17:612–614.

265. Hart, Z., Sahashi, K., Lambert, E. H., et al. (1979): A congenital, familial myasthenic syndrome caused by a presynaptic defect of transmitter resynthesis or mobilization (Abstr.). *Neurology (NY)*, 29:556.

266. Hashimoto, I. (1977): Familial intracranial aneurysms and cerebral vascular anomalies. *J. Neurosurg.*, 46:419–427.

267. Hassin, G. B. (1920): Histopathology and histogenesis of syringomyelia. *Arch. Neurol. Psychiatr.*, 3:130.

268. Hassin, G. B., and Harris, T. H. (1936): Olivopontocerebellar atrophy. *Arch. Neurol. Psychiatry*, 35:43–63.

269. Hausman, L. (1929): Macrosoma in a case of syringomyelia. *Arch. Neurol. Psychiatry*, 21:227.

270. Healton, E., Brust, J., Kerr, D., Resor, S., and Penn, A. (1980): Presumably Azorean disease in a presumably non-Portuguese family. *Neurology*, 30:1084–1089.
271. Hecht, F., McCaw, B., and Koler, R. D. (1973): Ataxia-telangiectasia: Clonal growth of translocation lymphocytes. *N. Engl. J. Med.*, 289:286–297.
272. Hers, H. G. (1959): Etudes enzymatiques sur fragments hepatiques. *Rev. Int. Hepatol.*, 9:35.
273. Heston, L. L. (1980): Dementia associated with Parkinson's disease: A genetic study. *J. Neurol. Neurosurg. Psychiatry*, 43:846–848.
274. Hewer, R. L. (1968): Study of fatal cases of Friedreich's ataxia. *Br. Med. J.*, 3:649–652.
275. Hirano, A., Malamud, N., Elizan, T. S., and Kurland, L. T. (1966): Amyotrophic lateral sclerosis and parkinsonism-dementia complex on Guam: Further pathologic studies. *Arch. Neurol.*, 15:35–51.
276. Hirschhorn, R., Papgeorgiou, P., Kesarwala, H., and Taft, L. (1980): Amelioration of neurologic abnormalities after "enzyme replacement" in adenosine deaminase deficiency. *N. Engl. J. Med.*, 303:377–380.
277. Hizeidarsson, S. J., Thomas, G. H., Kihara, H., Fluharty, A. L., Kolodny, E. H., Moser, H. W., and Reynolds, L. W. (1983): Impaired cerebroside sulfate hydrolysis in fibroblasts of sibs with "pseudo" arylsulfatase A deficiency without metachromatic leukodystrophy. *Ped. Res.*, 17:701–704.
278. Hogan, E. L., Lo, H. S., Power, J. M., et al. (1978): Genetic deficiency of myoadenylate deaminase (Abstr.). *IV International Congress on Neuromuscular Diseases*, 517.
279. Holmes, G. (1907): A form of familial degeneration of cerebellum. *Brain*, 30:466.
280. Holowell, J., Coryell, M., Hall, W., Findley, J., and Thevoas, T. (1968): Homocystinuria as affected by pyridoxine, folic acid, and vitamin B$_{12}$. *Proc. Soc. Exp. Biol. Med.*, 129:327–333.
281. Homan, R. W., Vasko, M. R., and Blaw, M. (1980): Phenytoin plasma concentrations in paroxysmal kinesigenic choreoathetosis. *Neurology*, 30:673–676.
282. Hopkins, S. L. C., Jackson, J. A., and Elsas, L. J. (1982): Emery-Dreifuss humeroperoneal muscular dystrophy: An X-linked myopathy with unusual contractures and bradycardia. *Ann. Neurol.*, 10:230–237.
283. Horton, W. A., Eldridge, R., and Brody, J. (1976): Familial motor neuron disease. *Neurology (Minneap.)*, 26:460–465.
284. Horwich, A. L., Fenton, W. A., Williams, K. R., Kalousek, F., Kraus, J. P., Doolittle, R. F., Konigsberg, W., and Rosenberg, L. E. (1984): Structure and expression of a complementary DNA for the nuclear coded precursor of human mitochondrial ornithine transcarbamylase. *Science*, 224:1068–1074.
285. Howell, R. R. (1972): The glycogen storage diseases. In: *The Metabolic Basis of Inherited Disease*, edited by J. Stanbury, J. Wyngaarden, and D. Fredrickson, pp. 149–173. McGraw-Hill, New York.
286. Howell, R. R., Kaback, M. M., and Brown, B. I. (1971): Branching enzyme deficiency in skin fibroblasts and possible heterozygote detection: Type IV glycogen storage disease. *J. Pediatr.*, 78:638–642.
286a. Howell, R. R., and Williams, J. C. (1983): The glycogen storage diseases. In: *The Metabolic Basis of Inherited Diseases*, 5th ed., edited by J. Stanbury, J. Wyngaarden, D. Fredrickson, J. Goldstein, and M. Brown, pp. 141–166. McGraw-Hill, New York.
287. Hsia, D. Y. Y., Driscoll, K., Troll, W., and Knox, W. (1956): Detection by phenylalanine tolerance tests of heterozygous carriers of phenylketonuria. *Nature*, 178:1239–1240.
288. Hsia, D. Y. Y., and Walker, F. A. (1961): Variability in the clinical manifestations of galactosemia. *J. Pediatr.*, 59:872–883.
289. Hug, G., Schubert, W. K., and Chuck, G. (1969): Deficient activity of dephosphorylase kinase and accumulation of glycogen in the liver. *J. Clin. Invest.*, 48:704–715.
290. Hultberg, B. (1969): N-Acetylhexosaminidase activities in Tay-Sachs disease. *Lancet*, 2:1195.
291. Hunt, J. R. (1921): Dyssynergia cerebellaris myoclonica. *Brain*, 44:490–538.
292. Hunter, C. (1917): A rare disease in two brothers. *Proc. R. Soc. Med.*, 10:104–116.
293. Hurler, G. (1920): Ueber einen Typ multiplier Abartungen, vorwiegend am Skelettsystem. *Z. Kinderheilkd.*, 24:220.
294. Hyman, B. T., Van Hoesen, G. W., Damasio, A. R., and Barnes, C. L. (1984): Alzheimer's disease: Cell specific pathology isolates the hippocampal formation. *Science*, 225:1168–1170.
295. Igarashi, M., Schaumburg, H. H., Powers, J., Kishimoto, V., Kolodny, E., and Suzuki, K. (1976): Fatty acid abnormality in adrenoleukodystrophy. *J. Neurochem.*, 26:851–860.
296. Ikeda, S., Kondo, K., Oguchi, K., Yanagisawa, N., Horigome, R., and Murata, F. (1984): Adult fucosidosis. *Neurology*, 34:451–456.

297. Illingworth, B., and Cori, G. T. (1952): Structure of glycogens and amylopectins. III. Normal and abnormal human glycogen. *J. Biol. Chem.*, 199:653–660.

298. Isselbacher, K. J., Anderson, E. P., Kurahashi, K., and Kalchar, H. M. (1956): Congenital galactosemia, a single enzymatic block in galactose metabolism. *Science*, 123:635–646.

299. Ivy, G. O., Schottler, F., Wenzel, J., Baudry, M., and Lynch, G. (1984): Inhibitors of lysosomal enzymes: Accumulation of lipofuscin-like dense bodies in the brain. *Science*, 226:985–987.

300. Jackson, J., Currier, R., Terasaki, P., and Morton, N. (1977): Spinocerebellar ataxia and HLA linkage: Risk predictions by HLA typing. *N. Engl. J. Med.*, 296:1138–1141.

301. Jaffe, R., Crumrine, P., Hashiday, Y., and Moser, H. W. (1982): Neonatal adrenoleukodystrophy. Clinical, pathological and biochemical delineation of a syndrome affecting both males and females. *Am. J. Pathol.*, 108:100–111.

302. Jankovic, J., Kirkpatrick, J. B., Blomquist, K., Langlais, P., and Bird, E. (1985): Late-onset Hallervorden-Spatz disease presenting as familial parkinsonism. *Neurology*, 35:227–234.

303. Jersild, C., Dupont, B., Fog, T., Platz, P. J., and Svejgaard, A. (1975): Histocompatibility determinants in multiple sclerosis. *Transplant Rev.*, 22:148–163.

304. Jervis, G. (1953): Phenylpyruvic oligophrenia deficiency of phenylalanine-oxidizing system. *Proc. Soc. Exp. Biol. Med.*, 82:514–515.

305. Johnson, R. H., and Spalding, J. M. K. (1964): Progressive sensory neuropathy in children. *J. Neurol. Neurosurg. Psychiatry*, 27:125–130.

306. Johnson, W. G. (1981): The clinical spectrum of hexosaminidase deficiency diseases. *Neurology*, 31:1453–1456.

307. Johnson, W. G. (1982): Hexosaminidase deficiency: A cause of recessively inherited motor neuron diseases. In: *Human Motor Neuron Disease*, edited by L. P. Rowland. Raven Press, New York.

308. Johnson, W. G., Desnick, R. J., Long, D. M., Sharp, M. L., Krivit, W., Brady, B., and Brady, R. O. (1973): Intravenous injections of purified hexosaminidase A into a patient with Tay-Sachs disease. In: *Enzyme Therapy in Genetic Disease*, edited by R. W. Desnick, R. W. Bernloke, and W. Krivit. Birth Defects Original Article Series, Vol. IX, 120–124.

309. Johnson, W., Schwartz, G., and Barbeau, A. (1962): Studies on dystonia musculorum deformans. *Arch. Neurol.*, 7:301–313.

310. Johnson, W. G., Schwartz, R. C., and Chutorian, A. M. (1981): Artificial insemination by donors: The need for genetic screening. *N. Engl. J. Med.*, 304:755–757.

311. Jolly, D. J., Okayama, H., Berg, P., et al. (1983): Isolation and characterization of a full length expressible cDNA for human HGPRT. *Proc. Natl. Acad. Sci. USA*, 80:477–481.

312. Joynt, R. J., and Perret, G. E. (1961): Meningiomas in a mother and daughter. *Neurology*, 11:164–165.

313. Karpati, G., Carpenter, S., Engel, A., et al. (1975): The syndrome of systemic carnitine deficiency. *Neurology*, 25:16–24.

314. Kaufman, H. H., and Brisman, R. (1972): Familial gliomas. *J. Neurosurg.*, 37:110–112.

315. Kawamura, N., Moser, A. E., Moser, H. W., Ogino, T., Suzuki, K., Schaumburg, H., Milunsky, A., Murphy, J., and Kishimoto, Y. (1978): High concentration of hexacosanoate in cultured skin fibroblasts lipids from adrenoleukodystrophy patients. *Biochem. Biophys. Res. Commun.*, 82:114–120.

316. Kayser, B. (1902): Uber einen Fall von angeborener grunlicher Verfarbung der Kornea. *Klin. Monatsbl. Augenheilkd.*, 40(2):22–25.

317. Kelly, W. N., and Meade, J. C. (1971): Studies on hypoxanthine-guanine phosphoribosyltransferase in fibroblasts from patients with the Lesch-Nyhan syndrome. *J. Biol. Chem.*, 246:2953–2958.

318. Kelly, W., and Wyngaarden, J. (1983): Clinical syndromes associated with hypoxanthine-guanine phosphoribosyltransferase deficiency. In: *The Metabolic Basis of Inherited Disease*, 5th ed., edited by J. Stanbury, J. Wyngaarden, D. Fredrickson, J. Goldstein, and M. Brown, 1115–1143. McGraw-Hill, New York.

319. Kennaway, N. B., Buist, N. R. M., Darlen-Usmar, V. M., et al. (1984): Lactic acidosis and mitochondrial myopathy associated with deficiency of several components of complex III of the respiratory chain. *Ped. Res.*, 18:991–999.

320. Kennedy, R. M., Rowe, V., and Kepes, J. (1980): Cockayne syndrome: An atypical case. *Neurology*, 30:1268–1272.

321. Kilpatrick, C., Burns, R., and Blumbergs, P. C. (1983): Identical twins with Alzheimer's disease. *J. Neurol. Neurosurg. Psychiatry*, 46:421–425.

322. Kitahara, T., Ariga, N., Yamaura, A., Makino, H., and Maki, Y. (1979): Familial occurrence of

Moya-Moya disease; report of three Japanese families. *J. Neurol. Neurosurg. Psychiatry*, 42:208–214.

323. Klenk, E. (1939): Niemann-Picksche Krankheit und amaurotische Idiotie. *Hoppe Seylers Z. Physiol. Chem.*, 262:128–143.

324. Klenk, E. (1942): Uber die Ganglioside des Gehirns bei der infantilen amaurotischen Idiotie vom Typ Tay-Sachs. *Ber. Dtsch. Chem. Gas.*, 75:1632–1636.

325. Kolodny, E., Brady, R., and Volk, B. (1969): Demonstration of an alteration of ganglioside metabolism in Tay-Sachs disease. *Biochem. Biophys. Res. Commun.*, 37:526–531.

326. Komrower, G. M., Schwarz, V., Holzel, A., and Goldberg, L. (1956): A clinical and biochemical study of galactosemia. *Arch. Dis. Child.*, 31:254–264.

327. Konigsmark, B. W., and Weiner, L. P. (1970): The olivopontocerebellar atrophies: A review. *Medicine*, 49:227–241.

328. Kopits, S., Perovic, M. N., McKusick, V. A., Robinson, R. A., and Bailey, J. A. III (1972): Congenital atlantoaxial dislocation in various forms of dwarfism (Abstr.). *J. Bone Joint Surg.*, 54A:1349–1350.

329. Kornzweig, A. L. (1970): Bassen-Kornzweig syndrome: Present status. *J. Med. Genet.*, 7:271–276.

330. Krabbe, K. (1916): A new familial, infantile form of diffuse brain-sclerosis. *Brain*, 39:74–114.

331. Krebs, H. (1951): Urea synthesis. In: *The Enzymes, Vol. 2, Part 2*, edited by J. B. Sumner and K. Myrback, p. 866. Academic Press, New York.

332. Kresse, H. (1974): Mucopolysaccharidosis III A (Sanfilippo A disease): Deficiency of a heparin sulfamidase in skin fibroblasts and leukocytes. *Biochem. Biophys. Res. Commun.*, 54:1111–1118.

333. Krivit, W., Pierpont, M. E., Ayaz, K., Tsai, M., et al. (1984): Bone marrow transplantation in the Maroteaux-Lamy syndrome. *N. Engl. J. Med.*, 311:1606–1611.

334. Kugelberg, F., and Welander, L. (1954): Familial neurogenic (spinal?) muscular atrophy simulating ordinary proximal dystrophy. *Acta (Scand.) Psychiat.*, 29:42–43.

335. Kurland, L. T. (1958): Epidemiological investigations of amyotrophic lateral sclerosis: III. A genetic interpretation of incidence and geographic distribution. *Mayo Clin. Proc.*, 32:449–462.

336. Kuwert, E. K. (1977): Genetical aspects of multiple sclerosis with special regard to histocompatibility determinants. *Acta Neurol. Scand.*, 55(Suppl.)63:23–42.

337. Kuzuhara, S., Kanazawa, I., Sasaki, H., Nakanishi, T., and Shimamura, K. (1983): Gerstmann-Straussler-Scheinker's disease. *Ann. Neurol.*, 14:216–225.

338. LaDue, B., Howell, R., Jacoby, G., Seegmiller, J., Sober, E., Zannon, V., Canby, J., and Ziegler, L. (1963): Clinical and biochemical studies on two cases of histidinemia. *Pediatrics*, 32:216–227.

339. Lalley, P. A., Brown, J. A., Eddy, R. L., and Haley, L. L. (1975): Shows TB: Assignment of the gene for β-glucuronidase (BGUS) to chromosome 7 in man. *Gene Mapping Conference, Baltimore*, 3:184–187.

340. Landau, W. M., and Gitt, J. J. (1951): Hereditary spastic paraplegia and hereditary ataxia. A family demonstrating a variety of phenotypic manifestations. *Arch. Neurol. Psychiatry*, 66:346–354.

341. Landis, D. M., Rosenberg, R. N., Landis, S. C., Schut, L., and Nyhan, W. L. (1974): Olivopontocerebellar degeneration. Clinical and ultrastructural abnormalities. *Arch. Neurol.*, 31:295–307.

342. Larsen, T., Dunn, H., Jan, J., and Calne, D. (1985): Dystonia and calcification of the basal ganglia. *Neurology*, 35:533–537.

343. Laurence, K. M. (1983): The genetics and prevention of neural tube defects. In: *Principles and Practice of Medical Genetics, Vol. 1*, edited by A. E. H. Emery and D. L. Rimoin, pp. 231–245. Churchill-Livingstone, New York.

344. Layzer, R., Rowland, L., and Ranney, H. (1967): Muscle phosphofructokinase deficiency. *Arch. Neurol.*, 17:512–523.

345. Lebo, R. V., Gorin, F., Fletterick, R. J., Kao, F.-T., Cheung, M.-C., Bruce, B. D., and Kay, V. W. (1984): High resolution chromosome sorting and DNA spot-blot analysis assign McArdle's syndrome to chromosome II. *Science*, 225:57–59.

346. Leckman, J., Detlor, J., Harcherik, D., Ort, S., Shaywitz, B., and Cohen, D. (1985): Short- and long-term treatment of Tourette's syndrome with clonidine: A clinical perspective. *Neurology*, 35:343–351.

347. Ledley, F. D., Grenett, H., DiLella, A., Kwok, S., and Woo, S. (1985): Gene transfer and expression of human phenylalanine hydroxylase. *Science*, 228:77–79.

348. Lehmann, A. R., Francis, A., and Giannelli, F. (1985): Prenatal diagnosis of Cockayne's syndrome. *Lancet*, 1:486–488.

349. Leibel, R., Shih, V., Goodman, S., Bauman, M., McCabe, E., Zerdling, R., Bergman, I., and

Costello, C. (1980): Glutaric acidemia: A metabolic disorder causing progressive choreoathetosis. *Neurology*, 30:1163–1168.

350. Leigh, D. (1951): Subacute necrotizing encephalomyelopathy in an infant. *J. Neurol. Neurosurg.*, 14:216–221.

351. Lejeune, J., Lafourcase, J., Berger, R., Violatte, J., Boeswillwald, M., Seringe, P., and Turpin, R. (1963): Trois cas de deletion partielle du bras court d'un chromosome, 5. *C.R. Acad. Sci. Paris (D)*, 257:3098.

352. Lesch, M., and Nyhan, W. (1964): A familial disorder of uric acid metabolism and central nervous system function. *Am. J. Med.*, 36:561–570.

353. Lichtenstein, B. W. (1943): Cervical syringomyelia and syringomyelia-like states associated with Arnold-Chiari deformity and platybasia. *Arch. Neurol. Psychiatry*, 49:881–894.

354. Lidsky, A. S., Guttler, F., and Woo, S. (1985): Prenatal diagnosis of classic phenylketonuria by DNA analysis. *Lancet*, 1:549–555.

355. Lima, L., and Coutinho, P. (1980): Clinical criteria for diagnosis of Machado-Joseph disease: Report of a non-Azorean Portuguese family. *Neurology*, 30:319–322.

356. Linarelli, L. G., and Prichard, J. W. (1970): Congenital sensory neuropathy: Complete absence of superficial sensations. *Am. J. Dis. Child.*, 119:513–520.

357. Lindgren, V., de Martinville, B., Horwich, A. L., Rosenberg, L. E., and Francke, U. (1984): Human ornithine transcarbamylase locus mapped to band Xp21.1 near the Duchenne muscular dystrophy locus. *Science*, 226:698–700.

358. Louis-Barr, M. (1941): Sur un syndrome progressif comprenant des telangiectasies capillaires cutanees et conjunctivalis symmetriques, a disposition naevoide et des troubles cerebelleux. *Confin. Neurol.*, 4:32.

359. Love, J. G., and Olafson, R. A. (1966): Syringomyelia: A look at surgical therapy. *J. Neurosurg.*, 24:714–718.

360. Lowe, C. U., Terrey, M., and MacLachlan, E. A. (1952): Organic-aciduria decreased renal ammonia production, hydrophthalmos, and mental retardation. *Am. J. Dis. Child.*, 83:164–184.

361. Lucas, R. N. (1977): Migraine in twins. *J. Psychosom. Res.*, 21:147–156.

362. Lundberg, A., Lilja, L., Lundberg, P. O., and Try, K. (1972): Heredopathia atactica polyneuritiformis (Refsum's disease): Experiences of dietary treatment and plasmapheresis. *Eur. Neurol.*, 8:309–324.

363. Lyon, M. F. (1961): Gene action in the X chromosome of the mouse (*Mus musculus* L.). *Nature*, 190:372–373.

364. MacDonald, E. A., and Holden, J. A. (1985): Duplication 12q24-qter in an infant with Dandy-Walker syndrome. *J. Neurogenet.*, 2:123–129.

365. Mackay, R. P. (1963): Course and prognosis in amyotrophic lateral sclerosis. *Arch. Neurol.*, 8:117–127.

366. MacLeod, P. M., and Dolman, C. L. (1977): Neuronal ceroid-lipofuscinosis. *Arch. Neurol.*, 34:199.

367. Magee, K. R. (1960): Familial progressive bulbar-spinal muscular atrophy. *Neurology (Minneap.)*, 10:295–305.

368. Magee, K. R., and DeJong, R. N. (1965): Hereditary distal myopathy with onset in infancy. *Arch. Neurol.*, 13:387–390.

369. Mahloudji, M., and Chuke, P. O. (1968): Familial spastic paraplegia with retinal degeneration. *Johns Hopkins Med. J.*, 123:142–144.

370. Mabry, C. (1963): Maternal PKU: A cause of mental retardation in children without the metabolic defect. *N. Engl. J. Med.*, 269:1404.

371. Marie, P. (1893): Sur l'hérédoataxie cérébelleuse. *Sem. Med. (Paris)*, 13:444–447.

372. Maroteaux, P., and Lamy, M. (1966): La pseudo-polydystrophie de Hurler. *Presse. Med.*, 74:2889–2892.

373. Maroteaux, P., Leveque, B., Marie, J., and Lamy, M. (1963): Une nouvelle dysostose avec elimination urinaire de chondroitine-sulfate B. *Presse. Med.*, 71:1849–1852.

374. Martin, J. B. (1984): Huntington's disease: New approaches to an old problem. *Neurology*, 34:1059–1072.

375. Martin, W. E., Young, W. I., and Anderson, V. E. (1973): Parkinson's disease, a genetic study. *Brain*, 96:495–506.

376. Mason, H. H., and Turner, M. E. (1935): Chronic galactemia. *Am. J. Dis. Child.*, 50:359–374.

377. Masters, C. L., Gajdusek, D. C., and Gibbs, C. J., Jr. (1981): The familial occurrence of Creutz-feldt-Jakob disease and Alzheimer's disease. *Brain*, 104:535–558.

378. Masters, C. L., Gajdusek, D. C., and Gibbs, C. J., Jr. (1981): Creutzfeldt-Jakob disease virus isolations from the Gerstmann-Straussler syndrome with an analysis of the various forms of amyloid plaque deposition of the virus-induced spongiform encephalopathies. *Brain*, 104:559–588.

379. Matalon, R., and Dorfman, A. (1972): Hurler's syndrome, an alpha-L-iduronidase deficiency. *Biochem. Biophys. Res. Commun.*, 47:959–964.

380. Matalon, R., and Dorfman, A. (1974): Sanfilippo A syndrome: Sulfamidase deficiency in cultured skin fibroblasts and liver. *J. Clin. Invest.*, 54:907–912.

381. McArdle, B. (1951): Myopathy due to a defect in muscle glycogen breakdown. *Clin. Sci.*, 10:13–35.

382. McDonald, W. I. (1961): Cortical cerebellar degeneration with ovarian carcinoma. *Neurology (Minneap.)*, 11:328–334.

383. McFarlin, D. E., Strober, W., and Waldmann, T. A. (1972): Ataxia-telangiectasia. *Medicine*, 51:281–314.

384. McIlroy, W. J., and Richardson, J. C. (1965): Syringomyelia: A clinical review of 75 cases. *Can. Med. Assoc. J.*, 93:731–734.

384a. McKusick, V. A., and Neufeld, E. F. (1983): The mucopolysaccharide storage diseases. In: *The Metabolic Basis of Inherited Diseases*, 5th ed., edited by J. Stanbury, J. Wyngaarden, D. Fredrickson, J. Goldstein, and M. Brown. McGraw-Hill, New York.

385. McKusick, V. A., Howell, R. R., Hussels, I. E., Neufeld, E. F., and Stevenson, R. (1972): Allelism, non-allelism and genetic compounds among the mucopolysaccharidoses. *Lancet*, 1:993–996.

386. McKusick, V. A., et al. (1967): The Riley-Day syndrome. Observations genetics and survivorship. *Isr. J. Med. Sci.*, 3:372–379.

387. McKusick, V. A., Kaplan, D., Wise, D., et al. (1965): The genetic mucopolysaccharidoses. *Medicine*, 44:445–483.

388. McKusick, V. A. (1983): *Mendelian Inheritance in Man, 6th Ed.*, p. 183. The Johns Hopkins University Press, Baltimore.

389. McMurray, W., Mohyuddin, F., Rossiter, R., Rathbun, J., Valentine, G., Koegler, S., and Zarfas, D. (1962): Citrullinuria: A new aminoaciduria associated with mental retardation. *Lancet*, 1:138.

390. Meienhofer, M. C., Askanvas, V., Proux-Daegelen, J., et al. (1977): Muscle-type phosphorylase activity present in muscle cells cultured from three patients with myophosphorylase deficiency. *Arch. Neurol.*, 34:779–781.

391. Meir, M., et al. (1960): Acanthrocytosis, pigmentary degeneration of the retina and ataxic neuropathy: A genetically determined syndrome and associated metabolic disorder. *Blood*, 16:1586–1608.

392. Menkes, J. H., Alter, M., Steigleder, G. K., Weakley, D. R., and Sung, J. H. (1962): A sex-linked recessive disorder with retardation of growth, peculiar hair, and focal cerebral and cerebellar degeneration. *Pediatrics*, 29:764–779.

393. Menkes, J. H., and Corbo, L. M. (1977): Adrenoleukodystrophy: Accumulation of cholesterol esters with very long chain fatty acids. *Neurology*, 27:928–932.

394. Menkes, J. H., Hurst, P. L., and Craig, J. M. (1954): A new syndrome: Progressive familial infantile cerebral dysfunction associated with an unusual urinary substance. *Pediatrics*, 14:462–466.

395. Menkes, J. H., Schimschock, J., and Swanson, P. (1968): Cerebrotendinous xanthomatosi: The storage of cholestanol within the nervous system. *Arch. Neurol.*, 19:47–53.

396. Merritt, H., and Fremont-Smith, F. (1937): The cerebrospinal fluid. In *Syringomyelia*, pp. 173–175. W. B. Saunders, Co., Philadelphia.

397. Metrakos, J. D., and Metrakos, K. (1960): Genetics of convulsive disorders. I. *Neurology*, 10:228–240.

398. Metrakos, K., and Metrakos, J. D. (1961): Genetics of convulsive disorders. II. *Neurology*, 11:470–483.

399. Meyer, K., Hoffman, P., Linker, A., Grumbach, M., and Sampson, P. (1959): Sulfated mucopoly-saccharides of urine and organs in gargoylism (Hurler's syndrome). II. Additional studies. *Proc. Soc. Exp. Biol. Med.*, 102:587–590.

400. Miller, A. D., Jolly, D. J., Friedman, T., and Verma, I. M. (1983): A transmissible retrovirus expressing human HGPRT: Gene transfer cells obtained from humans deficient in HGPRT. *Proc. Natl. Acad. Sci. USA*, 80:4709–4713.

401. Miller, C., and Parker, W. (1985): Hypomelanosis of Ito: Association with a chromosomal abnormality. *Neurology*, 35:607–610.

402. Miranda, A., Shanske, S., Hays, A., and DiMauro, S. (1985): Immunocytochemical analysis of normal and acid maltase-deficient muscle cultures. *Arch. Neurol.*, 42:371–373.
403. Mitsumoto, H., Sliman, R., Schafer, I., Sternick, C., Kaufman, B., Wilbourn, A., and Horwitz, S. (1985): Motor neuron disease and adult hexosaminidase: A deficiency in two families. *Ann. Neurol.*, 17:378–385.
404. Mommaerts, W. F. H. M., Illingworth, B., Pearson, C. M., Guillory, P. J., and Seraydarian, K. (1959): A functional disorder of muscle associated with the absence of phosphorylase. *Proc. Natl. Acad. Sci. USA*, 45:791–797.
405. Monaco, S., Autilio-Gambetti, L., Zabel, D., and Gambetti, P. (1985): Giant axonal neuropathy: Acceleration of neurofilament transport in optic axons. *Proc. Natl. Acad. Sci. USA*, 82:920–924.
406. Moreadith, R. W., Batchaw, M. L., Ohnishi, T., et al. (1984): Deficiency of the iron-sulfur clusters of mitochondrial NADH-ubiquinone oxidoreductase (complex 1) in an infant with congenital lactic acidosis. *J. Clin. Invest.*, 74:685–697.
407. Morgan-Hughes, J. A., Hayes, D., Clark, J., Landon, D. N., Swash, M., Stark, R., and Rudge, P. (1982): Mitochondrial encephalomyopathies. *Brain*, 105:553–582.
408. Morquio, L., (1935): Sur une forme de dystrophie osseuse familiale. *Arch. Med. Enf.*, 38:5.
409. Morris, J. C., Cole, M., Banker, B. Q., and Wright, D. (1984): Hereditary dysplasic dementia and the Pick-Alzheimer spectrum. *Ann. Neurol.*, 16:455–466.
410. Morris, M., Lewis, B., Doolan, P., and Harper, H. (1961): Clinical and biochemical observations on an apparently nonfatal variant of branched chain ketoaciduria (maple syrup urine disease). *Pediatrics*, 28:918–923.
411. Morrison, M. (1985): Alzheimer's disease—Progress Report, Neurology Grand Rounds. University of Texas Health Science Center at Dallas, Jan. 23, 1985.
412. Morrison, M., and Rosenberg, R. N. (1983): Specific mRNA changes in Joseph disease cerebella. *Ann. Neurol.*, 14:73–79.
413. Moser, A. E., Singh, I., Brown, F. R., Solish, G. I., Kelly, R. I., Benke, P. J., Burton, B. K., and Moser, H. W. (1984): The cerebro-hepato-renal (Zellweger) syndrome and neonatal adrenoleukodystrophy. *N. Engl. J. Med.*, 310:1141–1146.
414. Moser, H. W., Moser, A. E., Singh, I., and O'Neill, B. P. (1984): Adrenoleukodystrophy: Survey of 303 cases: Biochemistry, diagnosis and therapy. *Ann. Neurol.*, 16:628–641.
415. Moser, H. W., Tutschka, P. J., Brown, F. R., Moser, A. E., Yeager, A. M., Singh, I., Mark, S. A., Kumar, A. A. J., McDonnell, J. M., White, C. L., Maumenee, I. H., Green, W. R., Powers, J. M., and Santos, G. W. (1984): Bone marrow transplant in adrenoleukodystrophy. *Neurology*, 34:1410–1417.
416. Msall, M., Batshaw, M. L., Sus, R., Brusilow, S. W., and Mellits, E. D. (1984): Neurologic outcome in children with inborn errors of urea synthesis. *N. Engl. J. Med.*, 310:1500–1505.
417. Mudd, S., Finkelstein, J., Irreverre, F., and Laster, L. (1964): Homocystinuria: An enzymatic defect. *Science*, 143:1443–1445.
418. Mulder, D. W., and Howard, F. M. (1976): Patient resistance and prognosis in amyotrophic lateral sclerosis. *Mayo Clin. Proc.*, 51:537–541.
419. Mulligan, L., Phillips, M., Forster-Gibson, C., Beckett, J., Partington, M., Simpson, N., Holden, J., and White, B. (1985): Genetic mapping of DNA segments relative to the locus for the fragile X syndrome in Xq27.3. *Am. J. Hum. Genet.*, 37:463–472.
420. Munch-Peterson, C. J. (1931): Studien uber erbliche Erkrankungen des Zentralnervensystems: Die familiare, amyotrophische Lateral-sclerose. *Acta Psychiatr. Neurol.*, 6:55.
421. Murray, J. M., Davies, K. E., Harper, P. S., Meredith, L., Mueller, C. R., and Williamson, R. (1982): Linkage relationship of a cloned DNA sequence on the short arm of the X chromosome to Duchenne muscular dystrophy. *Nature*, 300:69–71.
422. Myers, R., Cupples, L., Schoenfeld, M., D'Agostino, R., Terrin, N., Goldmakher, N., and Wolf, P. (1985): Maternal factors in onset of Huntington disease. *Am. J. Hum. Genet.*, 37:511–523.
423. Nakano, K., Dawson, D., and Spence, A. (1972): Machado disease; a hereditary ataxia in Portuguese immigrants to Massachusetts. *Neurology*, 22:49–55.
424. Namba, T., Aberfeld, D. C., and Grob, D. (1970): Chronic proximal spinal muscular atrophy. *J. Neurol. Sci.*, 11:401–423.
425. Naumann, G. (1985): Clearing of cornea after perforating keratoplasty in mucopolysaccharidosis Type VI (Maroteaux-Lamy syndrome). *N. Engl. J. Med.*, 312:995.
426. Nausieda, P. A., Grossman, B. J., Koller, W. C., Weiner, W. J., and Klawans, H. L. (1980): Sydenham chorea: An update. *Neurology*, 30:331–334.

427. Naylor, S. L., Klebe, R. J., and Shows, T. B. (1978): Argininosuccinic aciduria: Assignment of the argininosuccinate lyase gene to the pter-q22 region of human chromosome 7 by bioautography. *Proc. Natl. Acad. Sci. USA*, 75:6159–6162.

428. Nemeroff, C. B., Youngblood, W. W., Manberg, P. J., Prange, A. J., and Kizer, J. S. (1983): Regional brain concentrations of neuropeptides in Huntington's chorea and schizophrenia. *Science*, 221:972–974.

429. Netsky, M. G. (1953): Syringomyelia: A clincopathologic study. *Arch. Neurol. Psychiatry*, 70:741–777.

430. Neufeld, E. F. (1974): The biochemical basis for mucopolysaccharidoses and mucolipidoses. *Prog. Med. Genet.*, 10:81–101.

431. Niemann, A. (1914): Ein unbekanntes Krankheitsbild. *Jahrb. Kinderheilkd.*, 79:1.

432. Njaa, A. (1946): Sex-linked type of gargoylism. *Acta Paediatr.*, 33:267.

433. Norman, R. N. (1961): Cerebellar hypoplasia in Werdnig-Hoffman disease. *Arch. Dis. Child.*, 36:96–101.

434. Norman, R., Urich, H., Tingey, A., and Goodbody, R. (1959): Tay-Sachs disease with visceral involvement and its relationship to Niemann-Pick's disease. *J. Pathol. Bacteriol.*, 78:409–421.

435. Novotny, E., Dorfman, L., Louis, A., Sogg, R., and Steinman, L. (1985): A neurodegenerative disorder with generalized dystonia: A new mitochondriopathy. *Neurology (Suppl. 1)*, 35:273.

436. Nyhan, W. L., ed. (1974): *Heritable Disorders of Amino Acid Metabolism.* Wiley, New York.

437. Nyhan, W. L., Johnson, H. G., Kaufman, I. A., and Jones, K. L. (1980): Serotonergic approaches to the modification of behavior in the Lesch-Nyhan syndrome. *Appl. Res. Ment. Retard.*, 1:25–40.

438. Nyhan, W. L., and Sakati, N. O. (1976): *Genetic and Malformation Syndromes in Clinical Medicine.* Year Book, Chicago.

439. Oberholzer, V., Levin, B., Burgess, E., and Young, W. (1967): Methylmalonic aciduria: An inborn error of metabolism leading to chronic metabolic acidosis. *Arch. Dis. Child.*, 42:492–504.

440. Oelschlager, R., White, H. H., and Schinike, R. N. (1971): Levy-Roussy syndrome: Report of a kindred and discussion of the nosology. *Acta Neurol. Scand.*, 47:80.

441. Oesch, B., Westaway, D., Walchli, M., Kent, S., Aebersold, R., Barry, R., Tempst, P., Teplow, D., Hood, L., Prusiner, S., and Weissman, C. (1985): A cellular gene encodes scrapie PrP 27-30 protein. *Cell*, 40:735–746.

442. Old, J. M., Purvis-Smith, S., Wilcken, B., Pearson, P., Williamson, R., et al. (1985): Prenatal exclusion of ornithine transcarbamylase deficiency by direct gene analysis. *Lancet*, 1:73–75.

443. Oldstone, M. B. A., Perrin, L. H., Wilson, C. V., and Norris, F. H., Jr. (1976): Evidence for immune-complex formation in patients with amyotrophic lateral sclerosis. *Lancet*, i:169–172.

444. O'Neill, B. P., and Moser, H. W. (1982): Adrenoleukodystrophy. *Can. J. Neurol. Sci.*, 9:449–452.

445. O'Neill, B. P., Moser, H. W., Saxena, K. M., and Marmion, L. C. (1984): Adrenoleukodystrophy: Clinical and biochemical manifestations in carriers. *Neurology*, 34:798–801.

446. Opitz, J., Stiles, F., Wisc, D., vonGemmingen, G., Race, R., Sander, R., Cross, E., and deGroot, W. (1965): The genetics of angiokeratoma corporis diffusum (Fabry's disease) and its linkage with Xg(a) locus. *Amer. J. Hum. Genet.*, 17:325–342.

447. Ounsted, C. (1955): Genetic and social aspects of the epilepsies of childhood. *Eugen. Rev.*, 47:33–49.

448. Parker, H. L., and Kernohan, J. W. (1933): Parenchymatous cortical cerebellar atrophy (chronic atrophy of Purkinje cells). *Brain*, 56:191–212.

449. Patau, K., Smith, D., Therman, E., Inhorn, S., and Wagner, H. (1960): Multiple congenital anomaly caused by an extra autosome. *Lancet*, 1:790–793.

450. Patrick, A., and Lake, B. (1969): An acid lipase deficiency in Wolman's disease. *Biochem. J.*, 112:29p.

451. Pavlakis, S. G., Phillips, P. C., DiMauro, S., DeVivo, D., and Rowland, L. P. (1984): Mitochondrial myopathy, encephalopathy, lactic acidosis, and stroke like episodes. *Ann. Neurol.*, 16:481–488.

452. Pearson, J., Finegold, M. J., et al. (1970): The tongue and taste in familial dysautonomia. Ophthalmologic studies of familial dysautonomia. *Pediatrics*, 45:739–745.

453. Pedreira, F. A., and Long, R. E. (1971): Arthrogryposis multiplex congenita in one of congenital twins. *Am. J. Dis. Child.*, 121:64–66.

454. Peisach, J., Aisen, P., and Blumberg, W. E., eds. (1966): *The Biochemistry of Copper.* Academic Press, New York.

455. Penrose, L., and Quastel, J. (1937): Metabolic studies in phenylketonuria. *Biochem. J.*, 31:266–274.

456. Perry, T., Currier, R., Hansen, S., and MacLean, J. (1977): Aspartate-taurine imbalance in dominantly inherited olivopontocerebellar atrophy. *Neurology*, 27:257–261.

457. Perry, T. L., Kish, S. J., Hinton, D., Hansen, S., Becker, L. E., and Gelfand, E. W. (1984): Neurochemical abnormalities in a patient with ataxia-telangiectasia. *Neurology*, 34:187–191.
458. Perry, T., Wright, J., Hansen, S., and MacLeod, P. (1979): Isoniazid therapy of Huntington disease. *Neurology*, 29:370–375.
459. Philippart, M., and van Bogaert, L. (1969): Cholestanolosis (cerebrotendinous xanthomatosis). A follow-up study of the original family. *Arch. Neurol.*, 21:603–610.
460. Phillips, L., Kelly, T., Schnatterly, P., and Parker, D. (1985): Hereditary motor-sensory neuropathy (HMSN). Possible X-linked dominant inheritance. *Neurology*, 35:498–502.
461. Pick, L. (1922): Zur pathologischen Anatomie des Morbus Gaucher. *Med. Klin.*, 18:1408.
462. Pincus, J. H. (1972): Subacute necrotizing encephalomyelopathy (Leigh's disease): A consideration of clinical features and etiology. *Dev. Med. Child. Neurol.*, 14:87–101.
463. Pirskanen, R. (1976): Genetic associations between myasthenia gravis and the HLA system. *J. Neurol. Neurosurg. Psychiatry*, 39:23–33.
464. Plaitakis, A. (1984): Abnormal metabolism of neuroexcitatory amino acids. In: *Olivopontocerebellar Atrophies*, edited by R. C. Duvoisin and A. Plaitakis, pp. 225–243. Raven Press, New York.
465. Plaitakis, A., Nicklas, W. J., and Desnick, R. J. (1980): Glutamate dehydrogenase deficiency in 3 patients with spinocerebellar syndrome. *Ann. Neurol.*, 7:297–303.
466. Plaitakis, A., Whetsell, W. O., Jr., Cooper, J. R., and Yahr, M. D. (1980): Chronic Leigh disease: A genetic and biochemical study. *Ann. Neurol.*, 7:304–310.
467. Poll-The, B. T., Aicardi, J., Girot, R., and Rosa, R. (1985): Neurological findings in triosephosphate isomerase deficiency. *Ann. Neurol.*, 17:439–443.
468. Pompe, J. C. (1932): Ober idopatische hypertrophie van het hart. *Ned. Tijdschr. Geneeskd.*, 76:304.
469. Pompen, A., Ruiter, M., and Wyers, H. (1947): Angiokeratoma corporis diffusum (universale) Fabry, as a sign of an unknown internal disease; two autopsy reports. *Acta Med. Scand.*, 128:234–255.
470. Porter, M., Fluharty, A., and Kihara, H. (1971): Correction of abnormal cerebroside sulfate metabolism in cultured metachromatic leukodystrophy fibroblasts. *Science*, 172:1263–1265.
471. Posner, C. M. (1956): *The Relationship Between Syringomyelia and Neoplasm*. Charles C Thomas, Springfield.
472. Prick, M., Gareels, F., Renier, W., Trijbels, F., Jaspar, H., Lamars, K., and Kok, J. (1981): Pyruvate dehydrogenase deficiency restricted to brain. *Neurology*, 31:398–404.
473. Prusiner, S. B., McKinley, M. P., Bowman, K. A., Bolton, D. C., Bendheim, P. E., Groth, D. F., and Glenner, G. B. (1983): Scrapie prions aggregate to form amyloid-like birefringent rods. *Cell*, 35:349–358.
474. Purdy, A., Hahn, A., Barnett, H. J. M., Bratty, P., Ahmad, D., Lloyd, K. G., McGeer, E., and Perry, T. L. (1979): Familial fatal parkinsonism with alveolar hypoventilation and mental depression. *Ann. Neurol.*, 6:523–531.
475. Reeve, A., Shulman, S. A., Zimmerman, A. W., and Cassidy, S. B. (1985): Methylphenidate therapy for aggression in a man with ring 22 chromosome. *Arch. Neurol.*, 42:69–72.
476. Refsum, S., Stokke, O., Eldjarn, L., and Tardeu, M. (1975): Heredopathia atactica polyneuritiformis (Refsum's disease). In: *Peripheral Neuropathy*, edited by P. J. Dyck, P. K. Thomas, and E. M. Lambert, pp. 868–890. Saunders, Philadelphia.
477. Reimann, H. A., McKechnie, W. G., and Stanisavljevic, S. (1958): Hereditary sensory radicular neuropathy and other defects in a large family. *Am. J. Med.*, 25:573–579.
478. Relkin, R., (1965): Arthrogryposis multiplex congenita: Report of two cases; review of literature. *Am. J. Med.*, 39:871.
479. Rett, A. (1966): *Ueber ein Cerebral-Atrophisches Syndrom bei Hyperammonamie*. Bruder Hollinek, Vienna.
480. Rett, A. (1977): Cerebral atrophy associated with hyperammonemia. In: *Handbook of Clinical Neurology, Vol. 29*, edited by P. J. Vinken and G. W. Bruyn, pp. 3305–3329. North Holland, Amsterdam.
481. Riccardi, V. (1981): Von Recklinghausen neurofibromatosis. *N. Engl. J. Med.*, 305:1617–1627.
482. Rice, G. P. A., Boughner, D. R., Stiller, C., and Ebers, G. C. (1980): Familial stroke syndrome associated with mitral valve prolapse. *Ann. Neurol.*, 7:130–134.
483. Riggs, J. E., Schochet, S., Jr., Fadkadej, A., Papadimitriou, A., DiMauro, S., Crosby, T., Gutmann, L., and Moxley, R. T. (1984): Mitochondrial encephalomyopathy with decreased succinate-cytochrome c reductase activity. *Neurology*, 34:48–53.

484. Riley, C. M., Day, R. L., Greely, D. M., and Langford, N. S. (1949): Central autonomic dysfunction with defective lacrimation: I. Report of five cases. *Pediatrics*, 3:468–478.
485. Riley, C. M., and Moore, R. H. (1966): Familial dysautonomia differentiated from related disorders: Case reports and discussion of current concepts. *Pediatrics*, 37:435.
486. Rizzo, W. B., Avigan, J., Chemke, J., and Schulman, J. D. (1984): Adrenoleukodystrophy: Very long chain fatty acid metabolism in fibroblasts. *Neurology*, 34:163–169.
487. Roberts, G., Crow, T., and Polak, J. (1985): Location of neuronal tangles in somatostatin neurons in Alzheimer's disease. *Nature*, 314:92–94.
488. Robertson, E. E. (1953): Progressive bulbar paralysis showing heredofamilial incidence and intellectual impairment. *Arch. Neurol. Psychiatry*, 69:197–207.
489. Robison, S. H., Munzer, J. S., Tandan, R., et al. (1985): Repair of alkylated DNA is impaired in Alzheimer's disease cells. *Neurology (Suppl. 1)*, 35:217.
490. Roe, P. F. (1963): Hereditary spastic paraplegia. *J. Neurol. Neurosurg. Psychiatry*, 26:516–519.
491. Rogers, S., Lowenthal, A., Terheggen, H. G., and Columbo, J. P. (1973): Induction of arginase activity with the slope papilloma virus in tissue culture cells from an argininemic patient. *J. Exp. Med.*, 137:1091–1096.
492. Romano, J., Michael, M., Jr., and Merritt, H. H. (1940): Alcoholic cerebellar degeneration. *Arch. Neurol. Psychiatry*, 44:1230–1236.
493. Romanul, F., Fowler, H., Radvany, J., et al. (1977): Azorean disease of the nervous system. *N. Engl. J. Med.*, 296:1505–1508.
494. Rosenberg, L. E. (1976): Vitamin responsive inherited metabolic disorders. In: *Advances in Human Genetics, Vol. 6*, edited by H. Harris and K. Hirschhorn, pp. 1–74. Plenum Press, New York.
495. Rosenberg, L., Lilljeqvist, A., and Hsia, J. (1968): Methylmalonic aciduria: Metabolic block localization and vitamin B_{12} deficiency. *Science*, 162:805–807.
496. Rosenberg, R. N., Sassin, J., Zimmerman, E., et al. (1967): The interrelationship of neurofibromatosis and fibrous dysplasia. *Arch. Neurol.*, 17:174–179.
497. Rosenberg, R. N. (1979): Syringomyelia. In: *A Textbook of Neurology*, 6th ed., edited by H. H. Merritt, pp. 564–569. Lea and Febiger, New York.
498. Rosenberg, R. N. (1982): Amyotrophy. In: *Multisystem Genetic Diseases: Human Motor Neuron Diseases*, edited by L. P. Rowland, Raven Press, New York.
499. Rosenberg, R. N. (1984): Molecular genetics, recombinant DNA techniques and genetic neurological disease. *Ann. Neurol.*, 15:511–520.
500. Rosenberg, R. N., and Chutorian, A. (1967): Familial opticoacoustic nerve degeneration and polyneuropathy. *Neurology (Minneap.)*, 17:827–832.
501. Rosenberg, R. N., Ivy, N., Kirkpatrick, J., Bay, C., Nyhan, W. L., and Baskin, F. (1981): Joseph disease and Huntington disease, protein patterns in fibroblasts and brain. II. *Neurology*, 31:1003–1014.
502. Rosenberg, R. N., Nyhan, W. L., Bay, C., and Shore, P. (1976): Autosomal dominant striatonigral degeneration. *Neurology (Minneap.)*, 26:703.
503. Rosenberg, R. N., Nyhan, W. L., Coutinho, P., and Bay, C. (1978): Joseph disease: An autosomal dominant neurological disease in the Portuguese of the United States and the Azores Islands. In: *The Inherited Ataxias*, edited by P. Kark, R. N. Rosenberg, and L. Schut, pp. 33–57. Raven Press, New York.
504. Rosenberg, R. N., and Pettegrew, J. W. (1980): Genetic diseases of the nervous system. In: *Neurology, Vol. 5, Science and Practice of Clinical Medicine*, edited by J. M. Dietschy, pp. 165–243. Grune and Stratton, New York.
505. Rosenberg, R. N., and Pettegrew, J. W. (1983): Genetic neurological diseases. In: *The Clinical Neurosciences, Vol. 1*, edited by R. N. Rosenberg, pp. 33–165. Churchill-Livingstone, Inc., New York, London.
505a. Rosenberg, R. N., Robinson, A. B., and Partridge, D. (1975): Urine vapor pattern for olivopontocerebellar degeneration. *Clin. Biochem.*, 8:365–368.
506. Rosenberg, R. N., Thomas, L., Bay, C., Baskin, F., and Nyhan, W. L. (1979): Joseph disease. Fibroblast and brain proteins on acrylamide gels. *Neurology*, 29:917–926.
507. Rosing, H., Hopkins, L., Wallace, D., Epstein, C., and Weidenheim, K. (1985): Maternally inherited mitochondrial myopathy and myoclonic epilepsy. *Ann. Neurol.*, 17:228–237.
508. Roussy, G., and Levy, G. (1926): Sept cas d'une maladie familiale particuliere: Troubles de la marche, pieds bots et areflexie tendineuse generalisee, avec accessoirement legere maladresse des mains. *Rev. Neurol.*, 33:427.

509. Rowland, L. P. (1983): Molecular genetics, pseudogenetics and clinical neurology. *Neurology*, 33:1179–1195.

510. Rowland, L. P., Hays, A. P., DiMauro, S., DeVivo, D., and Behrens, M. (1983): Diverse clinical disorders associated with morphological abnormalities of mitochondria. In: *Mitochondrial Pathology in Muscle Disease*, edited by G. Scarlato and C. G. Cerri, pp. 141–158. Piccin, Padua.

511. Rowland, L., Lovelace, R., Schotland, D., Araki, S., and Carmel, P. (1966): The clinical diagnosis of McArdle's disease. Identification of another family with deficiency of muscle phosphorylase. *Neurology*, 16:93–100.

512. Rozen, R., Fox, J., Fenton, W., Horwich, A., and Rosenberg, L. (1985): Gene deletion and restriction fragment length polymorphisms at the human ornithine transcarbamylase locus. *Nature*, 313:815–817.

513. Rukavina, J. G., Block, W. D., Jackson, C. E., Falls, H. F., Carey, J. H., and Curtis, A. C. (1956): Primary systemic amyloidosis: A review and an experimental, genetic, and clinical study of 29 cases with particular emphasis on the familial form. *Medicine (Balt.)*, 35:239–334.

514. Rumpel, A. (1913): Uber das Wesen und die Bedeutung der Lebeveranderungen und der Pigmentierungen bei den damit verbunden Faalen von Pseudosklerose, Zugleich ein Beitrag zur Lehre von der Pseudosklerose (Westphal-Strumpell). *Dtsch. Z. Nervenheilkd.*, 49:54–73.

515. Sachs, B. (1896): A family form of idiocy, generally fatal, associated with early blindness (amaurotic family idiocy). *J. Nerv. Ment. Dis.*, 23:475–479.

516. Sackellares, J. C., and Swift, T. R. (1976): Shoulder enlargement as the presenting sign in syringomyelia. *JAMA*, 236:2878–2879.

517. Sajdel-Sulkowska, E. M., and Marotta, C. A. (1984): Alzheimer's disease brain: Alterations in RNA levels in a ribonuclease-inhibitor complex. *Science*, 225:947–949.

518. Sander, J., Malamud, N., Cowan, M., Packoran, S., Amman, A., and Wara, D. (1980): Intermittent ataxia and immunodeficiency with multiple carboxylase deficiencies: Abiotin-responsive disorder. *Ann. Neurol.*, 8:544–547.

519. Sandhoff, K. (1969): Variation of β-*n*-acetylhexosaminidase pattern in Tay-Sachs disease. *FEBS Lett.*, 4:351.

520. Sandhoff, K., Andreae, U., and Jatzkewitz, H. (1968): Deficient hexosaminidase activity in an exceptional case of Tay-Sachs disease with additional storage of kidney globoside in visceral organs. *Life Sci.*, 7:283–288.

521. Sandhoff, K., and Jatzkewitz, H. (1972): The chemical pathology of Tay-Sachs disease. In: *Sphingolipids, Sphingolipidoses, and Allied Disorders*, edited by B. W. Volk and S. M. Aronson, p. 305. Plenum Press, New York.

522. Sanfilippo, S. J., Podosin, R., Langer, L. O., Jr. and Good, R. A. (1963): Mental retardation associated with acid mucopolysacchariduria (heparitin sulfate type). *J. Pediatr.*, 63:837–838.

523. Sasaki, H., Sakaki, Y., Takagi, Y., Sahashi, K., et al. (1985): Presymptomatic diagnosis of heterozygosity for familial amyloidotic polyneuropathy by recombinant DNA techniques. *Lancet*, 1:100.

524. Schaumann, B., and Alter, B. (1976): *Dermatoglyphics in Medical Disorders*. Springer, New York.

525. Schaumburg, H. H., Powers, J. M., Raine, C. S., Johnson, A. R., Kolodny, E. H., Kishimoto, Y., Igarashi, M., and Suzuki, K. (1976): Adrenoleukodystrophy: A clinical pathological and biochemical study. *Adv. Exp. Med. Biol.*, 68:379–387.

526. Schaumburg, H. H., Powers, J. M., Raine, C. S., Spencer, P. S., Griffin, J. W., Prineas, J. W., and Boehmen, D. M. (1977): Adrenomyeloneuropathy: A probable variant of adrenoleukodystrophy. *Neurology*, 27:1114–1119.

527. Schaumburg, H. H., Powers, J. M., Raine, C. S., Suzuki, K., and Richardson, E. P. (1975): Adrenoleukodystrophy: A clinical and pathological study of 17 cases. *Arch. Neurol.*, 32:577–591.

528. Schaumburg, H. H., Richardson, E. P., Johnson, P. C., Cohen, R. B., Powers, J. M., and Raine, C. S. (1972): Schilder's disease: Sex linked recessive transmission with specific adrenal changes. *Arch. Neurol.*, 27:458–460.

529. Scheie, H. G., Hambrick, G. W., Jr., and Barnes, L. A. (1962): A newly recognized forme fruste of Hurler's disease (gargoylism). *Am. J. Ophthalmol.*, 53:753–769.

530. Scheinberg, I. H., and Gitlin, D. (1952): Deficiency of ceruloplasmin in patients' hepatolenticular degeneration (Wilson's disease). *Science*, 116:484–485.

531. Schenkein, I., Bucker, E., Helson, L., Axelrod, R., and Dancis, J. (1974): Increased nerve-growth stimulating activity in disseminated neurofibromatosis. *N. Engl. J. Med.*, 290:613–614.

532. Schmid, R., and Mahler, R. (1959): Chronic progressive myopathy with myoglobinuria: Demonstration of a glycogenolytic defect in the muscle. *J. Clin. Invest.*, 38:2044–2058.

533. Schmitt, H. P., Emser, W., and Heimes, C. (1984): Familial occurrence of amyotrophic lateral sclerosis, parkinsonism, and dementia. *Ann. Neurol.*, 16:642–648.
534. Schneider, A. S., Valentine, W. N., Hattori, M., et al. (1965): Hereditary hemolytic anemia with triosephosphate isomerase deficiency. *New Engl. J. Med.*, 272:229–235.
535. Schneider, C. (1936): Uber eine eigenartige Hirnerkrankung (Vaskulare Lipoidose). *Allg. Z. Psychiatr.*, 104:144.
536. Schoene, W. C., et al. (1970): Hereditary sensory neuropathy. *J. Neurol. Sci.*, 11:463–487.
537. Schuh, S., Rosenblatt, D. S., Cooper, B. A., Schroeder, M.-L., Bishop, A. J., Seargeant, L. E., and Haworth, J. C. (1984): Homocystinuria and megaloblastic anemia responsive to vitamin B_{12} therapy. *N. Engl. J. Med.*, 310:686–690.
538. Schut, J (1950): Hereditary ataxia: Clinical study through six generations. *Arch. Neurol. Psychiatry*, 63:535–568.
539. Schwartz, A. R. (1963): Charcot-Marie-Tooth disease: A 45-year follow-up. *Arch. Neurol.*, 9:623–634.
540. Schwartz, J. F., et al. (1963): Bassen-Kornzweig syndrome. *Arch. Neurol.*, 8:438–454.
541. Schwartz, O., and Jampel, R. (1962): Congenital blepharophimosis associated with a unique generalized myopathy. *Arch. Ophthalmol.*, 68:52–57.
542. Schwarz, G. A. (1952): Hereditary (familial) spastic paraplegia. *Arch. Neurol. Psychiatr.*, 68:655–682.
543. Schwarz, G. A., and Yanoff, M. (1965): Lafora's disease. *Arch. Neurol.*, 12:172–188.
544. Scriver, C., and Whelan, D. T. (1969): Glutamic acid decarboxylase in mammalian tissue outside the central nervous system and the possible relevance to hereditary vitamin B6 dependency with seizures. *Ann. N.Y. Acad. Sci.*, 166:83–96.
545. Seegmiller, J., Rosenbloom, F., and Kelly, W. (1967): An enzyme defect associated with a sex-linked human neurological disorder and excessive purine synthesis. *Science*, 155:1682.
546. Segal, S. (1983): Disorders of galactose metabolism. In: *The Metabolic Basis of Inherited Disease*, 5th ed., edited by J. Stanbury, J. Wyngaarden, D. Fredrickson, J. Goldstein and M. Brown, pp. 167–191. McGraw-Hill, New York.
547. Shapira, Y., Cederbaum, S. D., Cancilla, P., Nielsen, D., and Lippe, B. M. (1975): Familial poliodystrophy, mitochondrial myopathy and lactate acidemia. *Neurology*, 25:614–626.
548. Shapira, Y., Harel, S., and Russell, A. (1977): Mitochondrial encephalomyopathies. *Isr. J. Med. Sci.*, 13:161–164.
549. Shapiro, S. L., Sheppard, G. L., Jr., Dreifuss, F. E., and Newcombe, O. S. (1966): X-Linked recessive inheritance of a syndrome of mental retardation with hyperuricemia. *Proc. Soc. Exp. Biol. Med.*, 122:609–611.
550. Shih, V., and Efron, M., (1972): Urea cycle disorders. In: *The Metabolic Basis of Inherited Disease*, 3rd ed., edited by J. Stanbury, J. Wyngaarden, and D. Fredrickson, pp. 370–392. McGraw-Hill, New York.
551. Short, E., Conn, H., Snodgrass, P., Campbell, A., and Rosenberg, L. (1973): Evidence for X-linked dominant inheritance of ornithine transcarbamylase deficiency. *N. Engl. J. Med.*, 288:7–12.
552. Shy, G. M., Engel, W. K., Somers, J. E., et al. (1963): Nemaline myopathy, a new congenital myopathy. *Brain*, 86:793–810.
553. Shy, G. M., and Magee, K. R. (1956): A new congenital nonprogressive myopathy. *Brain*, 79:610–621.
554. Siekert, R. G., et al. (1959): Symposium on ataxia in childhood. *Proc. Mayo Clin.*, 34:659.
555. Siemerling, E., and Creutzfeldt, H. G. (1923): Bronzekrankheit und sklerosierende Encephalomyelitis (diffuse Sklerose). *Arch. Psychiatr. Nervenkr.*, 68:217–244.
556. Siemerling, E., and Oloff, H. (1922): Pseudosklerose (Westphal-Strumpell) mit Cornealring (Kayser-Fleischer) und doppelseitiger Scheinkatarakt, die nur bei seitlicher Beleuchtung sichtbar ist und die der nach Verletzung durch Kupfersplitter entstehenden Katarakt ahnlich ist. *Klin. Wochenschr.*, 1:1087–1089.
557. Siggers, D. C., Rogers, J. C., Boyer, S. H., Margolet, L., Dorkin, H., Banerjee, S. P., and Shooter, E. M. (1976): Increased nerve-growth factor beta chain cross-reacting material in familial dysautonomia. *N. Engl. J. Med.*, 295:629–634.
558. Silver, J. R. (1966): Familial spastic paraplegia with amyotrophy of the hands. *Ann. Hum. Genet.*, 30–75.
559. Singh, I., Moser, A. E., Moser, H. W., and Kishimoto, Y. (1984): Adrenoleukodystrophy: Im-

paired oxidation of very long chain fatty acids in white blood cells, cultured skin fibroblasts and amniocytes. *Ped. Res.*, 18:286–290.

560. Sipe, J. C. (1973): Leigh's syndrome: The adult form of subacute necrotizing encephalomyelopathy with predilection for the brain stem. *Neurology*, 23:1030–1038.

561. Skillicorn, S. A. (1955): Presenile cerebellar ataxia in chronic alcoholics. *Neurology*, 5:527–534.

562. Skre, H., and Loken, A. C. (1970): Myoclonus epilepsy and subacute presenile dementia in heredo-ataxia. *Acta Neurol. Scand.*, 46:42.

563. Sloan, H., and Fredrickson, D. (1972): Rare familial diseases with neutral lipid storage. In: *The Metabolic Basis of Inherited Disease*, 3rd ed., edited by J. Stanbury, J. Wyngaarden, and D. Fredrickson, pp. 808–832. McGraw-Hill, New York.

564. Slonim, A., and Goans, P. (1985): Myopathy in McArdle's syndrome: Improvement with a high-protein diet. *N. Engl. J. Med.*, 312:355–359.

565. Sly, W. S., Hewett-Emmett, D., Whyte, M. P., Yu, Y.-S. L., and Tashian, R. E. (1983): Carbonic anhydrase II deficiency identified as the primary defect in the autosomal recessive syndrome of osteoporosis with renal tubular acidosis and cerebral calcification. *Proc. Natl. Acad. Sci. USA*, 80:2752–2756.

566. Sly, W. S., Quinton, B. A., McAllister, W. H., and Rimoin, D. L. (1973): β-Glucuronidase deficiency: Report of clinical, radiologic, and biochemical features of a new mucopolysaccharidosis. *J. Pediatr.*, 82:249–257.

567. Sly, W. S., Whyte, M. P., Sundaram, V., Tashian, R., Hewett-Emmett, D., Guibaud, P., Vainsel, M., Baluarte, H., Gruskin, A., Al-Mosawi, M., Sakati, N., and Ohlsson, A. (1985): Carbonic anhydrase II deficiency in 12 families with the autosomal recessive syndrome of osteoporosis with renal tubular acidosis and cerebral calcification. *New Engl. J. Med.*, 313:139–145.

568. Smith, A. A., and Dancis, J. (1967): Catecholamine release in familial dysautonomia. *N. Engl. J. Med.*, 277:61–64.

569. Smith, A. A., Farbman, A., and Dancis, J. (1965): Tongue in familial dysautonomia. *Am. J. Dis. Child.*, 110:152.

570. Smith, A. A., Taylor, T., and Wortis, S. B. (1963): Abnormal catechol amine metabolism in familial dysautonomia. *N. Engl. J. Med.*, 268:705–707.

571. Smith, J. K., Gonda, V. E., and Malamud, N. (1958): Unusual form of cerebellar ataxia: Combined dentato-rubral and pallido-luysian degeneration. *Neurology*, 8:205–209.

572. Smith, M. (1960): Nerve fibre degeneration in the brain in amyotrophic lateral sclerosis. *J. Neurol. Neurosurg. Psychiatry*, 23:269–282.

573. Solitare, G. B., and Cohen, G. S. (1965): Peripheral autonomic nervous system lesions in congenital or familial dysautonomia. *Neurology*, 15:321–327.

574. Spellmann, G. G. (1962): Report of familial cases of parkinsonism: Evidence of a dominant trait in a patient's family. *JAMA*, 179:372.

575. Spencer-Peet, J., Norman, M., Lake, B., and McNamara, P. A. (1971): Hepatic glycogen storage disease: Clinical and laboratory findings in 23 cases. *Q. J. Med.*, 40:95–114.

576. Spiller, W. G. (1910): Friedreich's ataxia. *J. Nerv. Ment. Dis.*, 37:411.

577. Spiro, A. J., Shy, G. M., and Gonatas, N. K. (1966): Myotubular myopathy, persistence of fetal muscle in an adolescent boy. *Arch. Neurol.*, 14:1–14.

578. Stein, S., and Morrison, M. (1985): The molecular biology of Lesch-Nyhan syndrome. *Trends in Neurosci.*, 8:148–150.

579. Sternlieb, I., and Scheinberg, I. H. (1968): Prevention of Wilson's disease in asymptomatic patients. *N. Engl. J. Med.*, 278:352–359.

580. Sternlieb, I., and Scheinberg, I. H. (1972): Chronic hepatitis as a first manifestation of Wilson's disease. *Ann. Intern. Med.*, 76:59–64.

581. Stumpf, D. A., McAfee, J., Parks, J. K., and Eguren, L. (1980): Propionate inhibition of succinate:CoA ligase (GDP) and the citric acid cycle in mitochondria. *Pediatr. Res.*, 14:1127–1131.

582. Stumpf, D. A., Parker, W. D., Jr., and Angelini, C. (1985): Carnitine deficiency, organic acidemias, and Reye's syndrome. *Neurology*, 35:1041–1045.

583. Stumpf, D. A., Parks, J. K., E'quren, L. A., and Haas, R. (1982): Friedreich's ataxia. III. Mitochondrial malic enzyme deficiency. *Neurology*, 32:221–227.

584. Sulzberger, R. M., Frazer, J., and Hutner, L. (1938): Incontinentia pigmenti (Bloch-Sulzberger): Report of an additional case with comment on possible relation to a new syndrome of familial and congenital anomalies. *Arch. Dermatol. Syphilol.*, 38:57.

585. Suzuki, K., and Suzuki, Y. (1970): Globoid cell leucodystrophy (Krabbe's disease): Deficiency of galactocerebroside β-galactosidase. *Proc. Natl. Acad. Sci. USA*, 66:302–309.
586. Suzuki, K., Schneider, E., and Epstein, C. (1971): In utero diagnosis of globoid cell leukodystrophy (Krabbe's disease). *Biochem. Biophys. Res. Commun.*, 45:1363–1366.
587. Svennerholm, L., and Raal, A. (1961): Composition of brain gangliosides. *Biochim. Biophys. Acta*, 53:422–424.
588. Syllaba, L., and Henner, K. (1926): Contribution a l'independance de l'athetose double idiopathique et congenitale. *Rev. Neurol.*, 1:541–562.
589. Symonds, C. P., and Blackwood, W. (1962): Spinal cord compression in hypertrophic neuritis. *Brain*, 85:251–259.
590. Takashima, S., and Becker, L. (1985): Basal ganglia calcification in Down's syndrome. *J. Neurol. Neurosurg. Psychiatry*, 48:61–64.
591. Tanaka, K., Budd, M., Efron, M., and Isselbacher, K. (1966): Isovaleric acidemia: A new genetic defect of leucine metabolism. *Proc. Natl. Acad. Sci. USA*, 56:236–242.
592. Tarui, S., Okuno, G., Ikura, Y., Tanaka, T., Suda, M., and Nishikawa, M. (1965): Phosphofructokinase deficiency in skeletal muscle: A new type of glucogenosis. *Biochem. Biophys. Res. Commun.*, 19:517–523.
593. Tay, W. (1881): Symmetrical changes in the region of the yellow spot in each eye of an infant. *Trans. Ophthalmol. Soc. UK*, 1:155.
594. Tedesco, T., and Mellman, W. (1967): Argininosuccinate synthetase activity and citrulline metabolism in cells cultured from a citrullinemic subject. *Proc. Natl. Acad. Sci. USA*, 57:829–834.
595. Terheggen, H. G., Schwenk, A., Lowenthal, A., Van Sande, M., and Colombo, J. P. (1969): Arginineaemia with arginase deficiency. *Lancet*, 2:748–749.
596. Thilenius, O. G., and Grossman, B. J. (1961): Friedreich's ataxia with heart disease in children. *Pediatrics*, 27:246–254.
597. Thomas, P. K., Halpern, J. P., King, R. H. M., and Patrick, D. (1984): Galactosyl ceramide lipidosis: Novel presentation as a slowly progressive spinocerebellar degeneration. *Ann. Neurol.*, 16:618–620.
598. Thomas, P. K., and Lascalles, R. G. (1967): Hypertrophic neuropathy. *Q. J. Med.*, 36:223–238.
599. Thomson, A. F., and Alvarez, F. A. (1968): Hereditary amyotrophic lateral sclerosis. *J. Neurol. Sci.*, 8:101–110.
600. Todorov, A. (1965): Le syndrome de Marinesco-Sjogren: Premiere etude anatomoclinique. *J. Genet. Hum.*, 14:197.
601. Tomlinson, B. E., Irving, D., and Blessed, G. (1981): Cell loss in the locus coeruleus in senile dementia of the Alzheimer type. *J. Neurol. Sci.*, 49:419–428.
602. Tomlinson, S., and Westall, R. (1964): Argininosuccinic aciduria, argininosuccinase, and arginase in human blood cells. *Clin. Sci.*, 26:261–269.
603. Tonshoff, B., Lehnert, W., and Ropers, H. H. (1982): Adrenoleukodystrophy: Diagnosis and carrier detection by determination of long chain fatty acids in cultured fibroblasts. *Clin. Genet.*, 22:25–59.
604. Tooth, H. H. (1886): *The Peroneal Type of Progressive Muscular Atrophy*. H. K. Lewis, London.
605. Tuchman, L., Suma, H., and Cori, J. (1956): Elevation of serum acid phosphatase in Gaucher's disease. *J. Mt. Sinai Hosp.*, 23:277.
606. Tuchman, M., Stoeckler, J., Kiang, D., O'Dea, R., Ramnaraine, M., and Mirkin, B. (1985): Familial pyrimidinemia and pyrimidinuria associated with severe flurouracil toxicity. *N. Engl. J. Med.*, 313:245–249.
607. Turkington, R. W., and Stiefel, J. W. (1965): Sensory radicular neuropathy. *Arch. Neurol.*, 12:19–24.
608. Turner, G., Brookwell, R., Daniel, A., Selikowitz, M., and Zilibowitz, M. (1980): Heterozygous expression of X-linked mental retardation and X-chromosome marker fra(x) (q27). *N. Engl. J. Med.*, 303:662–664.
609. Urich, H., Norman, R. M., and Lloyd, O. C. (1957): Suprasegmental lesions in Friedreich's ataxia. *Confinia Neurol. Separatum*, 17:360.
610. van Bogaert, L. (1951): Sur ces formes d'heredoataxie de l'enfant et de l'adolescent qui comportent une atteinte grave des noyaux moteurs spino-bulbo-mesencephaliques. *Rev. Neurol.*, 84:121.
611. van Bogaert, I., Scherer, H. J., and Epstein, E. (1937): *Une Forme Cerebrale de la Cholesterinose Generalisee*. Masson, Paris.

612. van der Eecken, H., Adams, R., and van Bogaert, L. (1960): Striopallidal-nigral degeneration. An hitherto undescribed lesion in paralysis agitans. *J. Neuropathol. Exp. Neurol.*, 19:159–161.
613. van Epps, C., and Kerr, H. D. (1940): Familial lumbosacral syringomyelia. *Radiology*, 35:160–173.
614. van Hoff, F., and Hers, H. G. (1964): L'ultrastructure des cellules hepatiques dans la malade de Hurler (gargoylisme). *CR Acad. Sci. Paris (D)*, 259:1281.
615. Vejjajiva, A., Foster, J. B., and Miller, H. (1967): Motor neuron disease: A clinical study. *J. Neurol. Sci.*, 4:299–314.
616. Vestermark, B. (1966): Arthrogryposis multiplex congenita: A case of neurogenic origin. *Acta Paediatr. Scand.*, 55:117–120.
617. Victor, M., Adams, R. D., and Mancall, E. L. (1959): A restricted form of cerebellar cortical degeneration occurring in alcoholic patients. *Arch. Neurol.*, 1:579–688.
618. Visscher, B., Detels, R., Dudley, J. P., Haile, R. W., Malcgren, R. M., Terasaki, P. I., and Park, M. S. (1979): Genetic susceptibility to multiple sclerosis. *Neurology*, 29:1354–1360.
619. von Gierke, E. (1929): Hepato-nephromegalia glykogenia (Glykogenspeicherkrankheit der Leber und Nieren). *Beitr. Pathol.*, 82:497.
620. von Motz, I. P., Bots, G., and Endtz, L. J. (1977): Astrocytoma in three sisters. *Neurology*, 27:1038–1041.
621. Waaler, P., Garatun-Tjeldsto, O., and Moe, P. (1970): Genetic studies in glycogen storage disease type III. *Acta Paediatr. Scand.*, 59:529–535.
622. Wada, Y., Taka, K., Minagawa, A., Yoshida, T., Morikawa, T., and Okamura, T. (1963): Idiopathic hypervalinemia: Probably a new entity of inborn error of valine metabolism. *Tohoku J. Exp. Med.*, 81:46.
623. Walker, P. D., Blitzer, M., and Shapira, E. (1985): Marinesco-Sjögren syndrome: Evidence for a lysosomal storage disorder. *Neurology*, 35:415–419.
623a. Walser, M. (1983): Urea cycle disorders and other hereditary hyperammonemic syndromes. In: *The Metabolic Basis of Inherited Diseases*, 5th ed., edited by J. Stanbury, J. Wyngaarden, D. Fredrickson, J. Goldstein, and M. Brown, pp. 402–438. McGraw-Hill, New York.
624. Walshe, J. M. (1956): Wilson's disease: New oral therapy. *Lancet*, 1:25–26.
625. Wechsler, I. S., Brock, S., and Weil, A. (1929): Amyotrophic lateral sclerosis with objective and subjective (neuritic) sensory disturbances. *Arch. Neurol. Psychiatry*, 21:299–310.
626. Weinreb, H. J. (1985): Fingerprint patterns in Alzheimer's disease. *Arch. Neurol.*, 42:50–54.
627. Weinshilboum, R., and Axelrod, J. (1971): Reduced plasma dopamine-beta-hydroxylase activity in familial dysautonomia. *N. Engl. J. Med.*, 285:938–942.
628. Weiss, S., and Carter, S. (1959): Course and prognosis of acute cerebellar ataxia in children. *Neurology*, 9:711–721.
629. Weleber, R. G., Hecht, F., and Giblett, E. R. (1960): Ring G chromosome: A new G deletion syndrome. *Am. J. Dis. Child.*, 115:489–493.
630. Weller, R. O. (1967): Electron microscopic study of hypertrophic neuropathy of Dejerine and Sottas. *J. Neurol. Neurosurg. Psychiatry*, 30:111–125.
631. Wells, C. E. C., Spillane, J. D., and Bligh, A. S. (1959): The cervical spinal canal in syringomyelia. *Brain*, 82:23–40.
632. Wells, H., and Wells, W. (1967): Galactose toxicity and myoinositol metabolism in the developing rat brain. *Biochemistry*, 6:1168–1173.
633. Westall, R., Dancis, J., and Miller, S. (1957): Maple sugar urine disease. *Am. J. Dis. Child.*, 94:571–572.
634. White, R. (1984): Looking for epilepsy genes. *Ann. Neurol.*, 16 *(Suppl.)*:S12–S17.
635. Whitehouse, P. J., Price, D. L., Struble, R. G., Clark, A. W., Coyle, J. T., and DeLong, M. R. (1982): Alzheimer's disease and senile dementia: Loss of neurons in the basal forebrain. *Science*, 215:1237–1239.
636. Wigboldus, J. M., and Bruyn, G. W. (1968): Hallervorden-Spatz disease. In: *Handbook of Clinical Neurology, Vol. 6*, edited by P. J. Vinken and G. W. Bruyn, pp. 604–631. North Holland, Amsterdam.
637. Wilcken, D. E. L., Wilcken, B., Dudman, N. P. B., and Tyrrell, P. A. (1983): Homocystinuria— The effects of betaine in the treatment of patients not responsive to pyridoxine. *N. Engl. J. Med.*, 309:448–453.
638. Williams, J. C., Butler, I. J., Rosenberg, H. S., Verani, R., Scott, C. I., and Conley, S. B. (1984):

Progressive neurologic deterioration and renal failure due to storage of glutamyl-ribose-5-phosphate. *N. Engl. J. Med.*, 311:152–155.

639. Wilson, J. M., Young, A. B., and Kelly, W. N. (1983): Hypoxanthine-guanine phosphoribosyl transferase deficiency. *N. Engl. J. Med.*, 309:900–910.

640. Wilson, S. A. K. (1912): Progressive lenticular degeneration: A familial nervous disease associated with cirrhosis of the liver. *Brain*, 34:295–509.

641. Winters, P., Harrod, M., Molenich, S., Kirkpatrick, J., and Rosenberg, R. (1976): α-L-Iduronidase deficiency and possible Hurler-Scheie genetic compound. *Neurology*, 26:1003–1007.

642. Wisniewski, K. E., Dalton, A. J., McLahlan, C., Wen, G., and Wisniewski, H. M. (1985): Alzheimer's disease in Down's syndrome: Clinicopathologic studies. *Neurology*, 35:957–961.

643. Wohlfart, G., Jörgen, F., and Eliasson, S. (1955): Hereditary proximal spinal muscular atrophy— A clinical entity simulating progressive muscular dystrophy. *Acta Psychiatr. Neurol. Scand.*, 30:395–406.

644. Wolff, D. (1942): Microscopic study of temporal bones in dysostosis multiplex (gargoylism). *Laryngoscope*, 52:218–223.

645. Woo, S., Lidsky, A., Güttler, F., Chandra, T., and Robson, K. (1983): Cloned human phenylalanine hydroxylase gene allows prenatal diagnosis and carrier detection of classical phenylketonuria. *Nature*, 306:151–155.

646. Woods, B. T., and Schaumburg, H. (1972): Nigro-spino-dentatal degeneration with nuclear ophthalmoplegia. *J. Neurol. Sci.*, 17:149–166.

647. Woodworth, J. A., Bockett, R. S., and Netsky, M. G. (1959): A composite of hereditary ataxias. *Arch. Intern. Med.*, 104:594–606.

648. Yang, T. P., Patel, P. I., Chinault, A. C., Stout, J. T., Jackson, L. G., Hildebrand, B. M., and Caskey, C. T. (1984): Molecular evidence for new mutation at the HGPRT locus in Lesch-Nyhan patients. *Nature*, 310:412–414.

649. Yasuda, Y., Akiguchi, I., Shio, H., and Kameyama, M. (1984): Scanning electron microscopy studies of erythrocytes in spinocerebellar degeneration. *J. Neurol. Neurosurg. Psychiatry*, 47:269–274.

650. Yatsu, F., and Zussman, W. (1964): Familial dysautonomia (Riley-Day syndrome). Case report with postmortem findings of a patient at age 31. *Arch. Neurol.*, 10:459–463.

651. Zabel, B. U., and Baumann, W. A. (1982): Langer-Giedion syndrome with interstitial Sq-deletion. *Am. J. Med. Genet.*, 11:353–358.

652. Zang, K. D. (1983): Cytological and cytogenetical studies on human meningioma. *Cancer Genet. Cytogenet.*, 6:249–274.

653. Zang, K. D., and Singer, H. (1967): Chromosomal constitution of meningiomas. *Nature*, 216:84–85.

654. Zatz, M., Itskan, S. B., Sanger, R., et al. (1974): New linkage data for the X-linked types of muscular dystrophy and G6PD variants, colour blindness and Xg blood groups. *J. Med. Genet.*, 11:321–327.

655. Zellweger, H., et al. (1969): Heritable spinal muscular atrophies. *Helv. Pediatr. Acta*, 24:92–105.

656. Zeman, W., (1976): The neuronal ceroid-lipofuscinoses. In: *Progress in Neuropathology, Vol. III*, edited by H. M. Zimmerman, pp. 203–223. Grune and Stratton, New York.

657. Zeman, W., and Scarpelli, D. G. (1958): The non-specific lesions of Hallervorden-Spatz disease. *J. Neuropathol. Exp. Neurol.*, 17:622–630.

658. Ziegler, D. K., Hassanein, R. S., Harris, D., and Stewart, R. (1975): Headache in a non-clinic twin population. *Headache*, 14:213–218.

659. Ziegler, M. G., Lake, C. R., and Kopin, I. J. (1976): Deficient sympathetic nervous response in familial dysautonomia. *N. Engl. J. Med.*, 294:630–633.

7

The New Genetics: The New Neurology

There is a profound awakening just ahead in neurogenetics, both in acquiring molecular insights into brain development and behavior and in deciphering the main neurologic genetic diseases. Recombinant DNA techniques and genetic engineering promise a far-reaching revolution, an exponential accumulation of molecular insights. Look what has already been achieved in the past decade with mapping of neurologic genetic disorders to specific chromosomal loci by classic linkage and somatic cell hybrid methods (Table 1).

A new system of genetic markers detected by a direct analysis of DNA sequence polymorphism with restriction endonuclease enzymes has allowed the construction of a detailed genetic linkage map for the human (12). These new genetic loci are being identified and defined by complementary DNA (cDNA) segments that represent genes of known specific function or unique arbitrary loci without a known function. With family studies it has been possible to measure the linkage distances and gene sequence order that characterize these new markers (12).

It has been estimated that the entire human genome is about 3,300 centimorgans (cM), and that the localization of a new locus can be obtained if the marker loci for which cDNA probes exist are spaced about 30 to 50 cM apart. Thus only 70 to 130 evenly spaced genetic marker loci may be needed to cover the human genome entirely and allow an assignment of a new marker with precision and reliability (12).

As genetic disease loci are mapped, the adjacent polymorphic DNA markers can be used to determine the genotype of at risk presymptomatic individuals. This approach has been successful for several important genetic neurologic diseases in which these diseases have been linked with DNA markers. These diseases include Duchenne's (8) and Becker's (4) muscular dystrophy, Huntington's disease (3), X-linked retinitis pigmentosa (1), fragile X mental retardation (2), ornithine transcarbamylase deficiency (9), and autosomal dominant amyloid polyneuropathy (10). These achievements will rapidly be followed by many others so that by the end of the century it will be possible with probes and pedigrees to eliminate many disorders from selected families and determine the exact mutation responsible for the cause of disease. In turn these results will provide insight into what was the biological function of the normal gene product for brain development or its maintenance.

As White et al. point out (12), cDNA probes and their assignment on the linkage map will make it possible as well to evaluate the genetic or environmental basis of multifactorial disorders such as familial schizophrenia and inherited forms of epilepsy. The finding of the cosegregation of the disorder with a specific marker locus can make judgment possible about who might be susceptible to the disease in an at risk family. To date about 200 polymorphic DNA markers have been reported (12), and so progress to achieve this goal is clearly being realized.

Weatherall (11) has offered a possible time scale for developments in genetic engineering that will be applied to medicine. In the category of what is scientifically and technically possible to be achieved now, he includes the prenatal diagnosis of some common single gene disorders and commercial production with recombinant techniques of hormones (insulin, growth hormone), interferon, vaccines (hepatitis B), and blood products (factors 8 and 9). In the possible foreseeable future he suggests that recombinant techniques will be able to provide the following: an accurate restriction map of the human genome with adequate numbers of probes evenly spaced to provide linkage markers to prevent most common single-gene and several chromosomal disorders; the ability to predict risk rates for common polygenic disorders; and determination of the molecular basis of mutation or expression for important neurologic and psychiatric disorders with clear genetic predisposition such as manic-depressive disease, schizophrenia, multiple sclerosis, myasthenia gravis, and muscular dystrophy, and inherited degenerative diseases such as parkinsonism, spinocerebellar degeneration, and familial epilepsy. In the next decade or longer he speculates that somatic cell gene replacement therapy for single-gene disorders will probably be successful, including the thalassemias, sickle cell disease, purine nucleoside phosphorylase deficiency (the absence of which results in a severe immunodeficiency disease), adenosine deaminase deficiency (which produces severe combined immunodeficiency disease), and Lesch-Nyhan disease. As referred to in the formal discussion on Lesch-Nyhan disease (Chapter 6), it has already been possible to express the human gene for hypoxanthine guanine phosphoribosyl transferase (HGPRT), the enzyme defective in the disorder, after the gene has been trasfected into mouse bone marrow cells and retransplanted into the mouse bone marrow. The next step is to achieve the same result in patients. Some suggest that this remarkable form of gene therapy is already being planned in the near future for Lesch-Nyhan patients, which would be a major achievement for the field of molecular neurogenetics and for our patients. Bone marrow cell gene therapy would correct the purine metabolic disorders in nonbrain tissue, but the limitation of the blood-brain barrier for the enzyme would restrict its availability to the CNS.

Somatic cell gene therapy is one issue, and examples of its medical and biological benefits have been reviewed, but germ cell gene therapy is quite another issue medically, scientifically, and ethically. To alter the genome of the ovum, sperm, or zygote so as to change the species for a medical reason carries with it profound implications about maintenance and even survival of the human race. One obvious immediate attempt in this area of research would be to improve intelligence or other neurologic or behavioral abilities of the species, assuming behavioral genes

TABLE 1. *Neurogenetic disorders and functions and their chromosome map location*

Chromosome 1	
Charcot-Marie-Tooth	1q
Gaucher's disease	1q
Chromosome 2	
N-*myc* oncogene neuroblastoma	2p
Proopiomelanocortin (ACTH) gene	2p
Chromosome 3	
Generalized gangliosidosis	3p
Ceruloplasmin; Wilson's disease	3q
Somatostatin	3q
Chromosome 4	
Huntington's disease	4p
Atypical phenylketonuria (dihydropteridine reductase deficiency)	4
Chromosome 5	
Sandhoff's disease	5q
Maroteaux-Lamy syndrome	5q
Dihydrofolate reductase	5q
Chromosome 6	
Spinocerebellar degeneration	6p
Prolactin	6p
HLA complex	6p
Chromosome 7	
Argininosuccinic aciduria	7
Mucopolysaccharidosis, type 7	7
Marfan syndrome	7q
Chromosome 8	
Glutathione reductase deficiency	8p
Osteopetrosis syndrome	8q
Thyroglobulin (genetic cretinism)	8q
Chromosome 9	
Citrullinemia	9
Galactosemia	9p
Acute hepatic porphyria	9q
Chromosome 10	
Wolman's disease	10q
Cholesterol ester storage disease	10q
Chromosome 11	
Lactate dehydrogenase A	11p
Parathyroid hormone	11p
Lysosomal acid phosphatase deficiency	11p
Acute intermittent porphyria	11q
Chromosome 12	
Lactate dehydrogenase B	12p
Phenylketonuria	12q
Chromosome 13	
Retinoblastoma	13q
Chromosome 14	
Creatine phosphokinase, brain isoenzyme (BB)	14q
Chromosome 15	
Tay-Sachs disease	15q
Prader-Willi syndrome	15p
Chromosome 16	
Lecithin-cholesterol acyltransferase deficiency	16q
Chromosome 17	
Pompe's disease (glycogen storage disease, type II)	17q
Growth hormone	17q
Myosin, heavy chain cluster	17p
Galactokinase deficiency	17q

TABLE 1. *(continued)*

Chromosome 19	
Myotonic muscular dystrophy	19p
Poliovirus sensitivity	19q
Chromosome 20	
Adenosine deaminase deficiency	20q
Chromosome 21	
Superoxide dismutase	21q
Homocystinuria	21q
Chromosome 22	
Metachromatic leukodystrophy	22q
Hurler-Scheie syndrome	22q
X Chromsome	
Glucose-6-phosphate dehydrogenase	Xq
Color blindness	Xq
Ocular albinism	Xp
Duchenne's muscular dystrophy	Xp
Lesch-Nyhan syndrome	Xq
Fragile X syndrome	Xp

Adapted from ref. 6.

have been identified that influence cognition. Such an approach involves us immediately in the heated, controversial area of IQ theory and testing. Can a single number, the IQ, like the height, weight, or temperature of a person, completely define his or her intelligence or mental potential? The controversies surrounding Cyril Burt's and A. R. Jensen's statistical analyses of this point are profoundly disturbing and yet clear enough to cause doubt that such a simple quantification will do justice to defining the issue. Politicians, theologians, and strict biological determinists for their parochial reasons and prejudicial biases have conveniently used a genetic basis of behavior and ability as the sole determinant. A person's genetic composition makes his or her behavior, ability, and class rank immutable, they say. Environmental stimuli, cultural conditioning, and careful nuturing are minimized by biological determinists in their value to improve IQ and to improve one's mental functioning. Lewontin et al. in *Not in Our Genes* (5) strongly argue for the separation of the science from the politics and prejudices of biological determinism. Clearly there are genetic factors crucial for brain development, but I would argue individual conditioning also plays a major role in maximizing the human potential.

The point here is that germ cell gene therapy and potential behavior modification are not areas that will be easy to deal with and resolve. The ethics of germ line alteration, as well as somatic cell gene therapy, needs careful scrutiny by the recently established Recombinant DNA Advisory Committee of the National Institutes of Health in the United States and its potential equivalent in other countries. Further, the creation of a President's Commission on Human Applications of Genetic Engineering is a part of a bill sponsored by Senator Albert Gore. This bill when it becomes law would establish a commission that would outline matters of policy and procedure rather than review actual recombinant DNA proposals. This would be a beginning to ensure that a uniform policy be achieved with a consideration of broad ethical matters. As Motulsky points out in his fine review on this subject, "Impact of Genetic Manipulation on Society and Medicine" (7), "it is crucial in order to be able to make wise decisions on these matters that the public at large must become well informed. Medicine and genetics must be elevated at all levels of our society. The public in general and the scientific community in particular have not fully absorbed the full impact of recombinant DNA techniques and it is up to us to enlighten them for the ultimate good of us all."

"Enlightened democratic societies" (7) using the new DNA technology ethically and responsibly will provide better health and welfare for their people. The future looks bright indeed for molecular neurogenetics, which will bring us the "new neurology," and it is indeed a good time for medical and graduate students and neurology residents to join in and move this enterprise forward for all humanity.

REFERENCES

1. Bhattacharya, S., Wright, A., Clayton, J., Price, W., Phillips, C., McKeown, C., Jay, M., Bird, A., Pearson, P., Southern, E., Evans, H., et al. (1984): Close genetic linkage between X-linked retinitis pigmentosa and a restriction fragment length polymorphism identified by recombinant DNA probe LI.28. *Nature*, 309:253–255.
2. Camerino, G., Matlei, M., Matlei, J., Jaye, M., and Mandel, J. (1983): Close linkage of fragile X-mental retardation syndrome to haemophilia B and transmission through a normal male. *Nature*, 306:701–704.
3. Gusella, J., Wexler, N. S., Conneally, P. M., Naylor, S. L., Anderson, M. A., Tanzi, R. E., Watkins, P. C., Ottina, K., Wallace, M. R., Sakaguchi, A. Y., Young, A. B., Shoulson, I., Bonilla, E., and Marin, J. B. (1983): A polymorphic DNA marker genetically linked to Huntington's disease. *Nature*, 306:234–238.
4. Kingston, H., Thomas, N., Pearson, P., Sarfarazi, M., and Harper, P. (1983): Genetic linkage between Becker muscular dystrophy and a polymorphic DNA sequence on the short arm of the X chromosome. *J. Med. Genet.*, 20:255–258.
5. Lewontin, R. C., Rose, S., and Kamin, L. J. (1984): *Not in Our Genes*. Pantheon Books, New York.
6. McKusick, V. (1984): Diseases of the genome (an interview). *JAMA*, 252:1041–1048.
7. Motulsky, A. (1983): Impact of genetic manipulation on society and medicine. *Science*, 219:135–140.
8. Murray, J., Davies, K., Harper, P., Meredith, L., Mueller, C., and Williamson, R. (1982): Linkage relationship of a cloned DNA sequence on the short arm of the X chromosome to Duchenne muscular dystrophy. *Nature*, 300:69–71.
9. Old, J., Purvis-Smith, S., Wilcken, B., Pearson, P., Williamson, R., et al. (1985): Prenatal exclusion of ornithine transcarbamylase deficiency by direct gene analysis. *Lancet*, 1:73–75.
10. Sasaki, H., Sakaki, Y., Takagi, Y., Sahashi, K., et al. (1985): Presymptomatic diagnosis of heterozygosity for familial amyloidotic polyneuropathy by recombinant DNA techniques. *Lancet*, 1:100.
11. Weatherall, D. J., (1984): Implications for medical practice and human biology. *Lancet*, 2:1440–1444.
12. White, R., Leppert, M., Bishop, D., Barker, D., Berkowitz, J., Brown, C., Callahan, P., Holm, T., and Jerominski, L. (1985): Construction of linkage maps with DNA markers for human chromosomes. *Nature*, 313:101–105.

Subject Index